BRADY
Workbook

BOB ELLING • J. DAVID BERGERON

EMERGENCY CARE

EIGHTH EDITION

▶ MICHAEL F. O'KEEFE

▶ DANIEL LIMMER

▶ HARVEY D. GRANT

▶ ROBERT H. MURRAY, JR.

▶ J. DAVID BERGERON

Contributors
BETH LOTHROP ADAMS
BOB ELLING
DAVID M. HABBEN
FITZGERALD PETERSEN

Medical Editor
EDWARD T. DICKINSON, M.D., FACEP

BRADY/PRENTICE HALL
Upper Saddle River, New Jersey 07458

Dedicated to my two beautiful daughters: Laura and Caitlin. And to my lovely wife Kirsten. May you always maintain humility as your accomplishments meet the stars!

B.E.

NOTICE ON CARE PROCEDURES

This workbook reflects current EMS practices based on the 1994 U.S. Department of Transportation's EMT-Basic National Standard Curriculum. It is the intent of the authors and publisher that this workbook be used as part of a formal Emergency Medical Technician education program taught by qualified instructors and supervised by a licensed physician. The procedures described in this workbook are based upon consultation with EMS and medical authorities. The authors and publisher have taken care to make certain that these procedures reflect currently accepted clinical practice; however, they cannot be considered absolute recommendations.

The material in this workbook contains the most current information available at the time of publication. However, federal, state, and local guidelines concerning clinical practices, including, without limitation, those governing infection control and universal precautions, change rapidly. The reader should note, therefore, that new regulations may require changes in some procedures.

It is the responsibility of the reader to familiarize himself or herself with the policies and procedures set by federal, state, and local agencies as well as the institution or agency where the reader may be employed. The author and the publisher of this workbook disclaim any liability, loss, or risk resulting directly or indirectly from the suggested procedures and theory, from any undetected errors, or from the reader's misunderstanding of the text. It is the reader's responsibility to stay informed of any new changes or recommendations made by any federal, state, and local agency as well as by his or her employing institution or agency.

If when reading this workbook you find an error, have an idea for how to improve it, or simply want to share your comments with us, please send your letter to one of the following addresses below.

Brady Marketing Department
c/o Judy Streger
Prentice Hall
One Lake Street
Upper Saddle River, New Jersey 07458

elling1096@aol.com
Judy_Streger@prenhall.com

Prentice-Hall International (UK) Limited, London
Prentice-Hall of Australia Pty. Limited, Sydney
Prentice-Hall Canada, Inc., Toronto
Prentice-Hall Hispanoamericana, S.A., Mexico
Prentice-Hall of India Private Limited, New Delhi
Prentice-Hall of Japan, Inc., Tokyo
Simon & Schuster Asia Pte. Ltd., Singapore
Editora Prentice-Hall do Brasil, Ltda., Rio de Janeiro

Table of Contents

Module 5   Trauma

Module 6   Infants and Children

Module 7   Operations

Module 8   Advanced Airway Management

Appendices

Introduction

OVERVIEW

This workbook is designed to accompany the textbook *Emergency Care,* Eighth Edition. The workbook covers the course knowledge and U.S. Department of Transportation's skill objectives to which all standardized testing instruments are referenced. It is not meant to replace the text nor is it meant to substitute for a well-designed course in emergency care.

This is a self-instructional workbook. It has been designed to allow you to work at your own pace and to evaluate your progress. To benefit from this workbook, follow the procedures in this introduction. Thousands of EMT-B students before you have used prior editions of this workbook as part of their emergency medical training. The system works, having helped them to learn and excel on state and national certification and registration examinations. By doing your best on each chapter, you, as well as those patients to whom you deliver emergency care, will benefit.

A significant change in this edition, predicated on the 1994 change in the EMT curriculum, is the emphasis on patient assessment. The text devotes seven chapters directly to assessment and indirectly incorporates assessment into all other chapters. There is a strong emphasis on the pediatric patient in Chapters 13 and 29 and also throughout the book in a feature titled "Infants and Children." To correspond with changes in the textbook, the workbook incorporates information on hazardous materials and infection control in Chapter 2, "The Well-being of the EMT-Basic." It also includes new material in Chapter 13, "Pediatric, Adolescent, and Geriatric Assessment" and Appendix B, "Stress in EMS."

FEATURES

Each chapter in the workbook contains these specific elements:

- **Match Terminology/Definitions**—In this section, you are asked to match chapter terminology with appropriate definitions, which are included in the chapter's running text, appear in the chapter glossary, or both. The terms have been placed in alphabetical order so that after reading the definitions you can quickly select the appropriate term.

- **Multiple Choice Review**—This section provides some 25 to 45 questions (on average). Emphasis is placed on multiple choice questions, since this is the format of state and national exams used for certification or registration. Practice in answering multiple choice questions can help improve your understanding of the material as well as your course grades. These multiple choice questions appear in the sequential order that the topics appear in the textbook, enabling you to build on prior knowledge. When similar questions appear in the three Interim Exams, the order is scrambled, as is done on state and national exams.

- **Complete the Following**—This section focuses on your recalling and listing specific information on chapter objectives, such as the signs and symptoms of shock or the five stages of grief.

- **Label the Diagram/Photograph and Complete the Chart**—In some chapters, you are asked to study a visual and to identify its content or to complete a partially filled-in chart. These diagrams, photographs, and charts correspond to those in the textbook.

- **Case Study**—Each module includes a case study that requires you to synthesize information that you have learned up to that particular point in the course and to apply this knowledge to a real-life situation. As each step of the case is presented, you are asked a series of questions that build on the facts of the case.

- **Answer Key**—The Answer Key at the back of the workbook provide answers for all of the above-mentioned workbook elements. For the Multiple Choice Review questions, rationales appear for each answer along with the textbook page reference where each topic is discussed.

- **EMT-Basic Skills Performance Checklists**—In appropriate chapters, these checklists provide the key steps for each skill necessary for your performance as an EMT-Basic. These checklists are based on the American Heart Association standards, the National Registry testing standards, and the textbook. They offer a detailed but speedy review of each skill's steps in a checklist format.

▶ STEPS FOR SUCCESS

To get the most out of this workbook you should complete the following seven steps:

Step 1—Learn the Course Objectives

Each chapter of the textbook begins with objectives—objectives that were developed as a part of the U.S. Department of Transportation's EMT-B 1994 training curriculum. Most state and national certifying examinations are based on these course objectives. To score well on these exams, you must learn the objectives of the course. Use the objectives in the textbook in the following way:

1. Read them over.
2. Read the text.
3. Re-read the objective in the form of a question.
4. Write down your answer to each question on a blank piece of paper.
5. Perform a self assessment or ask your instructor to assess how well you understand the material in the chapter.

Step 2—Learn the Language of the EMT-Basic

Emergency Medical Services is clearly a medical field and as such it is necessary for the EMT-Basic to learn and understand the language of medicine. This will help you communicate with the other members of the health care team in a clear, concise, and accurate manner. In addition, learning the language of medicine will facilitate your understanding of medical and trade journal articles as you work to keep current in the constantly changing EMS field.

First, review the medical terminology in the text and then put aside the text. Next, test your understanding of the terminology by completing the Match Terminology/Definitions exercise in each workbook chapter. Complete the entire matching exercise before checking your answers with the Answer Key. For those terms you were unable to match, write down the word on one side of a 3″ × 5″ card and write the definition on the other side of the card. Carry these cards in your pocket and refer to them frequently to help you learn the terms.

Step 3—Learn the Structure of the Body

The language of medicine also includes learning the names and locations of the structures of the human body. Can you imagine being unable to control serious bleeding because you could not find the pressure point in the arm! To help you learn the structures of the body, in workbook chapters in which it is appropriate, anatomical drawings and diagrams are lifted directly from the text. For example, the drawing of the respiratory system in the workbook has blank numbered lines that point to each of the system's different structures. Label each structure as requested and check your answers in the back of the workbook. For those you miss, go to the textbook page suggested and study the drawing again.

Step 4—Answer the Multiple Choice Questions

For each Multiple Choice Review, complete the entire exercise at one sitting. Read each question and all the answer choices before you mark your answer. If you jump to a conclusion without fully reading the question, you could answer incorrectly. Also watch out for questions with negative expressions or the word "except." You will notice that the author has minimized the use of "all of the above" as an answer to questions in this edition. This was done to ensure that exam items mirror those utilized in standardized tests. Once you have completed the exercise, refer to the Answer Key to check your performance. A textbook page reference has been provided for the theory or principle tested in each question. Many answers have an "author's comment" whenever it is appropriate to clarify the answer to a question.

You will need to practice reading, and not reading into, multiple choice questions. If it has been many years since you took a standardized test, leave extra time to review this section of each workbook chapter. If you notice any trends in your performance on these questions, you may wish to consult your instructor for "test-taking assistance."

Step 5—Review the EMT-Basic Skill Performance Checklists

Whenever a skill is introduced in the chapter, a checklist has been included in the workbook. Work in pairs and use these checklists to test each other.

Step 6—Take the Interim Exams

Once you have completed each individual chapter, move on to the next chapter and repeat steps one to five. Interim Exams appear after Modules 2, 4, and 7 and are similar to the interim exams your instructor may give in the EMT-Basic course. Each exam covers material in the chapters that precede it. Therefore, when you have completed all of the material preceding an exam, it's time to take the Interim Exam.

Also be sure to review the extra value-added material in the BCLS Review that appears at the end of the workbook.

Step 7—Pay Close Attention to the Case Studies

The case studies integrated in the workbook help you synthesize your knowledge and apply it to real-life situations. They actually put you at a scene and require you to think quickly and accurately. Answers at the back of the workbook will help you sort out any problems you confront.

So that's it in seven simple steps. It will take your time and commitment to work through each of the steps. Since this is a self-instructional workbook, it will be up to you to reward yourself for doing well on chapters. At the same time you need to be honest with yourself. If you are having difficulty with a chapter, let your instructor know immediately so he or she can offer additional assistance.

It is the hope of the *Emergency Care* authors and development team that using this Workbook as an integral part of your EMT-Basic training package will help you improve your understanding of the material and enhance your performance in the field. After all, isn't quality patient care what EMS is all about? See you in the streets!

▶ ACKNOWLEDGMENTS

The authors of the *Emergency Care Workbook*, Eighth Edition would like to thank the publishing team led by Susan B. Katz and Lois Berlowitz for all their hard work and support on the *Emergency Care* series. Appreciation is extended to the coauthors of the text for their friendship and confidence and the opportunity to partake in this important project! Gratitude is extended to Terse Stamos for her excellent manuscript editing. And last, but not least, a special thanks to the three reviewers whose years of experience helped to ensure content accuracy: David M. Habben, NREMT-P, EMS Instructor/Consultant, Boise, Idaho; Edward B. Kuvlesky, REMT-P, Battalion Chief, Indian River County EMS, Indian River, FL; and Craig N. Story, REMT-P, Polk Community College, Winter Haven, FL.

▶ ABOUT THE EIGHTH EDITION WORKBOOK AUTHOR

Bob Elling, MPA, REMT-P is Program Coordinator for the Hudson Valley Community College Institute of Prehospital Emergency Medicine in Troy, New York. He is also a paramedic with the Town of Colonie, EMS Department. Bob has served as a paramedic for NYC*EMS, Associate Director of the New York State EMS Program, Education Coordinator for Emergency Medical Update, and is a coauthor of *Essentials of Emergency Care* and *First Responder: Exam Preparation and Review.*

Introduction to Emergency Medical Care

MATCH TERMINOLOGY/DEFINITIONS

A. State laws that allow an EMS system to exist

B. An all out effort by EMS personnel to improve the service provided from the moment of contact to the moment of delivery to the most appropriate medical facility and personnel

C. The provision for physician input and direction of patient care, training, and quality assurance of an emergency medical service or system

D. A system designed to get trained personnel to the patient as quickly as possible and to provide emergency care on the scene, en route to the hospital, and in the hospital

E. Policy or protocol issued by a Medical Director that authorizes EMT-Basics or others to perform particular skills in certain situations

F. Lists of steps, such as assessment and interventions, to be taken in different situations that are developed by the Medical Director of an EMS system

G. A communications system that has the capability of automatically identifying the caller's phone number and location

H. A system for telephone access to report emergencies in which a dispatcher answers the call, takes the information, and alerts EMS or the fire or police departments as needed

I. An EMT-B or other person authorized by a Medical Director to give medications and provide emergency care

J. A physician who assumes the ultimate responsibility for the patient care aspects of the EMS system

___I___ **1.** Designated agent

___D___ **2.** EMS System

___A___ **3.** Enabling legislation

___G___ **4.** Enhanced 911

___C___ **5.** Medical direction

___J___ **6.** Medical Director

___H___ **7.** 911 system

___F___ **8.** Protocols

___B___ **9.** Quality improvement

___E___ **10.** Standing order

MULTIPLE CHOICE REVIEW

B **1.** The earliest documented emergency medical service was in
- **A.** England in the 1890s.
- **B.** France in the 1790s.
- **C.** Seattle in the 1970s.
- **D.** Miami in the 1960s.

C **2.** In 1966, the _____ charged the United States _____ with developing EMS standards.
- **A.** Uniform Traffic Act : Department of Transportation
- **B.** President : Fire Academy
- **C.** National Highway Safety Act : Department of Transportation
- **D.** American Medical Association : Department of Health & Human Services

B **3.** Of the following, which is not a major component in the National Highway Traffic Safety Administration's EMS system assessment standards?
- **A.** transportation
- **B.** computerization
- **C.** communications
- **D.** evaluation

C **4.** An example of a "specialty" hospital in the EMS System is a(n)
- **A.** emergency department.
- **B.** correctional facility.
- **C.** poison control center.
- **D.** primary care center.

A **5.** National levels of EMS training include all of the following except
- **A.** advanced first aid.
- **B.** First Responder.
- **C.** EMT-Intermediate.
- **D.** EMT-Paramedic.

C **6.** The major emphasis of the curriculum for the EMT-B deals with _____ of the ill or injured patient in the prehospital setting.
- **A.** immediate life-threatening care
- **B.** interpretation of electrocardiograms
- **C.** assessment and care
- **D.** techniques of advanced airway care

B **7.** Patient care provided by the EMT-B should be
- **A.** delayed until transportation.
- **B.** based on assessment findings.
- **C.** guided by the service's attorney.
- **D.** based upon your diagnosis of the patient.

A **8.** An example of assuring continuity during the transfer of care of the patient would be
- **A.** providing pertinent patient information to the hospital staff.
- **B.** performing more hospital procedures in the field.
- **C.** only giving a report directly to a physician.
- **D.** None of the above.

D **9.** Patient advocacy is
- **A.** assessing your patient.
- **B.** abandoning your patient.
- **C.** executing your primary responsibility as an EMT-B.
- **D.** speaking up for your patient.

A **10.** Good personality traits are very important to the EMT-B. You should be
- **A.** cooperative and resourceful.
- **B.** cunning and inventive.
- **C.** respectful and condescending.
- **D.** emotionally stable and shy.

D **11.** If an EMT-B is not in control of personal habits, he/she might
- **A.** contaminate the patient's wounds.
- **B.** make inappropriate decisions.
- **C.** render improper care.
- **D.** All of the above.

C **12.** To prevent violating patient confidentiality, the EMT-B should
   A. communicate with medical direction.
   B. perform an accurate interview.
   C. avoid inappropriate conversation.
   D. develop the ability to listen to others.

C **13.** Way(s) in which an EMT-B may further his/her EMS education include
   A. re-reading the EMT-B textbook.   C. attending EMS conferences.
   B. repeating the EMT-B course.   D. All of the above.

C **14.** A system of continuous self-review of all aspects of an EMS system for the purpose of identifying and correcting aspects of the system that require improvement is called
   A. off-line medical direction.   C. quality improvement.
   B. patient advocacy.   D. continuing education.

B **15.** Obtaining feedback from patients and the hospital staff is a means of
   A. obtaining on-line medical direction.
   B. providing quality improvement.
   C. determining what is wrong with patients.
   D. avoiding charges of negligence.

C **16.** Participation in continuing education and keeping careful written documentation are examples of the EMT-B's role in
   A. patient advocacy.   C. quality improvement.
   B. medical direction.   D. transfer of care.

D **17.** Every EMS system should have a
   A. minimum of three EMT-Bs on each vehicle.
   B. call review on a monthly basis.
   C. contract with the local hospital.
   D. Medical Director.

C **18.** An EMT-B is operating as the Medical Director's _____ .
   A. employee   C. designated agent
   B. replacement   D. peer

D **19.** The difference between on-line (direct) and off-line (indirect) medical direction is that
   A. off-line does not need protocols.
   B. off-line orders are given by the on-duty physician, usually over the radio or phone.
   C. on-line uses standing orders.
   D. on-line orders are given by the on-duty physician, usually over the radio or phone.

B **20.** An example of a medication carried by EMT-Bs that may require a physician consult to administer is
   A. lidocaine.   C. oxygen.
   B. activated charcoal.   D. aspirin.

COMPLETE THE FOLLOWING

1. List at least six of the categories and standards of an EMS system as established by the National Highway Traffic Safety Administration.

   trauma systems

   Communication

   transportation

   facilities

   evaluation

   medical direction

2. List the four types of specialty hospitals.

   trauma

   burn

   Pediatic

   Poison center

3. List the four levels of EMS certification.

   First Responder

   EMT-B

   EMT-I

   EMT-P

2

The Well-being of the EMT-Basic

MATCH TERMINOLOGY/DEFINITIONS

A. Infection control based on the presumption that all body fluids are infectious

B. Mental health professionals and peer counselors who work as a team to provide emotional and psychological support to EMS personnel who are or have been involved in a highly stressful incident

C. The removal or cleansing of dangerous chemicals or other dangerous or infectious materials

D. Equipment such as eye wear, mask, gloves, gown, turnout gear, or helmet that protect the EMS worker from infection and/or from hazardous materials and the dangers of rescue operations

E. The organisms that cause infection, such as viruses and bacteria

F. An emergency involving multiple patients

G. When a patient mentally tries to postpone death for a short time

H. The release of a harmful substance into the environment

I. When a rescuer becomes overwhelmed by the stress of a scene

J. When a patient gets upset and questions, "Why me?"

K. Injections given to a rescuer that are designed to prevent him/her from getting a disease

L. When a patient puts off dealing with the inevitable end of the process of dying

M. A potentially infectious material

N. A high efficiency particulate air respirator or mask designed to reduce the spread of TB

O. Test that determines if a person has been exposed to TB

_J_ **1.** Anger

_G_ **2.** Bargaining

_M_ **3.** Biohazard

_A_ **4.** Body substance isolation (BSI)

_B_ **5.** Critical incident stress debriefing (CISD) teams

_C_ **6.** Decontamination

_L_ **7.** Denial

_I_ **8.** Distress

_H_ **9.** Hazardous material incident

_N_ **10.** HEPA

_K_ **11.** Immunizations

_F_ **12.** MCI

_E_ **13.** Pathogens

_D_ **14.** Personal protective equipment

_O_ **15.** PPD test

A **1.** The most important job of the EMT-B is to
   A. stay physically safe and emotionally well.
   B. immediately assess the patient and call the hospital.
   C. provide medical advice to friends and community members.
   D. check the unit at the end of each shift.

D **2.** The EMT-B can safeguard his/her well-being by
   A. understanding and dealing with job stress.
   B. ensuring scene safety.
   C. taking body substance isolation.
   D. All of the above.

B **3.** Each of the following is an example of a call that has a higher potential for causing excess stress on EMS providers except
   A. trauma to infants and children.
   B. an adult cardiac arrest.
   C. elderly abuse.
   D. death or serious injury of a coworker.

C **4.** Some warning signs that an EMT-B is being affected by stress include
   A. overeating and ringing in the ears.
   B. rapid urination and sweating.
   C. indecisiveness and guilt.
   D. increased sexual activity and sleep.

D **5.** All of the following are recommended life-style changes an EMT-B may take to deal with job stress except
   A. develop more healthful and positive dietary habits.
   B. devote time to relaxation.
   C. exercise.
   D. avoid talking about your feelings.

C **6.** A meeting held by a team of peer counselors and mental health professionals within 24 to 72 hours after a major incident is a
   A. incident critique.   **C.** critical incident stress debriefing.
   B. MCI.   **D.** quality circle.

D **7.** For a CISD to be effective,
   A. it must not be an investigation of the events of the call.
   B. information discussed must remain confidential.
   C. an EMT-B must feel open to discuss feelings, fears, and reactions.
   D. All of the above.

D **8.** A CISD can to be effective in returning personnel to work quicker because
   A. the debriefing can be combined with an incident critique.
   B. pressure from their peers is provided.
   C. it helps them suppress their feelings.
   D. it can accelerate the recovery process.

C **9.** When a patient finds out that he is dying he may go through which of the following emotional stages?
   A. anger and laughter   **C.** depression and acceptance
   B. denial and empathy   **D.** bargaining and elation

B **10.** A dying patient may go through emotional stages in the following order:
   A. acceptance, rage, depression, acceptance, bargaining.
   B. denial, anger, bargaining, depression, acceptance.
   C. bargaining, acceptance, denial, anger, depression.
   D. depression, bargaining, denial, acceptance, anger.

B **11.** An EMT-B will occasionally need to assist the patient who has a terminal illness. Experts suggest all of the following except
   A. listen empathetically to the patient.
   B. tell the patient that everything will be all right.
   C. be tolerant of angry reactions from the patient or family members.
   D. try to recognize the patient's needs.

D **12.** An organism that causes infection is referred to as a(n)
   A. airborne.   **C.** allergen.
   B. bloodborne.   **D.** pathogen.

C **13.** Precautions the EMT-B should take when dealing with all patients are known as
   A. universal precautions.   **C.** body substance isolation.
   B. general isolation.   **D.** quarantine isolation.

C **14.** To provide body substance isolation, the EMT-B may need to use
   A. handwashing and SCBA.
   B. HEPA mask and shoe covers.
   C. disposable gloves and eye protection.
   D. paper gown and leather gloves.

B **15.** An EMT-B should routinely wear a mask when treating a patient with
   A. hepatitis B.   **C.** AIDS.
   B. potential for blood or fluid spatter.   **D.** All of the above.

A **16.** When an EMT-B covers a patient's mouth and nose with a mask to prevent the spread of an airborne disease, he/she should
   A. monitor the respirations and airway closely.
   B. write "TB alert" on the patient's prehospital care report.
   C. wear a surgical mask to reduce the spread of TB.
   D. notify his/her supervisor prior to transporting the patient.

B **17.** Each of the following are ways the EMT-B can plan safety precautions in advance of the call except
   A. keeping your tetanus immunization current.
   B. maintaining a list of communicable patients.
   C. verifying immune status.
   D. obtaining hepatitis B vaccine.

C **18.** It is suggested that all EMT-Basics be immunized with all of the following vaccines except
   A. tetanus.   **C.** purified protein derivative.
   B. hepatitis B.   **D.** measles.

C **19.** A federal organization responsible for issuing guidelines for employee safety around biohazards is called the
   A. Food and Drug Administration.
   B. Federal Communications Commission.
   C. Occupational Safety and Health Administration.
   D. Public Health Service.

C **20.** Every employer of EMT-Bs must provide free of charge
   A. a yearly physical examination.   **C.** hepatitis B vaccination.
   B. an insurance policy.   **D.** universal health insurance.

B **21.** A federal act which establishes procedures by which emergency response workers can find out if they have been exposed to life-threatening infectious diseases is
   A. OSHA 1910.1030.   **C.** AZT Act.
   B. Ryan White CARE Act.   **D.** OSHA 1910.1200.

C __ 22. After contact with the blood or body fluids of a patient, an EMT-B may submit a request for a determination of exposure to his/her
   A. employer.   C. designated officer.
   B. Medical Director.   D. local hospital.

B __ 23. Always assume that a any person with
   A. a cold has a bloodborne disease.
   B. a productive cough has TB.
   C. a fever has typhoid.
   D. dehydration and sores has AIDS.

D __ 24. Which of the following is true about treating a contaminated patient at a hazardous material incident?
   A. Take the patient to the ambulance.
   B. Bring the patient to the hospital.
   C. Wear a SCBA when treating the patient.
   D. Delay treatment until the patient is decontaminated.

B __ 25. All of the following are part of the three "Rs" of reacting to danger <u>except</u>
   A. retreat.   C. radio.
   B. respond.   D. reevaluate.

COMPLETE THE FOLLOWING

1. List five types of calls with a high potential of stress for EMS personnel.
   - MCIs
   - Infants and Children
   - Severe injuries
   - abuse and neglect
   - death of a coworker

2. List at least five signs and symptoms of stress.
   - inability to concentrate
   - Change in daily activity
   - loss of interest in sexual activities
   - anxiety
   - isolation

3. List at least five of the critical elements of the infection control plan required by Title 29 Code of Federal Regulation 1910.1030.

°infection exposure control plan

• education and training

• hepatitis-B shot

• PPE

• methods of control

EMT-BASIC SKILLS PERFORMANCE CHECKLIST

▶ **HAND-WASHING PROCEDURE**

❑ Remove watch and rings. Roll up sleeves.

❑ Adjust water flow and temperature.

❑ Wet hands and distal forearms.

❑ Dispense soap into hands.

❑ Wash lower arms and hands. Clean around and under the nails.

❑ Rinse thoroughly under running water to remove all soap. Do not touch the sink!

❑ Use a paper towel to shut off the faucet to avoid recontaminating hands.

Medical/Legal and Ethical Issues

MATCH TERMINOLOGY/DEFINITIONS

A. Permission to treat an unconscious patient until he/she becomes conscious

B. A written order given by the physician based upon a decision by a patient prior to his/her demise

C. Being held legally responsible

D. An obligation to provide emergency care to a patient

E. Permission given by adults who are of legal age and mentally competent to make a rational decision in regard to their medical well-being

F. Permission from the patient to treat him/her

G. A series of laws, varying in each state, designed to provide immunity from liability to individuals trying to help in emergencies

H. The collective medical, legal, and ethical guidelines that govern the EMT-Basic

I. Not providing the standard of care

J. A finding of failure to act properly in a situation in which there was a duty to act

K. A legal document, usually signed by the patient and his/her physician, to "do not resuscitate"

L. The obligation not to reveal information obtained about a patient except to other health care professionals involved in the patient's care, or under subpoena, or in a court of law

M. Leaving a patient after care has been initiated without assuring the patient has been turned over to someone with equal or greater medical training

N. Child who is married or of a specific age who, in certain states, can make his/her own legal decisions

O. Subjecting a patient to unwanted care and transport can be considered this in a court of law

M	**1.** Abandonment
B	**2.** Advance directive
O	**3.** Battery
I	**4.** Breach of duty
L	**5.** Confidentiality
F	**6.** Consent
K	**7.** DNR order
D	**8.** Duty to act
N	**9.** Emancipated minor
E	**10.** Expressed consent
G	**11.** Good Samaritan laws
A	**12.** Implied consent
C	**13.** Liability
J	**14.** Negligence
H	**15.** Scope of practice

B   **1.** The collective set of regulations and ethical considerations governing the EMT-B is called
     A. duty to act.   **C.** advance directives.
     B. scope of practice.   **D.** Good Samaritan laws.

B   **2.** Legislation that governs the skill and medical interventions that may be performed by an EMT-B is
     A. uniform throughout the country.
     B. different from state to state.
     C. uniform for regions within a state.
     D. governed by the U.S. Department of Transportation.

C   **3.** When the EMT-B makes the physical/emotional needs of the patient a priority, this is considered a(n) _____ of the EMT-B.
     A. advance directive   **C.** ethical responsibility
     B. protocol   **D.** legal responsibility

C   **4.** Which of the following is <u>not</u> a type of consent required for any treatment or action by an EMT-B?
     A. child and mentally incompetent adult
     B. implied
     C. applied
     D. expressed

A   **5.** When you inform the adult patient of a procedure you are about to perform and its associated risks, you are looking for
     A. expressed consent.   **C.** implied consent.
     B. negligence.   **D.** applied consent.

C   **6.** Consent which is based on the assumption that an unconscious patient would approve the EMT-B's life-saving interventions is called
     A. expressed.   **C.** implied consent.
     B. negligence.   **D.** applied consent.

C   **7.** Your record of a patient's refusal of medical aid or transport should include all of the following <u>except</u>
     A. informing the patient of the risks and consequences of refusal.
     B. documenting the steps you took.
     C. signing of the form by the Medical Director.
     D. obtaining a "release" form with the patient's witnessed signature.

B   **8.** Forcing a competent adult patient to go to the hospital against his will may result in _____ charges against the EMT-Basic.
     A. abandonment   **C.** implied consent
     B. assault and battery   **D.** negligence

C   **9.** Which of the following is an action you should <u>not</u> take if a patient refuses care?
     A. Leave phone stickers with emergency numbers.
     B. Recommend that a relative call the family physician to report the incident.
     C. Tell the patient to call his family physician if the problem reoccurs.
     D. Call a relative or neighbor who can stay with the patient.

D   **10.** Another name for a DNR order is
     A. deviated nervous response.   **C.** refusal of treatment.
     B. duty not to react.   **D.** advance directive.

A 11. There are varying degrees of DNR orders, expressed through a variety of detailed instructions that may be part of the order, such as
   A. allowing for CPR only if cardiac or respiratory arrest was observed.
   B. allowing comfort care measures such as intravenous feeding.
   C. disallowing the use of long-term life-support measures.
   D. specifying only five minutes of artificial respiration will be attempted.

B 12. In a hospital, long-term life-support and "comfort care" measures would consist of intravenous feeding and
   A. routine inoculations.
   B. the use of a respirator.
   C. infection control by the health care providers.
   D. hourly patient documentation.

B 13. If an EMT-B with a duty to act fails to provide the standard of care, and if this failure causes harm or injury to the patient, the EMT-B may be accused of
   A. breach of promise.   **C.** abandonment.
   B. negligence.   **D.** assault.

C 14. Termination of care of the patient without assuring the continuation of care at the same level or higher is called
   A. liability infraction.   **C.** abandonment.
   B. battery.   **D.** breach of duty.

D 15. The EMT-B should not discuss information about a patient outside of relaying pertinent information to the physician at the Emergency Department. Information considered confidential includes
   A. patient history gained through interview.
   B. assessment findings.
   C. treatment rendered.
   D. All of the above.

D 16. The EMT-B can release confidential patient information in all of the following circumstances except
   A. to inform other health care professionals who need to know information to continue care.
   B. to report incidents required by state law, such as rape or abuse.
   C. to comply with a legal subpoena.
   D. to protect the other victims of a motor vehicle collision.

D 17. Medical identification insignia that indicate serious patient medical conditions come in the form of all of the following except
   A. bracelets.   **C.** cards.
   B. necklaces.   **D.** patches.

B 18. When treating a critical patient who has an organ donor card, the EMT-Basic should
   A. transport without delay and document a DNR.
   B. treat the patient the same as any other patient and inform the ED physician.
   C. withhold oxygen therapy from the patient to keep the organ hypoxic.
   D. All of the above.

A 19. At a crime scene, the EMT-B should
   A. avoid disturbing any evidence at the scene unless emergency care requires.
   B. immediately remove the patient from the scene.
   C. move all obstacles from around the patient to make more room to work.
   D. search the house for clues to the cause of the crime.

B 20. Commonly required reporting situations include all of the following except
   A. child and elderly abuse.   **C.** sexual assault.
   B. crimes in public places.   **D.** domestic abuse.

COMPLETE THE FOLLOWING

1. In order for a patient to refuse care or transport what three conditions must be fulfilled?

   • Patient must be mentally competent and oriented
   • fully informed
   • must sign a "release" form

2. A finding of negligence, or failure to act properly, requires all of the following circumstances be proven:

   • The EMT had a duty to the patient
   • The EMT did not provide the standard of care
   • The action of the EMT in not providing the SOC caused harm

3. Four examples of conditions that may be listed on a medical identification device (such as a necklace, bracelet, or card) include:

   • Heart conditions
   • Allergies
   • Diabetes
   • Epilepsy

EMT-BASIC SKILLS PERFORMANCE CHECKLIST

▶ PATIENT REFUSAL PROCEDURE*

❏ Spend time effectively communicating with the patient (includes reasoning, persistence, and "dealing" strategies to convince the patient to go to the hospital).

❏ Clearly inform the patient of the consequences of not going to the hospital.

❏ Consult with medical direction and/or supervision.

❏ Contact family members to help convince the patient.

❏ Call law enforcement who may be able to order or "arrest" the serious patient to force the patient to go to the hospital.

❏ Try to determine why the patient is refusing care (i.e., may be solely a financial reason).

❏ Complete thorough documentation of the refusal checklist including a patient refusal release, an initialed description of the process of the refusal, and what the patient was told by the EMT-B.

*Procedure may differ by state and jurisdiction. Always follow your local protocol.

CASE STUDY

▶ A WITNESSED COLLISION: FIRST ON THE SCENE

It's a summer morning and you are traveling on the interstate highway with your family to the lake. Although the speed is posted at 55 mph, traffic has been moving along at least 10 mph faster. All of a sudden you observe the station wagon a few cars in front of you goes from the center lane to the passing lane, cutting off a car, and then veers off the center of the road down a ravine and rolls over numerous times. The vehicle comes to rest on its roof.

1. If you are an EMT-B, must you legally stop to offer assistance?

No, except if your State requries you to Stop

2. Are you protected from a lawsuit?

Yes and No! Anyone can be sued. Most states have Good Samariton Laws

3. Are you protected from a liability suit provided your treatment is appropriate?

Yes, in most States

As you secure your vehicle off the shoulder and assign another helper to set out some flares, your spouse uses a cellular phone to call for emergency assistance.

4. In most communities, what is the universal emergency phone number?

911

5. What types of questions would you expect the dispatcher to ask about the collision?

A) *exact location of patient*

B) *What is your call back number*

C) *How old is the patient*

D) *What's the problem*

E) *What's the patients sex*

F) *IS the patient breathing*

6. What emergency response agencies would you expect to be sent?

The Police, Fire Dept., EMS

As you carefully climb down through the brush to the car, you notice there are two patients who were ejected from the vehicle. Another citizen arrives and she identifies herself as an EMT-B. You ask her to check out the two ejected patients while you check the car for additional patients. She reports one ejected patient is dead, and the other is unconscious and has an obvious head injury.

7. As additional help arrives, how can they help with this patient?

Manual Stabilization of Head and Neck

8. What types of injuries could the patient have?

broken bones, internal bleeding a head on neck

9. Do you need permission to treat the patient?

No, Consent is implied because patient is unconscious

Inside the car there is a conscious male patient approximately 40 years old who appears to have injured his abdomen in the left upper quadrant on the steering wheel. He also has a broken upper left leg. You also notice that the car continues to leak gasoline from the dented fuel tank. After obtaining some additional help, you decide to carefully move this patient out of the car.

10. What potential injuries might this patient have?

ruptured spleen, fractured ribs, back and neck injuries, as well as the obvious fractured leg

11. How can you help minimize further injury to the leg?

Assign Someone to lift patients injured leg and hold it still

12. Do you need permission to treat this patient?

Yes, he is conscious and must give actual Consent

Once the patient is out of the car, an ambulance arrives as well as the fire department with an engine and a rescue truck. Meanwhile the police have arrived and are dealing with the traffic congestion that has developed.

13. Since there is now plenty of help, can you leave?

No, check with the EMT-B in charge to see if help is needed

14. What would be the problem if you left prior to help arriving?

Gross negligence due to Abandonment

The Human Body

MATCH TERMINOLOGY/DEFINITIONS

▶ **PART A**

A. Main branch of the respiratory system that enters each of the lungs

B. Upper chambers of the heart

C. Muscle that divides the chest cavity from the abdominal cavity

D. The carotid and this pulse are considered central pulses

E. Tiny blood vessels

F. Pulse in the neck at the side of the larynx

G. Body system that transports blood throughout the body

H. Area directly posterior to the mouth

I. Pulse in the arm used to take a blood pressure

J. Area directly posterior to nose

K. Ring-shaped structure that forms the lower larynx

L. Structure that contains the vocal cords

M. Structure that closes to prevent food from going into the trachea during swallowing

N. Pulse on the top of the foot

O. Vessels that carry blood away from the heart

_O_ **1.** Arteries

_B_ **2.** Atria

_I_ **3.** Brachial pulse

_A_ **4.** Bronchi

_E_ **5.** Capillaries

_G_ **6.** Cardiovascular system

_F_ **7.** Carotid pulse

_K_ **8.** Cricoid cartilage

_C_ **9.** Diaphragm

_N_ **10.** Dorsalis pedis pulse

_M_ **11.** Epiglottis

_D_ **12.** Femoral pulse

_L_ **13.** Larynx

_J_ **14.** Nasopharynx

_H_ **15.** Oropharynx

PART B

A. Area that includes the oropharynx and nasopharynx

B. Parts of the blood needed to form blood clots

C. Watery, salty fluid that makes up over one half of the blood's volume

D. Pulse that may be palpated on the posterior aspect of the medial malleolus

E. Structure that carries inhaled air from the larynx to the bronchi, also called the windpipe

F. Vessels that carry blood from the capillaries back to the heart

G. Maximum pressure exerted on the arteries when the heart pumps

H. Body system that takes in oxygen and eliminates carbon dioxide

I. Socket that holds the ball of the femur

J. Lower chambers of the heart

K. Muscle type that works without the patient thinking about its operation

L. Two large veins that return blood to the heart

M. Long bone in the upper leg

N. Pulse on the thumb side of the wrist

O. Bone at the back of the lower leg

I	1. Acetabulum
M	2. Femur
O	3. Fibula
K	4. Involuntary muscle
A	5. Pharynx
B	6. Platelets
C	7. Plasma
D	8. Posterior tibial pulse
N	9. Radial pulse
H	10. Respiratory system
G	11. Systolic
E	12. Trachea
F	13. Veins
L	14. Venae cavae
J	15. Ventricles

PART C

A. Medial anterior portion of the pelvis

B. Vertebrae that form the back of the pelvis

C. Standing face forward with palms facing forward

D. Inferior most division of the spine that is referred to as the tailbone

E. Towards or closer to the midline

F. Lower jaw bone

G. Round ball of bone on the inside of the ankle

H. Wide bony ring that can be felt near the waist

I. System that consists of sensory and motor nerves

J. Round ball of bone on the outside of the ankle

K. Facial bone that surrounds each of the eyes

L. Breastbone

M. Seven vertebrae in the neck

N. Bones of the ankle

O. Medial and larger of the two bones of the lower leg

C	1. Anatomical position
M	2. Cervical spine
D	3. Coccyx
H	4. Iliac crest
J	5. Lateral malleolus
F	6. Mandible
E	7. Medial
G	8. Medial malleolus
K	9. Orbit
I	10. Peripheral nervous system
A	11. Pubis
B	12. Sacral spine
L	13. Sternum
N	14. Tarsals
O	15. Tibia

▶ PART D

A. Inferior tip of the sternum

B. Upper arm bone

C. Away from the midline

D. Nerves that transmit information from the body to the spinal cord and brain

E. When two points on the extremities are compared, the point closer to the torso

F. Outermost layer of the skin

G. When two points on the extremities are compared, the point further away from the torso

H. Nerves that carry messages from the brain to the body

I. Above or towards the head end of the torso

J. Layer of the skin in which the hair follicles, sweat glands, and oil glands are located

K. Bones in the fingers and toes

L. Joint where three bones of upper arm and forearm are connected

M. Front side of the torso

N. Heel bone

O. Back side of the torso

M	1. Anterior
N	2. Calcaneus
J	3. Dermis
G	4. Distal
L	5. Elbow
F	6. Epidermis
B	7. Humerus
C	8. Lateral
H	9. Motor nerves
K	10. Phalanges
O	11. Posterior
E	12. Proximal
D	13. Sensory nerves
I	14. Superior
A	15. Xiphoid process

▶ PART E

A. Body system that regulates metabolic functions such as sugar absorption by the cells

B. Body system that governs sensations, movement, and thought

C. Lateral bone of the forearm aligned with the thumb

D. Bones that make up the hand

E. Highest portion of the shoulder joint

F. Medial bone of the forearm

G. Bones that make up the wrist

H. Shoulder blade

I. Bone in the front of the shoulder

J. The body less the extremities and the head

K. Lying on the back

L. An imaginary line drawn vertically from the center of the clavicle to the nipple below

M. Sitting position on a stretcher with the body at a 45-to-60 degree angle

N. Similar on both sides of the body

O. Lying supine with the legs elevated a few inches

E	1. Acromion
N	2. Bilaterally
G	3. Carpals
I	4. Clavicle
A	5. Endocrine system
M	6. Fowler's
D	7. Metacarpals
L	8. Mid-clavicular
B	9. Nervous system
C	10. Radius
H	11. Scapula
K	12. Supine
J	13. Torso
O	14. Trendelenburg
F	15. Ulna

▶ PART F

A. Muscle under conscious control of the brain

B. Four divisions of the abdomen used to pinpoint the location of pain

C. Referring to the sole of the foot

D. Blood vessels that supply the muscle of the heart

E. Referring to the back of the body

F. Upper jaw bone

G. Body system that provides protection and movement

H. Pressure exerted on the arteries when the heart is at rest

I. Knee cap

J. Vertebrae of the lower back

K. Rib area of the spinal column

L. Imaginary line drawn vertically through the middle of the body

M. Anatomical term for the armpit

N. Patient's left side

O. Lying on the stomach or face down

_B_ 1. Abdominal quadrants

_M_ 2. Axilla

_D_ 3. Coronary arteries

_H_ 4. Diastolic

_E_ 5. Dorsal

_N_ 6. Left side

_J_ 7. Lumbar spine

_F_ 8. Maxilla

_L_ 9. Midline

_G_ 10. Musculoskeletal system

_I_ 11. Patella

_C_ 12. Plantar

_O_ 13. Prone

_K_ 14. Thoracic spine

_A_ 15. Voluntary muscle

MULTIPLE CHOICE REVIEW

_C_ 1. All of the following are body systems except
A. respiratory.
B. cardiovascular.
C. abdominal.
D. musculoskeletal.

_B_ 2. If a patient is lying on his left side, this position is called the _____ position.
A. Fowler's
B. recovery
C. left supine
D. left prone

_C_ 3. When a patient is placed in a sitting-up position on a stretcher, this position is called
A. prone.
B. supine.
C. Fowler's.
D. Trendelenburg.

_D_ 4. When a patient is lying flat with head lower than legs, this position is called
A. prone.
B. supine.
C. Fowler's.
D. Trendelenburg.

_B_ 5. The musculoskeletal system has three main functions. It gives the body shape, provides for body movements, and
A. gives the body sensation.
B. protects vital internal organs.
C. provides for the body's outer covering.
D. allows transport of oxygen into the cells.

_C_ 6. The upper jaw is also called the
A. mandible.
B. orbit.
C. maxillae.
D. nasal bone.

A 7. The spinal column includes the _____ vertebrae.
    A. thoracic and coccyx   **C.** lumbar and sternal
    B. cervical and orbit   **D.** sacrum and pelvic

C 8. An injury to the spinal cord at the _____ level may be fatal because control of the muscles of breathing arise from the spinal cord at this level.
    A. lumbar   **C.** cervical
    B. sacral   **D.** thoracic

A 9. Bones in the lower extremities include the
    A. femur, calcaneus, and phalanges.
    B. ischium, tibia, and ulna.
    C. orbit, lumbar, and shin.
    D. radius, fibula, and metatarsals.

A 10. Bones in the upper extremities include the
    A. humerus and radius.   **C.** phalanges and tibia.
    B. humerus and calcaneus.   **D.** ulna and cervical.

D 11. The types of muscle tissue include
    A. voluntary.   **C.** cardiac "automaticity."
    B. involuntary.   **D.** All of the above.

A 12. The type of muscle that allows body movement such as walking is called
    A. voluntary.   **C.** cardiac.
    B. involuntary.   **D.** smooth.

B 13. Involuntary, or smooth, muscle is found in the
    A. trachea.   **C.** heart.
    B. walls of the blood vessels.   **D.** quadriceps and biceps.

B 14. The structure in the throat that is described as the voice box is called the
    A. pharynx.   **C.** trachea.
    B. larynx.   **D.** sternum.

B 15. A leaf-shaped valve that prevents food and foreign objects from entering the trachea is called the
    A. pharynx.   **C.** larynx.
    B. epiglottis.   **D.** bronchi.

C 16. The normal order of passage of oxygen from the environment to the lungs is
    A. nose, bronchi, larynx, trachea, lung.
    B. larynx, esophagus, trachea, bronchi, alveoli.
    C. mouth, pharynx, trachea, bronchi, alveoli.
    D. epiglottis, trachea, cricoid, bronchi, alveoli.

C 17. When the diaphragm and intercostal muscles relax, the size of the chest cavity
    A. increases causing inhalation.   **C.** decreases causing exhalation.
    B. increases causing exhalation.   **D.** decreases causing inhalation.

D 18. The difference between the adult airway and the pediatric airway is that
    A. the adult's tongue takes up proportionately more space in the mouth than the child's.
    B. the trachea is softer and more flexible in an adult.
    C. the cricoid cartilage is softer in an adult.
    D. all structures are smaller and more easily obstructed in a child.

A 19. The right atrium
    A. receives blood from the venae cavae.
    B. receives blood from the pulmonary veins.
    C. pumps blood to the lungs.
    D. pumps blood to the body.

_A_ **20.** The aorta
    A. is the major artery originating from the heart.
    B. divides at the level of the nipples into the iliac arteries.
    C. supplies only the vessels of the lower body with blood.
    D. supplies only the vessels of the upper body with blood.

_B_ **21.** The major artery in the thigh is called the
    A. carotid.   **C.** radial.
    B. femoral.   **D.** brachial.

_C_ **22.** The vessel that carries oxygen-poor blood from the portions of the body below the heart and back to the right atrium is called the
    A. posterior tibial.   **C.** inferior vena cava.
    B. internal jugular.   **D.** aorta.

_B_ **23.** The left atrium
    A. receives blood from the veins of the body.
    B. receives blood from the pulmonary veins.
    C. pumps blood to the lungs.
    D. pumps blood to the body.

_D_ **24.** The fluid that carries the blood cells and nutrients is called
    A. platelets.   **C.** lymph.
    B. urine.   **D.** plasma.

_B_ **25.** The blood component that is essential to the formation of blood clots is called
    A. plasma.   **C.** white blood cells.
    B. platelets.   **D.** red blood cells.

_A_ **26.** The pressure on the walls of an artery when the left ventricle contracts is called the _____ pressure.
    A. systolic   **C.** diastolic
    B. arterial   **D.** residual

_A_ **27.** The two main divisions of the nervous system are
    A. central and peripheral.   **C.** brain and skin.
    B. bones and muscles.   **D.** spinal cord and brain.

_D_ **28.** Nerves which carry information from throughout the body to the brain are _____ nerves.
    A. motor   **C.** spinal
    B. cardiac   **D.** sensory

_C_ **29.** One of the functions of the skin is to
    A. eliminate excess oxygen into the atmosphere.
    B. regulate the diameter of the blood vessels in the circulation.
    C. protect the body from the environment, bacteria, and other organisms.
    D. allow environmental water to carefully enter the body.

_C_ **30.** The system that secretes hormones, such as insulin and adrenaline, and which is responsible for regulating many body activities, is called the _____ system.
    A. integumentary (skin)   **C.** endocrine
    B. nervous   **D.** gastrointestinal

COMPLETE THE FOLLOWING

1. List the names of nine arteries in the body.

Coronary	Brachial
Aorta	Radial
Pulmonary	Posterior tibial
Carotid	Dorsalis pedis
Femoral	

2. List five functions of the skin.

Protection	Excretion
Water Balance	Shock absorption
Temperature regulation	

LABEL THE DIAGRAMS

Fill in the name of each anatomical position on the line provided.

▶ **ANATOMICAL POSTURES**

1. Supine

2. Prone

3. Recovery

Fill in the appropriate directional term or landmark on the line provided.

▶ **DIRECTIONAL TERMS AND LANDMARKS**

Diagram 1

Diagram 2

1. Distal
2. Proximal
3. Midline
4. Mid-clavicular
5. Medial
6. Lateral
7. Palmar
8. Left
9. Dorsal
10. Right

11. Anterior (ventral)
12. Posterior (Dorsal)
13. Superior
14. Mid-axillary
15. Inferior

Fill in the name of each body region or structure on the line provided.

▶ **TOPOGRAPHY OF THE TORSO**

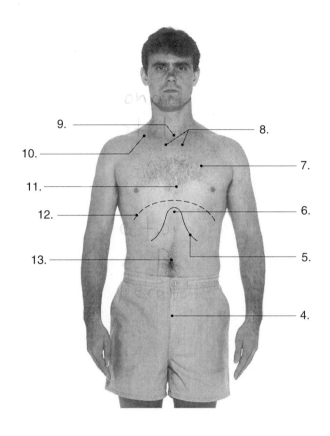

9.
8.
10.
11.
7.
12.
13.
6.
5.
4.

1.
2.
3.

1. Scapular region
2. Lumbar region
3. Iliac crest
4. Pubis
5. Costal arch (margin)
6. Xiphoid process
7. Pectoral region

8. Sternoclavicular joints
9. Suprasternal (jugular) notch
10. Clavicle
11. Sternum
12. Diaphragm
13. Umbilicus

CHAPTER 5

Lifting and Moving Patients

MATCH TERMINOLOGY/DEFINITIONS

A. Stretcher, made of a steel wire mesh and tubular steel rim or plastic and steel rim, used to transport patients from one level to another or over rough terrain

B. Portable folding chair with wheels used to transport the patient in a sitting position up or down stairs

C. Aluminum stretcher that splits in halves that can be pushed together under the patient

D. Method of transferring a patient from bed to stretcher in which two or more rescuers curl the patient to their chests, then reverse the process to lower the patient to the stretcher

E. Patient move that can be made if speed is not priority

F. Method of lifting and carrying a patient in which one rescuer slips hands under the patient's armpits and grasps the wrists, while another rescuer grasps the patient's knees

G. Also called the squat-lift position; a lift is made from a squatting position with weight to be lifted close to the body, feet apart and flat on the ground, body weight on or just behind balls of feet, back locked in.

H. Proper use of the body to facilitate lifting and moving and to prevent injury

I. Gripping with as much hand surface as possible the object being lifted, with all fingers bent at the same angle

J. Patient move that should be done quickly yet without any compromise of spinal integrity

K. Method of transferring a patient from bed to stretcher by grasping and pulling the loosened bottom sheet of the bed

L. Line that runs down the center of the body from the top of the head and along the spine

M. Method of lifting and carrying a patient from ground level to a stretcher in which two or more rescuers kneel, curl the patient to their chests, stand, then reverse the process to lower the patient to the stretcher

N. Removal of a patient from a hazardous environment in which safety is the first priority and spinal integrity is second priority

O. Procedure done by three or four rescuers that is designed to move a supine patient onto a long backboard without compromising spinal integrity

_A_	**1.** Basket stretcher
_H_	**2.** Body mechanics
_D_	**3.** Direct carry
_M_	**4.** Direct ground lift
_K_	**5.** Draw sheet method
_N_	**6.** Emergency move
_F_	**7.** Extremity lift
_O_	**8.** Log roll
_L_	**9.** Long axis
_E_	**10.** Non-urgent move
_I_	**11.** Power grip
_G_	**12.** Power lift
_C_	**13.** Scoop (orthopedic) stretcher
_B_	**14.** Stair chair
_J_	**15.** Urgent move

_C_   **1.** To assure your own safety when lifting a patient, it is important to
  A. always wear a back brace.
  B. keep the weight as far away from your body as possible.
  C. use your legs, not your back, to lift.
  D. avoid lifting a patient that weighs more than you do.

_B_   **2.** When lifting a patient you should do all of the following except
  A. communicate clearly with your partner.
  B. twist while you lift the patient.
  C. know your physical ability and limitations.
  D. communicate frequently with your partner.

_A_   **3.** When lifting a cot or stretcher,
  A. use an even number of people so that balance is maintained.
  B. keep both of your feet together and flat on the ground.
  C. use a third person positioned on the heaviest side.
  D. if you must use one hand only, compensate by using your back.

_A_   **4.** When placing all fingers and the palm in contact with the object being lifted, you are using a
  A. power grip.   C. lock grip.
  B. power lift.   D. grip lift.

_A_   **5.** When you must push an object,
  A. keep the line of pull through the center of your body by bending your knees.
  B. push from an overhead position, keeping your knees locked.
  C. keep the weight you are pushing at least 20 inches away from your body.
  D. keep the elbows straight with arms close to your sides.

_D_   **6.** The situations in which an emergency move would be used include all of the following except
  A. fire or danger of fire.
  B. explosives or other hazardous chemicals.
  C. inability to protect the patient from other hazards at the scene.
  D. dispatcher is holding another more serious call.

_C_   **7.** If the patient is on the floor or ground and the EMT-B has decided that an emergency move is appropriate, the patient can be moved by
  A. rolling him/her like a log.
  B. using a spine board and strapping him/her down.
  C. pulling on his/her clothing in the neck and shoulder area.
  D. using one rescuer on each extremity.

_B_   **8.** If the patient has an altered mental status, the EMT-B should consider a(n) _____ move.
  A. emergency   C. non-urgent
  B. urgent   D. immediate

_C_   **9.** When doing a log roll, lean from your hips and
  A. keep your back curved only while leaning over the patient.
  B. position yourself at least ten inches from the patient.
  C. use your shoulder muscles to help with the roll.
  D. roll the patient as fast as possible.

B 10. An urgent move for the patient found in the sitting position in an automobile is called the
   A. rapid takedown.
   B. rapid extrication procedure.
   C. application of a short backboard or vest.
   D. blanket-roll technique.

A 11. The final step in packaging a patient on a wheeled stretcher is
   A. securing the patient to the stretcher.
   B. placing a towel under the patient's head.
   C. covering the patient with a top sheet.
   D. adjusting the position of the back rest.

D 12. If you are carrying a patient down stairs, when possible
   A. flex at the waist with bent knees.
   B. keep your lower back muscles loose.
   C. place one hand on the railing for balance.
   D. use a stair chair instead of a stretcher.

C 13. Each of the following is a device used for patient lifting except
   A. stair chair.   C. direct carry stretcher.
   B. scoop stretcher.   D. portable stretcher.

B 14. Which of the following is not recommended for moving a patient with a suspected spinal injury?
   A. wheeled stretcher   C. short spine board
   B. scoop stretcher   D. long spine board

A 15. You have a patient positioned on a scoop-style stretcher and wish to lower the patient from a roof top. You should
   A. place the stretcher and patient in a plastic basket stretcher.
   B. transfer the patient to a wire basket stretcher.
   C. place the patient in a short spine board.
   D. lower the patient in the scoop stretcher.

A 16. To avoid trauma to a patient with an injured spine, the best patient-carrying device would be the
   A. long spine board.   C. Stokes basket.
   B. wheeled stretcher.   D. portable ambulance stretcher.

D 17. The direct ground lift is an example of a(n) _____ move for a patient who has no spine injury.
   A. emergency   C. immediate
   B. urgent   D. non-urgent

C 18. A common method for transferring a bed-level patient to a wheeled stretcher is the
   A. extremity carry.   C. draw sheet method.
   B. side carry method.   D. slide transfer method

C 19. When positioning a patient who has chest pain or discomfort and high blood pressure, the EMT-B should
   A. lay him flat on his stomach.
   B. lay him flat on his back.
   C. put him in a semi-sitting position.
   D. lay him flat on his back with his legs elevated.

D 20. When positioning a patient with no suspected spine injury who has hypoperfusion (shock), the EMT-B should
   A. lay her flat on her stomach.
   C. place her in a sitting position.
   B. lay her flat on her back.
   D. lay her flat on her back with her legs elevated.

COMPLETE THE FOLLOWING

1. List seven patient carrying devices.

wheeled Ambo. Stretcher

portable Ambo. stretcher

Stair chair

Scoop Stretcher

long spine board

basket Stretcher

flexible Stretcher

2. List at least four body mechanic principles that will help you lift efficiently and prevent injury.

Position your feet properly

Use legs, not back

never twist

Carrying Pt's on stairs, use a stair chair

LABEL THE PHOTOGRAPHS

Fill in the name of each lift, move, or drag on the line provided.

1. _Shoulder Drag_

2. _Incline Drag_

3. _Foot Drag_

4. _Clothes Drag_

5. _firefighter's Drag_

6. _Blanket Drag_

7. One-Rescuer Assist

8. Cradle Carry

9. Pack Strap Carry

10. Piggy Back Carry

11. Firefighter's Carry

12. Two-Rescuer Assist

EMT-BASIC SKILL PERFORMANCE CHECKLISTS

▶ **THE FIREFIGHTER'S DRAG**

❑ Place the patient in the supine position.

❑ Tie patient's hands together with something that will not cut into the skin.

❑ Straddle the patient, facing his/her head.

❑ Crouch and pass your head through the patient's trussed arms and then raise your body to raise the patient's head, neck, and upper trunk.

❑ Crawl on your hands and knees, dragging the patient and keeping the patient's head as low to the ground as possible.

▶ **THE BLANKET DRAG**

❑ Gather half of the blanket up against the patient's side.

❑ Roll the patient toward your knees so that you can place the blanket under the patient.

❑ Gently roll the patient back onto the blanket.

❑ Roll up the blanket by the patient's head, neck, and shoulders and drag this rolled material, keeping the patient's head as low to the ground as possible.

▶ **THE ONE-RESCUER ASSIST**

❑ Place the patient's arm around your neck.

❑ Grasp the patient's hand in your hand.

❑ Place your other arm around the patient's waist.

❑ Help the patient walk to safety, communicating with him/her about obstacles or uneven terrain.

▶ **THE CRADLE CARRY**

❑ Place one arm across the patient's back with your hand under his/her arm.

❑ Place your other arm under his/her knees and lift.

❑ If the patient is conscious, have him/her place the near arm over your shoulder.

▶ **THE PACK STRAP CARRY**

❑ Have the patient stand.

❑ Turn your back to the patient, bringing his/her arms over your shoulders to cross your chest.

❑ Keep his/her arms as straight as possible, his/her armpits over your shoulders.

❑ Hold the patient's wrists, bend, and pull the patient onto your back.

▶ THE PIGGY BACK CARRY

❏ Assist the patient to a standing position.

❏ Turn your back to the patient, placing the patient's arms over your shoulders so they cross your chest.

❏ While the patient holds on with his/her arms, crouch and grasp the patient's thighs.

❏ Use a lifting motion to move the patient onto your back.

❏ Pass your forearms under the patient's knees and grasp his/her wrists.

▶ THE FIREFIGHTER'S CARRY

❏ Place your toes against the patient's toes and pull the patient toward you.

❏ Bend at the waist and flex your knees.

❏ Duck and pull the patient across your shoulder, keeping hold of one of his/her wrists.

❏ Use your free arm to reach between his/her legs and grasp his/her thigh.

❏ Let the weight of the patient fall onto your shoulders.

❏ Stand up, transferring your grip on the patient's thigh to his/her wrist.

▶ TWO-RESCUER ASSIST

❏ The patient's arms are placed around the shoulders of both EMT-Bs.

❏ Both EMT-Bs place their free arm around the patient's wrist.

❏ Help the patient walk to safety.

▶ LOADING THE WHEELED STRETCHER INTO THE AMBULANCE

❏ Lift the rear step of the ambulance if necessary.

❏ Move the stretcher as close to the ambulance as possible.

❏ Make sure the stretcher is locked in its lowest level before lifting (depends on local procedure and type of stretcher).

❏ Position EMT-Bs on opposite sides of the stretcher, bend at the knees, and grasp the lower bar of the stretcher frame.

❏ Both EMT-Bs should come to a full standing position with their backs straight.

❏ Use oblique stepping movements to move the stretcher to the ambulance.

❏ Secure the stretcher into the ambulance securing device.

❏ Engage both forward and rear catches to hold the stretcher in place.

▶ EXTREMITY CARRY

❑ EMT-B #1 places the patient on his/her back with his/her knees flexed.

❑ EMT-B #1 kneels at the patient's head.

❑ EMT-B #1 places his/her hands under the patient's shoulders.

❑ EMT-B #2 kneels at the patient's feet and grasp his/her wrists.

❑ EMT-B #2 lifts patient forward while EMT-B #1 slips his/her arms under the patient's armpits and grasps patient's wrists.

❑ EMT-B #2 grasps the patient's knees while facing the patient or turns and grasps patient's knees while facing away from the patient.

❑ EMT-B #1 and EMT-B #2 both crouch, then stand at the same time and move as a unit when carrying the patient.

▶ DIRECT GROUND LIFT

❑ Set the stretcher in its lowest position and place opposite the patient.

❑ The EMT-Bs drop to one knee facing the patient.

❑ Place patient's arms on his/her chest if possible.

❑ EMT-B #1 at the head-end cradles the patient's head and neck by sliding one arm under the patient's neck to grasp shoulder; the other arm is placed under the patient's lower back.

❑ EMT-B #2 at the foot-end slides one arm under the patient's knees and the other under the patient above the buttocks.

❑ If a third rescuer is available, he/she should place both arms under the patient's waist while the two slide their arms up to the mid-back or down to the buttocks as appropriate.

❑ On a signal, the crew lifts the patient to their knees.

❑ On a signal, the crew stands and carries the patient to the stretcher, drop to one knee, and roll forward to place the patient onto the mattress.

▶ DIRECT CARRY

❑ EMT-B #1 at the head-end cradles the patient's head and neck by sliding one arm under the patient's neck to grasp the shoulder.

❑ EMT-B #2 at the foot-end slides hand under the patient's hip and lifts slightly.

❑ EMT-B #1 at the head-end slides his/her other arm under the patient's back.

❑ EMT-B #2 at the foot-end places his/her arms under the patient's hips and calves.

❑ EMT-Bs slide the patient to the edge of the bed and bend toward him/her with their knees slightly bent.

❑ They lift and curl the patient to their chests and return to a standing position.

❑ They rotate and slide the patient gently onto the stretcher.

CHAPTER

Airway Management

MATCH TERMINOLOGY/DEFINITIONS

▶ PART A

A. The flap of tissue that caps the trachea as you swallow

B. A means of correcting blockage of the airway by the tongue by tilting the head back and lifting the chin

C. The area inside the mouth joining the nasal passageways and the throat

D. The two large tubes that bring air to and from the lungs

E. The voicebox, which contains the epiglottis and vocal cords

F. The ring-shaped structure that forms the lower portion of the trachea

G. The process of breathing in

H. The muscle of breathing that separates the abdomen from the thorax

I. The process of breathing out

J. A means of correcting blockage of the airway by moving the jaw forward without tilting the head or neck

D 1. Bronchi

F 2. Cricoid cartilage

H 3. Diaphragm

A 4. Epiglottis

I 5. Exhalation

B 6. Head-tilt, chin-lift maneuver

G 7. Inhalation

J 8. Jaw-thrust maneuver

E 9. Larynx

C 10. Pharynx

▶ PART B

A. A device that uses oxygen under pressure to deliver artificial ventilations

B. A hand-held device with a face mask and self-refilling bag that can be squeezed to provide artificial ventilations to a patient

C. Expansion of the stomach caused by too forceful ventilation pressures that cause excess air to enter the stomach instead of the lungs

D. Another word for breathing

E. A permanent surgical opening in the neck through which the patient breathes

F. A device connected to the flowmeter to add moisture to the dry oxygen coming from an oxygen cylinder

G. The passageway by which air enters or leaves the body

H. Forcing air or oxygen into the lungs when a patient has stopped breathing or has inadequate breathing

I. A blue or gray skin color resulting from lack of oxygen in the body

J. The breathing in of air or oxygen

G 1. Airway

H 2. Artificial ventilation

B 3. Bag-valve mask (BVM)

I 4. Cyanosis

A 5. Flow-restricted, oxygen-powered ventilation device

C 6. Gastric distention

F 7. Humidifier

D 8. Respiration

E 9. Stoma

J 10. Ventilation

▶ **PART C**

A. A flexible breathing tube inserted through the patient's nose into the pharynx to help maintain an open airway

B. A face mask and reservoir bag device that delivers high concentrations of oxygen. The patient's exhaled air escapes through a valve.

C. A device that delivers low concentrations of oxygen through two prongs that rest in the patient's nostrils

D. A device connected to an oxygen cylinder to reduce cylinder pressure to a safe pressure for delivery of oxygen to a patient

E. A device, usually with a one-way valve, to aid in artificial ventilation. A rescuer breathes through the valve when the device is placed over the patient's face. It also acts as a barrier to prevent contact with a patient's breath or body fluids and can be used with supplemental oxygen when fitted with an oxygen inlet.

F. When breathing completely stops

G. To provide ventilations at a higher rate to compensate for oxygen not delivered during suctioning

H. Container filled with oxygen under pressure

I. Use of a vacuum device to remove blood, vomitus, and other secretions or foreign materials from the airway

J. A rigid curved device inserted through the patient's mouth into the pharynx to help maintain an open airway

K. Vomiting or retching that results when something is placed in the pharynx

L. The reduction of breathing to the point where not enough oxygen is being taken in to sustain life

M. An insufficiency of oxygen in the body's tissues

N. A valve that indicates the flow of oxygen in liters per minute

O. A valve on a BVM designed to blow off excessive pressure; this valve is no longer allowed per AHA standards on any BVM due to the danger of under inflation of the lungs.

N 1. Flowmeter
K 2. Gag reflex
G 3. Hyperventilate
M 4. Hypoxia
C 5. Nasal cannula
A 6. Nasopharyngeal airway
B 7. Nonrebreather mask
J 8. Oropharyngeal airway
H 9. Oxygen cylinder
E 10. Pocket face mask
O 11. Pop-off valve
D 12. Pressure regulator
F 13. Respiratory arrest
L 14. Respiratory failure
I 15. Suctioning

MULTIPLE CHOICE REVIEW

A 1. During respiration
    A. oxygen enters the body during each inspiration.
    B. carbon dioxide enters the body during each expiration.
    C. oxygen exits the body on each expiration.
    D. carbon dioxide does not enter the body.

B 2. Respiratory failure is
    A. the cessation of breathing.
    B. the reduction of breathing to a point where oxygen intake is not sufficient to support life.
    C. the same as respiratory arrest.
    D. caused by electrocution.

__C__ 3. Which of the following is <u>not</u> a sign of adequate breathing?
   A. air moving out of the nose and mouth.
   B. equal expansion of both sides of the chest.
   C. breathing limited to abdominal movement.
   D. absence of blue or gray skin coloration.

__D__ 4. Signs of inadequate breathing in children may include
   A. cyanotic skin, lips, tongue, or earlobes.
   B. retractions between the ribs.
   C. nasal flaring.
   D. All of the above.

__B__ 5. Each of the following are signs of inadequate breathing <u>except</u>
   A. inspirations or expirations that are prolonged.
   B. breathing rate in an adult of 14–18 breaths per minute.
   C. breathing is very shallow, very deep, or appears labored.
   D. the patient is unable to speak in full sentences.

__B__ 6. Additional signs of inadequate breathing include all of the following <u>except</u>
   A. absent chest movement.
   B. air that can be felt at the nose or mouth.
   C. diminished breath sounds.
   D. noises such as wheezing or crowing.

__C__ 7. Inadequate breathing in a child is defined as
   A. less than 15 breaths per minute.
   B. more than 30 breaths per minute.
   C. Both of the above.
   D. Neither of the above.

__A__ 8. When at rest, the normal adequate breathing rate for an adult is _____ times a minute.
   A. 12 to 20   C. 60 to 80
   B. 30 to 40   D. 75 to 100

__D__ 9. Cyanosis can be checked by observing the patient's
   A. tongue.   C. nail beds.
   B. ear lobes.   D. All of the above.

__C__ 10. If a patient's inspirations are prolonged, this may indicate a possible
   A. cardiac problem.   C. upper airway obstruction.
   B. history of asthma.   D. lower airway obstruction.

__C__ 11. One indication that a patient is experiencing inadequate breathing is that he
   A. has a headache.   C. talks in short choppy sentences.
   B. complains of nausea.   D. is dizzy when standing.

__D__ 12. The very first step to aid a patient who is not breathing is to
   A. clear the mouth.   C. apply positive ventilation.
   B. administer oxygen.   D. open the airway.

__B__ 13. What is the importance of mechanism of injury to airway care?
   A. An injured patient will need more oxygen.
   B. The procedure for opening the patient's airway is different in trauma.
   C. Patients without a mechanism of injury will have an open airway.
   D. An injury can make airway care easier to manage than a medical emergency.

__B__ 14. To open the airway of a patient with no suspected neck trauma, the EMT-B should use a
   A. jaw-thrust maneuver.   C. head-tilt, neck-lift maneuver.
   B. head-tilt, chin-lift maneuver.   D. modified jaw-thrust maneuver.

A 15. When performing the head-tilt, chin-lift maneuver, the EMT-B should
   A. not allow the patient's mouth to close.
   B. position himself at the top of the patient's head.
   C. tilt the head by applying pressure to the patient's chin.
   D. use fingertips to lift the neck.

D 16. When performing the jaw thrust, the EMT-B should do each of the following except
   A. kneel at the top of the patient's head.
   B. stabilize the patient's head with forearms.
   C. use the index fingers to push the angles of the patient's lower jaw forward.
   D. tilt the head by applying gentle pressure to the patient's forehead.

B 17. The main purpose of the jaw-thrust maneuver is to
   A. open the mouth with only one hand.
   B. open the airway without moving the head or neck.
   C. create an airway for the medical patient.
   D. create an airway when it is not possible to jut the jaw.

C 18. Examples of various techniques the EMT-B can use to provide artificial ventilation are:
   1) one-person bag-valve mask
   2) flow restricted, oxygen-powered ventilation device
   3) two-person bag-valve mask with high flow supplemental oxygen at 15 lpm
   4) mouth-to-mask with high flow supplemental oxygen at 15 lpm

   What is the order of preference of these techniques?
   A. 1, 2, 3, 4   C. 4, 3, 2, 1
   B. 2, 4, 1, 3   D. 4, 1, 2, 3

C 19. Each of the following are signs of inadequate artificial ventilations except
   A. the chest does not rise and fall with ventilation.
   B. the rate of ventilation is too slow or too fast.
   C. the patient's color changes from cyanotic to pink.
   D. the patient's heart rate does not return to normal with ventilations.

A 20. When performing mouth-to-mask ventilation on an adult patient, ventilations should be delivered over _____ seconds.
   A. 1½ to 2   C. 5 or 6
   B. 2½ to 3   D. 10

B 21. The bag-valve mask on your ambulance should have
   A. a non-refilling shell that is easily cleaned.
   B. a non-jam valve with an oxygen inlet.
   C. a standard 9/12 mm fitting.
   D. manual disabling pop-off valve.

A 22. The bag-valve mask should be capable of
   A. withstanding cold temperatures.
   B. providing a high pressure in the chest and airway.
   C. blowing off at pressures above 40 mm of water pressure.
   D. receiving an oxygen inlet flow of 25 liters per minute.

D 23. When ventilating a patient with a bag-valve mask when trauma is suspected, it is most effective to do all of the following except
   A. use a device with a volume of 1,000–1,600 ml.
   B. use two EMT-Bs to perform the procedure.
   C. position the EMT-B maintaining the mask seal at the top of the patient's head.
   D. maintain the head-tilt, chin lift.

___D___ 24. When ventilating an unconscious patient, a bag-valve mask is incomplete if it is <u>not</u> used with a(n)
A. reservoir bag.
B. oral airway.
C. oxygen tank and liter flow regulator.
D. All of the above.

___C___ 25. When using the bag-valve mask device by yourself, place the top part of the mask over the bridge of the patient's nose, then
A. use both hands to seal the mask.
B. raise the chin to close the mouth.
C. lower the mask over the mouth and upper chin.
D. All of the above.

___D___ 26. If the patient's chest does not rise and fall when using a bag-valve mask, the EMT-B should do all of the following <u>except</u>
A. reposition the head and re-attempt ventilations.
B. check for escape of air around the mask.
C. use an alternative method of artificial ventilation.
D. increase the rate at which the bag is squeezed.

___C___ 27. If the patient has a _____ and needs ventilatory assistance, the best device to use is a _____ .
A. stoma : pocket mask
B. tracheotomy : positive-pressure ventilator
C. stoma : bag-valve mask
D. tracheotomy : nasal airway

___D___ 28. The flow-restricted, oxygen-powered ventilation device should
A. operate in both ordinary and extreme environmental conditions.
B. have an audible alarm when the relief valve is activated.
C. have a trigger so two hands can be used to seal the mask.
D. All of the above.

___C___ 29. An oral or nasal airway should be
A. cleaned for re-use after the call.
B. inserted in all critically injured patients.
C. used to keep the tongue from blocking the airway.
D. used in order to prevent the need for suctioning.

___C___ 30. If something is placed in the patient's throat, the gag reflex causes the patient to
A. take deep breaths.   C. vomit or retch.
B. pass out.   D. All of the above.

___A___ 31. An oropharyngeal airway of proper size will extend from the
A. corner of the patient's mouth to the tip of the earlobe.
B. lips to the larynx.
C. nose to the angle of the jaw.
D. None of the above.

___C___ 32. An oral airway should be inserted
A. upside down, with the tip toward the roof of the mouth, then flipped 180 degrees over the tongue.
B. right side up, using a tongue depressor to press the tongue down and forward to keep it from obstructing the airway.
C. Both of the above.
D. Neither of the above.

B 33. A nasopharyngeal airway should be
  A. inserted with the bevel on the lateral side of the nostril.
  B. measured from the patient's nostril to the earlobe.
  C. inserted in the left nostril when possible.
  D. turned 180 degrees with the tip facing the roof of the mouth.

D 34. When inserting a nasopharyngeal airway, lubricate the outside of the tube with
  A. petroleum jelly.   C. a silicone-based lubricant.
  B. an oil-based lubricant.   D. a water-based lubricant.

C 35. The purpose(s) of suctioning include removal of
  A. teeth and large pieces of solid material.
  B. excess oxygen from the patient.
  C. blood, vomitus, and other secretions.
  D. All of the above.

A 36. When a patient begins to vomit, it is essential that you have a _____ ready to go at the patient's side.
  A. suction unit   C. blood pressure cuff
  B. oxygen tank   D. pocket mask

C 37. Which of the following is not true of the Yankauer suction tip?
  A. It has a rigid tip.
  B. It allows for excellent control over the distal end of the device.
  C. It is most successfully used with responsive patients.
  D. It has a larger bore than flexible catheters.

D 38. When using a soft flexible tip catheter,
  A. measure so that it is inserted only as far as the base of the tongue.
  B. never pass the catheter through a nasal tube.
  C. insert the device with the suction turned on.
  D. None of the above.

C 39. When suctioning an adult patient who is unconscious, never suction for longer than _____ seconds at a time.
  A. 5   C. 15
  B. 10   D. 20

A 40. When inserting a rigid tip suction catheter,
  A. insert the device only as far as you can see.
  B. measure from the nose to the ear lobe.
  C. slide the device along the palate in children.
  D. insert the device with the suction on.

C 41. Atmospheric air contains _____ oxygen.
  A. 10%   C. 21%
  B. 16%   D. 25%

C 42. A fully pressurized oxygen tank should have approximately _____ psi.
  A. 1,000   C. 2,000
  B. 1,500   D. 2,500

B 43. Which portable oxygen cylinder, when full, will last the longest?
  A. D   C. A
  B. E   D. M

B 44. Before connecting a regulator to an oxygen supply cylinder, the EMT-B should
  A. remove the protective seal and then open the valve.
  B. stand to the side of the main valve opening and crack the cylinder valve slightly.
  C. attach the nonrebreather to the flow meter; then attach to the tank.
  D. All of the above.

__C__ **45.** Humidified oxygen is
  A. not possible in an ambulance.
  B. not used for patients on chronic oxygen therapy.
  C. not needed in adult patients being transported for short distances.
  D. habit forming.

__A__ **46.** Concerns about the dangers of giving too much oxygen to patients with COPD
  A. are invalid in the prehospital setting.
  B. have been understated and proven with research.
  C. are invalid when the patient is over the age of 60.
  D. are dealt with by using a nonrebreather mask at low flow rates.

__D__ **47.** The best method for EMT-Bs to use when giving a high concentration of oxygen to breathing patients is a
  A. nasal cannula.
  B. venturi mask.
  C. simple face mask
  D. nonrebreather mask.

__D__ **48.** The oxygen concentration of a nonrebreather mask is between
  A. 20% and 40%.
  B. 40% and 60%.
  C. 60% and 80%.
  D. 80% and 100%.

__B__ **49.** The flow rate of a nonrebreather mask should be
  A. adjusted so that when the patient inhales the bag deflates by two-thirds.
  B. 12 to 15 liters per minute.
  C. adjusted to 6 liters per minute.
  D. All of the above.

__C__ **50.** The oxygen concentration of a nasal cannula is between
  A. 4% and 6%.
  B. 8% and 20%.
  C. 24% and 44%.
  D. 50% and 65%.

COMPLETE THE FOLLOWING

1. List at least six of the signs of inadequate breathing.

- Chest movements are Absent, minimal, or uneven
- Breath Sounds are diminished or Absent
- Noises; wheezing, crowing, stridor, snoring, gurgling
- Nasal flaring; in children and infants
- Pt's skin, Lips, tongue, ear lobes, or nail beds are blue or grey
- Breathing; very Shallow, very deep, labored

2. List in order of preference the four techniques available to the EMT-B to provide artificial ventilations.

- Mouth to Mask
- 2 person bag-value mask
- Flow restricted, O₂ powered ventilation device
- 1 person bag-value Mask

LABEL THE DIAGRAM

Write the name of each part of the respiratory system on the line provided.

1. Pharynx
2. Nasopharynx
3. Oropharynx
4. Epiglottis
5. Larynx
6. Thyroid Cartilage
7. Cricord Cartilage
8. Trachea
9. Bronchiole
10. Left main bronchus
11. Right main bronchus
12. Diaphragm
13. Lungs

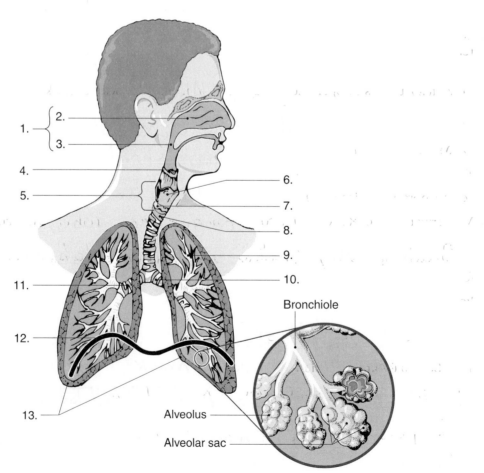

1.
2.
3.
4.
5.
6.
7.
8.
9.
10.
11.
12.
13.

Bronchiole

Alveolus

Alveolar sac

▶ HEAD-TILT, CHIN-LIFT MANEUVER

❑ Take body substance isolation.

❑ Once patient is supine, place one hand on the forehead and place the finger-tips of the other hand under the bony area at the center of the patient's lower jaw.

❑ Tilt the head by applying gentle pressure to the patient's forehead.

❑ Use your fingertips to lift the chin and to support the lower jaw. Move the jaw forward to a point where the lower teeth are almost touching the upper teeth. Do not compress the soft tissues under the lower jaw.

❑ Do not close the patient's mouth. It is best to insert an oral airway if the patient does not have a gag reflex.

▶ JAW-THRUST MANEUVER

❑ Take body substance isolation.

❑ Carefully keep the patient's head, neck, and spine aligned, moving him as a unit as you place him in the supine position.

❑ Kneel approximately 18 inches above the supine patient's head.

❑ Reach forward and gently place one hand on each side of the patient's lower jaw. Run your fingers along the jaw until you just pass the angle of the jaw.

❑ Stabilize the patient's head with your palms and forearms.

❑ Using your index fingers, push the angles of the patient's lower jaw forward.

❑ To keep the mouth open, use an oral airway on any patient without a gag reflex.

❑ Do not tilt or rotate the patient's head. Remember the purpose of the jaw-thrust maneuver is to open the airway without moving the head or neck from the neutral position.

▶ OROPHARYNGEAL AIRWAY INSERTION

❑ Take body substance isolation.

❑ Select appropriate size airway.

❑ Measure airway (center of mouth to angle of jaw or corner of mouth to ear lobe).

❑ Insert airway without pushing the tongue posteriorly (upside down and flip 180 degrees over the tongue, or straight in with a tongue blade holding tongue forward).

❑ Remove oropharyngeal airway if patient gags.

▶ NASOPHARYNGEAL AIRWAY INSERTION

❑ Take body substance isolation.

❑ Select appropriate size airway (diameter of patient's little finger).

❑ Measure airway (nostril to ear lobe).

❑ Verbalize lubrication of the nasal airway (water soluble jelly).

❑ Fully insert the airway with the bevel facing the nasal septum.

▶ MOUTH-TO-MASK WITH SUPPLEMENTAL OXYGEN

❏ Take body substance isolation.

❏ Connect one-way valve to mask.

❏ Connect oxygen to the inlet on the face mask. Oxygen should be run at 15 liters per minute. If oxygen is not immediately available, do not delay mouth-to-mask ventilations.

❏ Kneel about 18 inches above the supine patient's head.

❏ Opens airway (manually or with adjunct).

❏ Position the mask on the patient's face so that the apex is over the bridge of the nose and the base is between the lower lip and the prominence of the chin.

❏ Establish and maintain a proper mask-to-face seal (jaw-thrust maneuver) by placing both thumbs on the sides of the mask and the index, third, and fourth fingers of each hand grasping the lower jaw on each side, between the angle of the jaw and the ear lobe, to jut the jaw forward.

❏ Ventilate the patient at the proper volume and rate (800–1200 ml per breath, 10 to 20 breaths per minute, 1½ to 2 seconds for each adult breath).

❏ Remove your mouth from the port to allow for passive exhalation.

▶ TECHNIQUES OF SUCTIONING

❏ Take body substance isolation.

❏ Position yourself at the patient's head and turn the patient on his side.

❏ Measure flexible suction catheter: the distance between the patient's ear lobe and the corner of the mouth, or center of the mouth to the angle of the jaw. A rigid tip (Yankauer) does not need to be measured. This is the preferred device. But do not lose sight of the tip.

❏ Turn unit on. Attach a catheter and test for suction.

❏ Open and clear the patient's mouth.

❏ Place the rigid pharyngeal tip so that the convex (bulging-out) side is against the roof of the patient's mouth. Insert the tip just to the base of the tongue. Do not push the tip down into the throat or into the larynx.

❏ Apply suction only after the tip of the catheter or the rigid tip is in place, suctioning on the way out, moving the tip from side to side.

❏ Hyperventilate the patient.

► BAG-VALVE-MASK VENTILATION

(Two-Rescuer Medical Technique*)

❑ Take body substance isolation.

❑ Open the patient's airway using the head-tilt, chin-lift technique.

❑ Suction and insert an oral airway adjunct.

❑ Select the correct bag-valve-mask size (adult, child, or infant). A pop-off valve is unacceptable!

❑ Kneel approximately 18 inches above the supine patient's head.

❑ Position the mask on the patient's face so that the apex is over the bridge of the nose and the base is between the lower lip and the prominence of the chin.

❑ Position thumbs over the top half of the mask, index and middle fingers over the bottom half.

❑ Use the ring and middle fingers to bring the patient's jaw up to the mask and maintain the head-tilt, chin-lift. Tilt the head back as if you were trying to stand the patient on his head!

❑ The second EMT-B should connect the bag to mask, if not already done. While you maintain the mask seal, second EMT-B should squeeze the bag with two hands until the patient's chest rises. Ventilate the patient at the proper volume and rate (800-1200 ml per breath, 10 to 20 breaths per minute, 1 1/2 to 2 seconds for each adult breath **).

❑ The second EMT-B should release pressure on the bag and let the patient exhale passively. While this occurs, the bag from the oxygen reservoir is refilling.

*This technique can be used for a trauma patient by incorporating the combination jaw-thrust, manual-neck stabilization maneuver.

**The patient can be hyperventilated if his medical or traumatic condition warrants this method of treatment.

► PREPARING THE OXYGEN DELIVERY SYSTEM

❑ Select desired cylinder. Check label and hydrostat date.

❑ Place the cylinder in an upright position and stand to one side.

❑ Remove the plastic wrapper or cap protecting the cylinder outlet.

❑ Keep the plastic washer (some set-ups).

❑ Crack the main valve for one second to clean out valve.

❑ Select the correct pressure regulator and flowmeter.

❑ Place cylinder valve gasket on regulator oxygen port.

❑ Make certain that the pressure regulator is closed.

❑ Align pins or thread by hand.

❑ Tighten T-screw for pin yoke.

❑ Tighten with a wrench for a threaded outlet.

❑ Attach tubing and delivery device.

▶ Oxygen Administration—Nonrebreather Mask

- ❑ Take body substance isolation.
- ❑ Assemble regulator onto tank.
- ❑ Open main valve on tank.
- ❑ Check for leaks.
- ❑ Check tank pressure.
- ❑ Attach nonrebreather mask.
- ❑ Adjust liter flow to 12 to 15 liters per minute.
- ❑ Prefill reservoir.
- ❑ Apply and adjust mask to the patient's face. Make sure you explain the need for oxygen to the patient.
- ❑ Secure tank during transport.

▶ Oxygen Administration—Nasal Cannula

- ❑ Take body substance isolation.
- ❑ Assemble regulator onto tank.
- ❑ Open main valve on tank.
- ❑ Check for leaks.
- ❑ Check tank pressure.
- ❑ Attach nasal cannula.
- ❑ Adjust liter flow to 1 to 6 liters per minute.
- ❑ Secure tank during transport.

▶ Discontinuing Oxygen Administration

- ❑ Remove delivery device.
- ❑ Turn off the liter flow rate.
- ❑ Close the main valve.
- ❑ Remove the delivery tubing.
- ❑ Bleed the flowmeter.
- ❑ Change the tank before the volume reaches 200 psi.

▶ Repositioning the Patient for Basic Life Support*

- ❑ Take body substance isolation.
- ❑ Straighten the patient's legs and position the closest arm above his head.
- ❑ Cradle the patient's head and neck. Grasp under the distal armpit.
- ❑ Move the patient as a unit onto his side.
- ❑ Move the patient onto his back and reposition the extended arm.

* Note: This maneuver is used to initiate airway evaluation, artificial ventilation, or CPR when the EMT-Basic must act alone. When trauma is suspected, the four rescuer log-roll is the preferred technique.

CASE STUDY

▶ THE COMPLICATED AIRWAY: THE SELF-INFLICTED SHOOTING

Your unit and the police are dispatched to the scene of an attempted suicide with shots fired. Apparently the call was received by a family member who was called by the patient threatening to do harm to himself with a handgun. The police arrive before you and advise that the scene is secure (safe) and that you should respond directly to the scene, which is a private home in a suburban community. Upon arrival, you find a 45-year-old male lying with his face covered with blood. He is moaning, and his chest and abdomen appear to be moving as he breathes. After donning protective gloves, mask, and goggles, both you and your partners carefully provide manual stabilization of the neck and log roll the patient onto a long backboard.

What you reveal is a mandible and tongue that are severely lacerated, and the mouth and nose are bubbling with blood as the patient attempts to breathe.

1. How should you open the airway of this patient?

   Open the Pt airway but jutting the jaw, If possible
   or pulling the tongue forward away from the back
   of the throat

2. **A)** Does this patient need to be suctioned? **B)** If so, what is the maximum amount of time to accomplish this procedure?

   A) _Yes, The Pt needs Suctioned_

   B) _Max, Time is about 15 Seconds per attempt_

3. Should an airway adjunct be used on this patient?

   Yes, a oral or nasal

Once the patient's airway is opened and cleared, you need to oxygenate this patient. He has no other obvious injuries, yet you are treating him for a possible spinal injury due to the impact of the bullet and his backward fall from his desk chair during the incident. The police think that this is why he shot his chin instead of his brain during the suicide attempt. You evaluate the patient's breathing rate as 28, shallow and labored, and his pulse as 120, weak and regular.

4. What device should be used to administer oxygen to this patient?

   A Bag-Value Mask to assist the Pts
   ventilation

5. What is the proper liter flow to set the regulator for the device you choose in Number 4?

   12-15 Liters

6. Your portable D cylinder was full at the beginning of the shift and this is your first call. **A)** How many liters are in the tank? **B)** How much pressure in it? **C)** How much time can you expect to get out of the tank considering your service's policy is to refill tanks at 200 psi?

A) 350 Liters

B) 2,000 to 2,200 psi

C) 19 mins.

7. As you prepare to transport the patient, you continue to suction him making sure not to exceed **A)** _____ seconds per attempt because as you suction you are also removing **B)** _____ . **C)** Which would be better to use, a rigid tip or a flexible catheter?

A) 15 Seconds

B) Oxygen

C) rigid Yan Kauer

8. The patient has a BP of 100/70 so you decide his priority is **A)** [high or low?]. The major problem with this patient is his **B)** _____ . He should be transported **C)** [right away, in a few minutes] to the **D)** [local hospital or trauma center?].

A) high priority

B) Complicated airway

C) transported right away

D) trauma Center

9. From your knowledge of your EMS system, what ALS treatment might be helpful to this patient if you can arrange for an ALS intercept?

endotracheal intubation

10. What should you do if you hear hissing or bubbling around the mask as you ventilate?

Check Seal, airway possibly a not open

INTERIM EXAM 1

Use the answer sheet on pages 59–60 to complete this exam. It is perforated so it can be easily removed from this book.

1. The basis for most EMT-B training programs is the EMS standards and training developed by the
   A. American Red Cross (ARC).
   B. American Heart Association (AHA).
   C. United States Department of Transportation (DOT).
   D. National Institute of Health (NIH).

2. An EMT-B can inspire patient confidence and cooperation by
   A. transporting the patient from the scene to a hospital.
   B. providing patient care without regard for his own personal safety.
   C. telling the patient that everything will be all right.
   D. being pleasant, cooperative, sincere, and a good listener.

3. If an on-duty EMT-B fails to provide the standard of care and if this failure causes harm or injury to the patient, the EMT-B may be accused of
   A. assault.
   B. abandonment.
   C. negligence.
   D. breach of promise.

4. A conscious and mentally competent adult patient has the right to refuse care. This refusal must be _____ and documented.
   A. implied   C. involuntary
   B. actual   D. informed

5. The EMT-B can treat and transport an unconscious patient because of the legal consideration known as _____ consent.
   A. applied   C. triage
   B. implied   D. immunity

6. A child falls off the trampoline at elementary school and twists her ankle. Since the parents are not present, the child's consent is
   A. not needed.   C. implied.
   B. actual.   D. meaningless.

7. _____ help protect the off-duty EMT-B from lawsuits when stopping at the scene of a collision to offer assistance.
   A. Professional associations
   B. Blanket insurance policies
   C. Good Samaritan laws
   D. Abandonment laws

8. Each of the following is the responsibility of an EMT-B at a hazardous material incident except
   A. entering hazmat scenes with SCBA.
   B. protecting yourself and others.
   C. recognizing potential problems.
   D. notifying hazardous materials response team.

9. The form of infection control that assumes that all body fluids should be considered potentially infectious is
   A. infectious disease.
   B. body substance isolation.
   C. immunity.
   D. universal precautions.

10. When planning to lift, all of the following are important considerations except
    A. the weight of the object.
    B. one's physical characteristics.
    C. communicating with one's partner.
    D. the distance the object is to be carried.

11. When lifting, the EMT-B should
    A. keep the back loose and knees locked.
    B. twist or attempt to make moves other than the lift.
    C. use the leg muscles to do the lift.
    D. try not to communicate with his/her partner.

12. When carrying a conscious patient on the stairs, the EMT-B should
    A. keep the stretcher as level as possible.
    B. use a long backboard at all times.
    C. use a stair chair whenever possible.
    D. All of the above.

13. Ways an EMT-B can avoid a potential back injury include all the following except
    A. push, rather than pull, a load whenever possible.
    B. keep back locked-in while lifting.
    C. keep arms straight when pushing or pulling.
    D. push or pull from a kneeling position if the weight is below waist level.

14. An emergency move is required in each of the following situations except when
    A. the scene is hazardous.
    B. care of life-threatening conditions requires repositioning.

C. other patients must be reached who have life threats.

D. the patient is unconscious.

15. Which of the following is the greatest danger to the patient in an emergency move?
    A. A spinal injury may be aggravated.
    B. Bleeding may increase after movement.
    C. The airway may become obstructed.
    D. There is no danger associated with an emergency move.

16. A method of lifting and carrying a patient in which one EMT-B slips hands under the patient's armpits and grasps the wrists while another EMT-B grasps the patient's knees is called the
    A. direct ground lift.
    B. extremity lift.
    C. draw sheet method.
    D. direct carry method.

17. When moving a patient from the ambulance stretcher to the hospital stretcher, you probably will use the
    A. cradle carry
    B. modified draw sheet method
    C. direct ground lift.
    D. extremity lift.

18. To load the wheeled ambulance stretcher into the ambulance the two EMT-Bs should position themselves _____ of the stretcher.
    A. on opposite sides
    B. on opposite ends
    C. on the same side
    D. on one end and one side

19. A technique used to move a patient without broken bones or spinal injury from the floor to a stair chair is called the
    A. indirect carry.   **C.** slide transfer.
    B. extremity lift.   **D.** chair lift.

20. Drags are used only in emergencies because they
    A. do not protect the patient's neck and spine.
    B. require excessive energy from the EMT-B.
    C. may injure the EMT-B's back.
    D. provide full immobilization.

21. In order to maintain balance when lifting a patient carrying device, it is best to use _____ rescuers to carry the device.
    A. three
    B. an even number of
    C. an odd number of
    D. bystanders and

22. The driver of a vehicle involved in an accident requires immediate airway and bleeding control. You are unable to provide this treatment in the vehicle. You should
    A. check the patient's vital signs.
    B. make an urgent move.
    C. remove the patient on a short backboard.
    D. All of the above.

23. Which carry is considered very difficult to use with an unconscious person?
    A. cradle   **C.** shoulder
    B. three-rescuer   **D.** piggyback

24. Which carry must be performed in one unbroken sweep?
    A. pack strap carry
    B. front piggyback carry
    C. firefighter's carry
    D. four-rescuer carry

25. A canvas or rubberized stretcher that can be used to move a patient through a narrow hallway or restricted area is called a _____ stretcher.
    A. basket
    B. portable
    C. flexible
    D. wheeled-ambulance

26. A victim with obvious spinal injuries is found on the floor of a burning building. The EMT-B rates the situation hazardous, but not yet dire. Alone and without special equipment, the EMT-B should use the
    A. cradle carry.
    B. clothes drag.
    C. firefighter's carry.
    D. pack-strap method.

27. You wish to transfer a patient without spinal injury. Movement is unrestricted. The patient carrying device of choice is the
    A. portable ambulance stretcher.
    B. wire basket stretcher.
    C. wheeled ambulance stretcher.
    D. slat stretcher.

28. If you are an EMT-B with a service that does not provide the appropriate protective equipment, you should serve as an advocate for this equipment because
    A. your crew members could be injured unnecessarily.
    B. you could be seriously injured.
    C. an injured EMT-B is of little help to the patient.
    D. All of the above.

29. During an EMS call a lethal threat is recognized. The EMT-B should first
    A. retreat to a safe area.
    B. radio for assistance.
    C. re-evaluate the situation.
    D. remedy the situation.

30. Of the different types of stress, which is a positive form that helps the EMT-B work under pressure and respond effectively?
    A. cumulative stress
    B. eustress
    C. distress
    D. critical incident stress

31. When responding to a violent situation, observation begins when you
    A. enter the scene.
    B. exit the ambulance.
    C. enter the neighborhood.
    D. arrive at the patient's side.

32. To ensure crew safety, one member of the crew should always
    A. remain in the ambulance.
    B. carry a portable radio.
    C. wear a bulletproof vest.
    D. carry a canister of "pepper gas."

33. While treating a patient with a severely bleeding forearm, the patient's pet dog appears. The patient states, "He won't hurt you. He's very friendly." Your best course of action would be to
    A. have your partner observe the dog closely while you treat the patient.
    B. quickly control the bleeding; then have the dog locked in another room.
    C. ignore the dog since the patient assures it is friendly and will not harm you.
    D. All of the above.

34. If a patient refuses care and then becomes unconscious, it is best for the EMT-B to
    A. refuse to treat or transport the patient.
    B. ask a family member for permission to treat.
    C. treat life-threatening problems and transport.
    D. contact medical direction for advice.

35. An advantage to the "advanced directive" is that
    A. the patient is not involved in making a decision about his treatment.
    B. the patient's expressed wishes may be followed.
    C. no matter what the family says, CPR is not given.
    D. it protects the EMT-B from charges of negligence.

36. In most cases, the oral wishes of the patient's family to withhold care are
    A. all that is needed to stop CPR from being initiated.
    B. all that is needed to stop CPR once it is initiated.
    C. not a reason to withhold medical care.
    D. not sufficient unless they are given in writing.

37. You can prevent most lawsuits if you
    A. practice within the scope of your practice.
    B. properly document your care.
    C. are courteous and respectful to all your patients.
    D. All of the above.

38. The negligent EMT-B may be required to pay for all of the following except
    A. the patient's lost wages.
    B. the patient's medical expenses.
    C. the patient's pain and suffering.
    D. the patient's health insurance costs.

39. Which of the following is not a function of the musculoskeletal system?
    A. It gives the body shape.
    B. It protects the internal organs.
    C. It provides for body movement.
    D. It regulates body temperature.

40. The superior portion of the sternum is called the
    A. xiphoid process.   C. manubrium.
    B. sternal body.   D. clavicle.

41. A young girl fell while ice skating, injuring the protrusion on the inside of the ankle. The medical term for this location is the
    A. acromion.   C. lateral malleolus.
    B. medial malleolus.   D. calcaneus.

42. The heart muscle has a property called _____ . This means that the heart has the ability to generate and conduct electrical impulses on its own.
    A. contractility
    B. automaticity
    C. involuntary contraction
    D. conductibility

43. A division of the peripheral nervous system that controls involuntary motor functions is called the _____ nervous system.
    A. autonomic   C. sensory
    B. central   D. motor

44. When in the anatomical position, the person will be facing
    A. away from you.   C. face down.
    B. forward.   D. face up.

45. In the anatomical position, the person's palms will be facing
  A. forward.　　**C.** upward.
  B. backward.　　**D.** downward.

46. An anatomical term that is occasionally used to refer to the sole of the foot is
  A. calcaneus.　　**C.** dorsal.
  B. ventral.　　**D.** plantar.

47. The bones of the cheek are called the _____ bones.
  A. orbit　　**C.** zygomatic
  B. maxillae　　**D.** mandible

48. The heart is _____ to the stomach.
  A. distal　　**C.** proximal
  B. medial　　**D.** superior

49. When comparing body structure positions, the knees are said to be _____ to the toes, and the toes are _____ to the knees.
  A. inferior : superior
  B. proximal : distal
  C. distal : proximal
  D. superior : inferior

50. A patient found lying on his back is in the _____ position.
  A. anatomical　　**C.** supine
  B. prone　　**D.** lateral recumbent

51. To assist in describing the location of abdominal pain, we divide the abdomen into _____ parts.
  A. two　　**C.** four
  B. three　　**D.** five

52. The torso of the body is composed of the abdomen, pelvis, and the
  A. thorax.
  B. upper arms and legs.
  C. extremities.
  D. head.

53. The heart is located in the center of the _____ cavity.
  A. thoracic　　**C.** pelvic
  B. cranial　　**D.** cardiac

54. The structure that divides the chest cavity from the abdominal cavity is the
  A. meninges.　　**C.** diaphragm.
  B. duodenum.　　**D.** spinal column.

55. The anatomical name for the knee cap is the
  A. ilium.　　**C.** patella.
  B. malleolus.　　**D.** phalange.

56. The cranium consists of the
  A. facial bones.
  B. mandible and maxillae.
  C. top, back, and sides of the skull.
  D. zygomatic bones.

57. The highest point in the shoulder is the
  A. acromion process.　　**C.** metatarsal.
  B. humerus.　　**D.** clavicle.

58. At the scene of an accident, an off-duty EMT-B provides care to the patient, acting in good faith and to the best of his/her abilities. In many states this EMT-B is protected from care-related lawsuits by _____ laws.
  A. applied consent　　**C.** Good Samaritan
  B. total immunity　　**D.** jeopardy

59. When confronted with an unconscious minor without parents or a legal guardian present, the EMT-B should
  A. seek a physician's approval before beginning care.
  B. consider consent for care to be implied and begin care.
  C. ask the child for consent and begin care.
  D. consider consent to be applied and begin care.

60. The legal concept of negligence requires that three circumstances must be demonstrated. Which of the following is <u>not</u> one of the three circumstances?
  A. The EMT had a duty to act.
  B. The EMT committed a breach of duty.
  C. The EMT had a local duty.
  D. The breach of duty caused harm.

61. A person lying on his stomach with his face down is in the _____ position.
  A. supine　　**C.** coma
  B. prone　　**D.** recovery

62. In a trauma center, surgery teams are
  A. on call 12 hours a day.
  B. available most of the time.
  C. available 24 hours a day.
  D. supervised by the Medical Director.

63. In 1970, the _____ was founded to establish professional standards for EMS personnel.
  A. American Medical Association
  B. National Registry of Emergency Medical Technicians
  C. National Highway Traffic Safety Administration
  D. U.S. Department of Transportation

64. Safe, reliable transportation is a critical component of an EMS system. Most patients can be effectively transported by _____
  A. airplane.　　**C.** rescue vehicle.
  B. helicopter.　　**D.** ambulance.

65. An _____ is a national level EMT who has been trained to start IVs, perform advanced airway techniques, and administer some medicines beyond the EMT-B.

A. EMT-Responder
B. EMT-Intermediate
C. EMT-Critical Care
D. EMT-Paramedic

66. A continuous self-review with the purpose of identifying and correcting aspects of the EMS system that require improvement is called
   A. standing orders.
   B. quality improvement.
   C. protocols.
   D. medical direction.

67. A physician who assumes the ultimate responsibility for the patient care aspects of the EMS system is called the
   A. Designated Agent.
   B. Medical Director.
   C. Off-line Director.
   D. Primary Care Physician.

68. A common cause of lawsuits against EMS agencies is
   A. patients who refuse care.
   B. on-scene deaths.
   C. cardiac arrest cases.
   D. pedestrians struck by cars.

69. The legal extent or limits of the EMT-B's job are formally defined by the
   A. patient.
   B. DOT curriculum.
   C. state.
   D. scope of practice.

70. Which is not generally considered a sign or symptom of stress?
   A. decisiveness
   B. guilt
   C. loss of interest in work
   D. difficulty sleeping

71. All of the following are types of calls that have a high potential for causing excessive stress except
   A. calls involving infants and children.
   B. patients with severe injuries.
   C. cases of abuse and neglect.
   D. motor vehicle accidents.

72. Life style changes that can help the EMT-B deal with stress include all of the following except
   A. exercise to burn off tension.
   B. increased consumption of fatty foods.
   C. decreased caffeine consumption.
   D. decreased consumption of alcohol.

73. Changes in your professional life to reduce and prevent stress could include
   A. requesting a change of shift or location.
   B. requesting a busier location to make the shift go faster.
   C. working additional overtime shifts.
   D. taking on another part-time position.

74. After a CISD,
   A. management investigates the events of the call.
   B. performance appraisals are initiated.
   C. the peer team writes a detailed critique.
   D. a member of the peer team offers support and referrals.

75. Stress after a major EMS incident is
   A. unusual and unexpected.
   B. a sign of weakness.
   C. normal and to be expected.
   D. part of the grieving process.

76. Retreating to a world of one's own after hearing one is going to die is a result of the stage of grief called
   A. bargaining.   C. denial.
   B. depression.   D. anxiety.

77. All of the following communicable diseases should be of particular concern to the EMT-B except
   A. hepatitis B.   C. HIV/AIDS.
   B. tuberculosis.   D. PPD.

78. A disease which is spread by exposure to an open wound or sore of an infected individual is caused by a(n)
   A. universal precaution.
   B. airborne pathogen.
   C. bloodborne pathogen.
   D. infectious pathogen.

79. An infection that causes inflammation of the liver is called
   A. meningitis.   C. typhoid.
   B. tuberculosis.   D. hepatitis.

80. A disease spread by inhaling or absorbing droplets from the air through the eyes, nose, or mouth is considered
   A. bloodborne.
   B. noncommunicable.
   C. airborne.
   D. viral.

81. The communicable disease that kills the most health workers ever year in the United States is
   A. tuberculosis.   C. meningitis.
   B. HIV/AIDS.   D. hepatitis B virus.

82. Always assume that any patient with
   A. a cold has a bloodborne disease.
   B. a productive cough has TB.
   C. a fever has typhoid.
   D. All of the above.

83. Which of the following is not true about the human immunodeficiency virus (HIV)?
    A. It attacks the immune system.
    B. It doesn't survive well outside the human body.
    C. It can be introduced through puncture wounds.
    D. It is an airborne pathogen.

84. Your patient has hepatitis B. You are accidentally stuck with a needle that has some of this patient's infected blood on it. Your chance of contracting the disease is about
    A. 10%.   C. 30%.
    B. 20%.   D. 40%.

85. Your patient has HIV. You are accidentally stuck with a needle that has some infected blood on it. Your chance of contracting the disease is about
    A. 0.5%.   C. 10%.
    B. 5%.   D. 15%.

86. If you think your patient has TB, you should wear the normal personal protective equipment plus a
    A. surgeon's mask.   C. HEPA respirator.
    B. gown.   D. Tyvek suit.

87. When alone, instead of providing mouth-to-mouth ventilations on the non-breathing patient, the EMT-B should use a
    A. pocket mask with a one-way valve.
    B. one-way valve.
    C. bag-valve mask.
    D. endotracheal tube.

88. This method of infection control will reduce exposure to yourself, your crew, and your next patient.
    A. wearing a HEPA respirator
    B. taking universal precautions
    C. handwashing after each patient contact
    D. None of the above.

89. An act that establishes procedures through which emergency response workers can find out if they have been exposed to life-threatening infectious diseases is called
    A. OSHA 1910.1030.
    B. the Ryan White CARE act.
    C. AIDS Protection act.
    D. OSHA 1910.120.

90. Each emergency response employer must develop a plan that identifies and documents job classifications and tasks in which there is the possibility of exposure to potentially infectious body fluids. This is required by
    A. OSHA 1910.1030.
    B. The Ryan White CARE Act.
    C. AIDS Protection Act.
    D. OSHA 1910.120.

91. Every employer of EMT-Bs must provide free of charge
    A. a yearly physical examination.
    B. a life insurance policy.
    C. universal health insurance.
    D. hepatitis B vaccination.

92. Engineering controls that prevent the spread of bloodborne diseases include
    A. pocket masks.
    B. needle containers.
    C. disposable airway equipment.
    D. All of the above.

93. Which of the following is not required by the OSHA bloodborne pathogen standard?
    A. post-exposure evaluation and follow-up
    B. personal protective equipment
    C. HEPA respirator
    D. housekeeping controls and labeling

94. Which of the following is not considered a high risk area for TB?
    A. correctional facilities.
    B. daycare centers.
    C. homeless shelters.
    D. nursing home.

95. As you near an emergency scene, you should
    A. sound your siren to broadcast your arrival.
    B. go straight to the front door.
    C. secure the scene as quickly as possible.
    D. turn off your lights and siren.

96. If anyone at the scene is in possession of a weapon, the EMT-B should
    A. notify the police immediately.
    B. ask the person to give it to you.
    C. ignore the person with the weapon.
    D. advise the person to leave the scene.

97. The reduction of breathing to the point where oxygen intake is not sufficient to support life is called
    A. respiratory failure.
    B. anoxic metabolism.
    C. respiratory arrest.
    D. respiratory support.

98. Adequate signs of breathing include all of the following except
    A. equal expansion of both sides of the chest.
    B. air moving in and out of the nose.
    C. blue or gray skin coloration.
    D. present and equal breath sounds.

99. The widening of the nostrils of the nose with respirations is called
A. hyperventilating.   C. nasal gurgling.
B. nasal flaring.   D. wheezing.

100. When a patient's skin or lips are blue or gray this is called
A. stridor.   C. pallor.
B. cyanosis.   D. anemia.

101. If a patient is unable to speak in full sentences, this could be a sign of
A. complete airway blockage.
B. snoring.
C. shortness of breath.
D. respiratory arrest.

102. The procedures by which life-threatening respiratory problems are initially treated by the EMT-B include all of the following except
A. opening and maintaining the airway.
B. inserting an endotracheal tube immediately.
C. providing supplemental oxygen to the breathing patient.
D. assuring a clear airway with frequent suctioning.

103. Most airway problems are caused by
A. the tongue.   C. shock.
B. asthma.   D. the epiglottis.

104. Which maneuver is most appropriate for an unconscious patient found lying at the bottom of a stairwell?
A. head-tilt, chin-lift
B. head-tilt, neck-lift
C. jaw-pull lift
D. jaw-thrust

105. When choosing a means of ventilating a patient, your last choice would be
A. flow-restricted, oxygen-powered ventilation device.
B. one-person bag-valve mask.
C. two person bag-valve mask.
D. mouth to mask with high-flow supplemental oxygen.

106. Artificial ventilation may be inadequate if the
A. chest rises with each ventilation.
B. heart rate returns to normal.
C. rate of ventilation is too fast or too slow.
D. patient's color changes from blue to pale.

107. The standard respiratory fitting on a bag-valve mask that ensures a proper fit with other respiratory equipment is
A. 15/22 mm.   C. 5/20 mm.
B. 10/14 mm.   D. 20/26 mm.

108. A bag-valve mask should have all of the following except
A. self-refilling shell.
B. a clear face mask.
C. be easily cleared and sterilized.
D. a "pop-off" valve.

109. The proper oxygen flow rate when ventilating a patient with a BVM is _____ liters per minute.
A. 5   C. 15
B. 10   D. 20

110. According to the American Heart Association guidelines, at least _____ milliliters of air must be delivered to the patient when ventilating with a BVM.
A. 400   C. 800
B. 600   D. 1000

111. The first step in providing artificial ventilation of a stoma breather is to
A. leave the head and neck in a neutral position.
B. ventilate at the appropriate rate for the patient's age.
C. clear any mucus or secretions obstructing the stoma.
D. establish a seal using a pediatric-sized mask.

112. A flow-restricted, oxygen-powered ventilation device should have all of the following features except
A. an audible alarm when ventilation is activated.
B. a trigger that enables the rescuer to use both hands.
C. a peak flow rate of up to 40 liters per minute.
D. a rugged design and construction.

113. The two most common airway adjuncts for the EMT-B to use are the oropharyngeal airway and the
A. nasal cannula.
B. nasopharyngeal airway.
C. endotracheal tube.
D. Yankauer.

114. An oropharyngeal airway should be inserted in
A. all patients with inadequate breathing.
B. trauma patients with a gag reflex.
C. medical patients with a gag reflex.
D. all unconscious patients without a gag reflex.

115. When suctioning a patient, the EMT-B should
    A. suction on the way in and way out.
    B. avoid using eye wear or a mask.
    C. never suction for longer than 15 seconds.
    D. hypoventilate prior to suctioning.

116. The emergency situation in which there is a failure of the cardiovascular system to provide sufficient blood to all the vital tissues is called
    A. respiratory arrest.
    B. respiratory failure.
    C. shock.
    D. cardiac arrest.

117. An insufficiency in the supply of oxygen to the body's tissues is called
    A. anoxia.   C. hypoxia.
    B. no-oxia.   D. cyanosis.

118. Before the oxygen cylinder's pressure gauge reads _____ psi, you must switch to a fresh cylinder.
    A. 200   C. 800
    B. 400   D. 1000

119. When handling oxygen cylinders, the EMT-B should do all of the following except
    A. have the cylinders hypostatically tested every 5 years.
    B. ensure that valve seat inserts and gaskets are in good condition.
    C. store reserve cylinders in a warm, humid room.
    D. use medical grade oxygen in all cylinders.

120. The best way to deliver high concentration oxygen to a breathing patient is to use a
    A. nonrebreather mask.
    B. partial rebreather mask.
    C. bag-valve mask.
    D. nasal cannula.

121. A nasal cannula provides between _____ % and _____ % oxygen concentrations.
    A. 10:21   C. 36:58
    B. 24:44   D. 72:96

122. If the patient has dentures, during airway procedures the EMT-B should
    A. remove them right away.
    B. leave them in unless they are loose.
    C. remove the teeth one at a time.
    D. hold them in place with his/her free hands.

123. When managing an airway of a child, an airway consideration you should remember is
    A. the mouth and nose are smaller and more easily obstructed.
    B. the chest wall is firmer in a child.
    C. the trachea is wider and less easily obstructed.
    D. All of the above.

124. When breathing stops completely, the patient is in
    A. respiratory arrest.
    B. ventilatory reduction.
    C. artificial ventilation.
    D. respiratory failure.

125. Which ventilation device is contraindicated in infants and children?
    A. bag-valve mask
    B. pediatric pocket mask
    C. flow-restricted, oxygen-powered ventilation device
    D. nonrebreather mask

126. A device that allows the control of oxygen in liters per minute is called a _____ .
    A. flowmeter   C. humidifier
    B. G tank   D. reservoir

127. A type of flowmeter which has no gauge and allows for the adjustment of flow in liters per minute in stepped increments is called a
    A. Bourdon gauge flowmeter.
    B. constant flow selector valve.
    C. humidifier.
    D. pressure compensated flowmeter.

128. Why do some systems use humidified oxygen?
    A. Lack of humidity can dry out the patient's mucous membranes.
    B. It provides a reservoir for the oxygen.
    C. It limits the risk of infection.
    D. It is helpful when transporting patients short distances.

129. A patient in the end stage of a respiratory disease may have switched over to
    A. hyperventilation syndrome.
    B. hyperbaric therapy.
    C. hypoxic drive.
    D. carbon dioxide drive.

130. What is COPD?
    A. a type of shock
    B. a type of ventilation
    C. a mechanism of breathing
    D. a chronic pulmonary disease

INTERIM EXAM 1: ANSWER SHEET

Fill in the correct answer for each item. When scoring, note there are 150 questions valued at 0.666 points each.

1. [ ] A	[ ] B	[ ] C	[ ] D	
2. [ ] A	[ ] B	[ ] C	[ ] D	
3. [ ] A	[ ] B	[ ] C	[ ] D	
4. [ ] A	[ ] B	[ ] C	[ ] D	
5. [ ] A	[ ] B	[ ] C	[ ] D	
6. [ ] A	[ ] B	[ ] C	[ ] D	
7. [ ] A	[ ] B	[ ] C	[ ] D	
8. [ ] A	[ ] B	[ ] C	[ ] D	
9. [ ] A	[ ] B	[ ] C	[ ] D	
10. [ ] A	[ ] B	[ ] C	[ ] D	
11. [ ] A	[ ] B	[ ] C	[ ] D	
12. [ ] A	[ ] B	[ ] C	[ ] D	
13. [ ] A	[ ] B	[ ] C	[ ] D	
14. [ ] A	[ ] B	[ ] C	[ ] D	
15. [ ] A	[ ] B	[ ] C	[ ] D	
16. [ ] A	[ ] B	[ ] C	[ ] D	
17. [ ] A	[ ] B	[ ] C	[ ] D	
18. [ ] A	[ ] B	[ ] C	[ ] D	
19. [ ] A	[ ] B	[ ] C	[ ] D	
20. [ ] A	[ ] B	[ ] C	[ ] D	

1. [ ] A   [ ] B   [ ] C   [ ] D   37. [ ] A   [ ] B   [ ] C   [ ] D
2. [ ] A   [ ] B   [ ] C   [ ] D   38. [ ] A   [ ] B   [ ] C   [ ] D
3. [ ] A   [ ] B   [ ] C   [ ] D   39. [ ] A   [ ] B   [ ] C   [ ] D
4. [ ] A   [ ] B   [ ] C   [ ] D   40. [ ] A   [ ] B   [ ] C   [ ] D
5. [ ] A   [ ] B   [ ] C   [ ] D   41. [ ] A   [ ] B   [ ] C   [ ] D
6. [ ] A   [ ] B   [ ] C   [ ] D   42. [ ] A   [ ] B   [ ] C   [ ] D
7. [ ] A   [ ] B   [ ] C   [ ] D   43. [ ] A   [ ] B   [ ] C   [ ] D
8. [ ] A   [ ] B   [ ] C   [ ] D   44. [ ] A   [ ] B   [ ] C   [ ] D
9. [ ] A   [ ] B   [ ] C   [ ] D   45. [ ] A   [ ] B   [ ] C   [ ] D
10. [ ] A   [ ] B   [ ] C   [ ] D   46. [ ] A   [ ] B   [ ] C   [ ] D
11. [ ] A   [ ] B   [ ] C   [ ] D   47. [ ] A   [ ] B   [ ] C   [ ] D
12. [ ] A   [ ] B   [ ] C   [ ] D   48. [ ] A   [ ] B   [ ] C   [ ] D
13. [ ] A   [ ] B   [ ] C   [ ] D   49. [ ] A   [ ] B   [ ] C   [ ] D
14. [ ] A   [ ] B   [ ] C   [ ] D   50. [ ] A   [ ] B   [ ] C   [ ] D
15. [ ] A   [ ] B   [ ] C   [ ] D   51. [ ] A   [ ] B   [ ] C   [ ] D
16. [ ] A   [ ] B   [ ] C   [ ] D   52. [ ] A   [ ] B   [ ] C   [ ] D
17. [ ] A   [ ] B   [ ] C   [ ] D   53. [ ] A   [ ] B   [ ] C   [ ] D
18. [ ] A   [ ] B   [ ] C   [ ] D   54. [ ] A   [ ] B   [ ] C   [ ] D
19. [ ] A   [ ] B   [ ] C   [ ] D   55. [ ] A   [ ] B   [ ] C   [ ] D
20. [ ] A   [ ] B   [ ] C   [ ] D   56. [ ] A   [ ] B   [ ] C   [ ] D
21. [ ] A   [ ] B   [ ] C   [ ] D   57. [ ] A   [ ] B   [ ] C   [ ] D
22. [ ] A   [ ] B   [ ] C   [ ] D   58. [ ] A   [ ] B   [ ] C   [ ] D
23. [ ] A   [ ] B   [ ] C   [ ] D   59. [ ] A   [ ] B   [ ] C   [ ] D
24. [ ] A   [ ] B   [ ] C   [ ] D   60. [ ] A   [ ] B   [ ] C   [ ] D
25. [ ] A   [ ] B   [ ] C   [ ] D   61. [ ] A   [ ] B   [ ] C   [ ] D
26. [ ] A   [ ] B   [ ] C   [ ] D   62. [ ] A   [ ] B   [ ] C   [ ] D
27. [ ] A   [ ] B   [ ] C   [ ] D   63. [ ] A   [ ] B   [ ] C   [ ] D
28. [ ] A   [ ] B   [ ] C   [ ] D   64. [ ] A   [ ] B   [ ] C   [ ] D
29. [ ] A   [ ] B   [ ] C   [ ] D   65. [ ] A   [ ] B   [ ] C   [ ] D
30. [ ] A   [ ] B   [ ] C   [ ] D   66. [ ] A   [ ] B   [ ] C   [ ] D
31. [ ] A   [ ] B   [ ] C   [ ] D   67. [ ] A   [ ] B   [ ] C   [ ] D
32. [ ] A   [ ] B   [ ] C   [ ] D   68. [ ] A   [ ] B   [ ] C   [ ] D
33. [ ] A   [ ] B   [ ] C   [ ] D   69. [ ] A   [ ] B   [ ] C   [ ] D
34. [ ] A   [ ] B   [ ] C   [ ] D   70. [ ] A   [ ] B   [ ] C   [ ] D
35. [ ] A   [ ] B   [ ] C   [ ] D   71. [ ] A   [ ] B   [ ] C   [ ] D
36. [ ] A   [ ] B   [ ] C   [ ] D   72. [ ] A   [ ] B   [ ] C   [ ] D

73.	[ ] A	[ ] B	[ ] C	[ ] D		102.	[ ] A	[ ] B	[ ] C	[ ] D
74.	[ ] A	[ ] B	[ ] C	[ ] D		103.	[ ] A	[ ] B	[ ] C	[ ] D
75.	[ ] A	[ ] B	[ ] C	[ ] D		104.	[ ] A	[ ] B	[ ] C	[ ] D
76.	[ ] A	[ ] B	[ ] C	[ ] D		105.	[ ] A	[ ] B	[ ] C	[ ] D
77.	[ ] A	[ ] B	[ ] C	[ ] D		106.	[ ] A	[ ] B	[ ] C	[ ] D
78.	[ ] A	[ ] B	[ ] C	[ ] D		107.	[ ] A	[ ] B	[ ] C	[ ] D
79.	[ ] A	[ ] B	[ ] C	[ ] D		108.	[ ] A	[ ] B	[ ] C	[ ] D
80.	[ ] A	[ ] B	[ ] C	[ ] D		109.	[ ] A	[ ] B	[ ] C	[ ] D
81.	[ ] A	[ ] B	[ ] C	[ ] D		110.	[ ] A	[ ] B	[ ] C	[ ] D
82.	[ ] A	[ ] B	[ ] C	[ ] D		111.	[ ] A	[ ] B	[ ] C	[ ] D
83.	[ ] A	[ ] B	[ ] C	[ ] D		112.	[ ] A	[ ] B	[ ] C	[ ] D
84.	[ ] A	[ ] B	[ ] C	[ ] D		113.	[ ] A	[ ] B	[ ] C	[ ] D
85.	[ ] A	[ ] B	[ ] C	[ ] D		114.	[ ] A	[ ] B	[ ] C	[ ] D
86.	[ ] A	[ ] B	[ ] C	[ ] D		115.	[ ] A	[ ] B	[ ] C	[ ] D
87.	[ ] A	[ ] B	[ ] C	[ ] D		116.	[ ] A	[ ] B	[ ] C	[ ] D
88.	[ ] A	[ ] B	[ ] C	[ ] D		117.	[ ] A	[ ] B	[ ] C	[ ] D
89.	[ ] A	[ ] B	[ ] C	[ ] D		118.	[ ] A	[ ] B	[ ] C	[ ] D
90.	[ ] A	[ ] B	[ ] C	[ ] D		119.	[ ] A	[ ] B	[ ] C	[ ] D
91.	[ ] A	[ ] B	[ ] C	[ ] D		120.	[ ] A	[ ] B	[ ] C	[ ] D
92.	[ ] A	[ ] B	[ ] C	[ ] D		121.	[ ] A	[ ] B	[ ] C	[ ] D
93.	[ ] A	[ ] B	[ ] C	[ ] D		122.	[ ] A	[ ] B	[ ] C	[ ] D
94.	[ ] A	[ ] B	[ ] C	[ ] D		123.	[ ] A	[ ] B	[ ] C	[ ] D
95.	[ ] A	[ ] B	[ ] C	[ ] D		124.	[ ] A	[ ] B	[ ] C	[ ] D
96.	[ ] A	[ ] B	[ ] C	[ ] D		125.	[ ] A	[ ] B	[ ] C	[ ] D
97.	[ ] A	[ ] B	[ ] C	[ ] D		126.	[ ] A	[ ] B	[ ] C	[ ] D
98.	[ ] A	[ ] B	[ ] C	[ ] D		127.	[ ] A	[ ] B	[ ] C	[ ] D
99.	[ ] A	[ ] B	[ ] C	[ ] D		128.	[ ] A	[ ] B	[ ] C	[ ] D
100.	[ ] A	[ ] B	[ ] C	[ ] D		129.	[ ] A	[ ] B	[ ] C	[ ] D
101.	[ ] A	[ ] B	[ ] C	[ ] D		130.	[ ] A	[ ] B	[ ] C	[ ] D

7

Scene Size-up

MATCH TERMINOLOGY/DEFINITIONS

A. Force or forces that may have caused injury

B. Injury caused by an object that passes through the skin and other body tissues

C. Steps taken by EMS crew when approaching, arriving, and attending at the scene of an emergency call to ensure the safety of the crew, the patient, and bystanders

D. Area around the wreckage of a vehicle collision or other accident within which special safety precautions should be taken

E. Principle that a body in motion will remain in motion unless acted on by an outside force

F. Keen awareness that a person may have injuries

G. Agency that provides advice on hazardous materials via a hotline

H. Injury caused by a blow that does not penetrate through the skin or body tissues

I. Material available for first responder agencies to obtain quick information about hazardous materials

J. Violence in the home

_H_ **1.** Blunt force trauma

_G_ **2.** CHEMTREC

_D_ **3.** Danger zone

_J_ **4.** Domestic violence

_F_ **5.** High index of suspicion

_E_ **6.** Law of inertia

_A_ **7.** Mechanism of injury

_I_ **8.** *North American Emergency Response Guidebook*

_B_ **9.** Penetrating trauma

_C_ **10.** Scene size-up

MULTIPLE CHOICE REVIEW

_B_ **1.** Your top priority when conducting a scene size-up is determining
    A. patient safety.
    B. personal safety.
    C. number of injured.
    D. mechanism of injury.

_D_ **2.** Which of the following is the most accurate statement about scene size-up?
    A. It takes place as you are approaching the scene.
    B. It is replaced by patient care once you arrive at the scene.
    C. It is confined to the first part of the assessment process.
    D. It is an ongoing process throughout the call.

_B_ **3.** If you arrive at a collision scene where there are police, fire vehicles, and other ambulance already present, you should
    A. immediately begin patient care.
    B. conduct your own scene size-up.
    C. ensure that no bystanders are injured.
    D. All of the above.

D 4. Which of the following is an inappropriate action when you near the scene of a traffic collision?
  A. Look and listen for other EMS units as you near intersections.
  B. Look for signs of collision-related power outages.
  C. Observe traffic flow to anticipate blockage at the scene.
  D. Attempt to park your vehicle downhill from the scene.

A 5. When you are in sight of the collision scene, you should watch for the signals of police officers and other emergency service personnel because
  A. they may have information about hazards or the location of injured persons.
  B. the first ones on the scene are considered to be in charge.
  C. federal law requires you to follow the command of first responders.
  D. they are considered the medical-care experts on the scene.

B 6. When there are no apparent hazards, consider the danger zone to extend _____ feet in all directions from the wreckage.
  A. 25   C. 100
  B. 50   D. 200

C 7. When a collision vehicle is on fire, consider the danger zone to extend at least _____ feet in all directions, even if the fire appears small and limited to the engine compartment.
  A. 25   C. 100
  B. 50   D. 200

A 8. A good scene size-up should identify the
  A. potential for a violent situation.
  B. name and amount of toxic substances.
  C. number of patients and their diagnoses.
  D. All of the above.

D 9. The EMT-B's body substance isolation equipment during the scene size-up may include all of the following except
  A. eye protection.   C. mask.
  B. disposable gloves.   D. oxygen mask.

B 10. The key element of body substance isolation is to
  A. always wear all the protective clothing.
  B. always have personal protective equipment readily available.
  C. place equipment on the patient as well as the rescuer.
  D. determine which body fluids are a danger to the EMT-B.

B 11. Injuries to bones and joints are usually associated with
  A. fights and drug usage.   C. fires and explosions.
  B. falls and vehicle collisions.   D. bullet wounds.

C 12. Knowing the mechanism of injury assists the EMT-B in
  A. immobilizing the patient's spine.
  B. determining which BSI precautions to use.
  C. predicting various injury patterns.
  D. All of the above.

C 13. The law of inertia states that
  A. the faster you enter a turn the more your vehicle will be pulled straight.
  B. the slower the speed the greater the energy loss.
  C. a body in motion will remain in motion unless acted upon by an outside force.
  D. the mass or weight of an object is the most important contributor to an injury.

A 14. An unrestrained driver involved in a head-on, up-and-over collision is likely to sustain injuries to the
  A. skull.
  C. knees.
  B. fibula.
  D. femur.

C 15. Which of the following is least likely to be considered a mechanism of injury in up-and-over and down-and-under head-on collisions?
  A. steering wheel
  C. brake pedal
  B. windshield
  D. dashboard

C 16. Knee, leg, and hip injuries are common in a _____ collision.
  A. head-on, up-and-over
  C. head-on, down-and-under
  B. rear-end collision.
  D. rotational impact.

D 17. Which type of collision is most serious because it has the potential for multiple impacts?
  A. side impact
  C. head-on, up-and-over
  B. rear-end impact
  D. roll-over

D 18. All of the following are examples of mechanisms of injury except a
  A. patient who fell three times his height.
  B. spiderweb crack in the windshield.
  C. broken steering column in a collision.
  D. flat rear tire.

A 19. A severe fall for an adult is
  A. over 15 feet.
  B. often accompanied by an amputation.
  C. less than 10 feet.
  D. always fatal.

A 20. A penetrating injury that is usually limited to the penetrated area is called a _____ injury.
  A. low-velocity
  C. high-velocity
  B. medium-velocity
  D. super-velocity

C 21. The pressure wave around the bullet's tract through the body is called
  A. exsanguination.
  C. cavitation.
  B. gas penetration.
  D. pressure damage.

C 22. An injury caused by a blow that strikes the body but does not penetrate the skin is called
  A. inertia trauma.
  C. blunt-force trauma.
  B. cavitation.
  D. rotational impact.

B 23. In which of the following situations would it be necessary for you and your partner to call for additional assistance?
  A. You are treating a patient who has flu-like symptoms who also has a toddler with similar symptoms.
  B. Your patient is a 350-pound male who fell down the stairs and has a broken leg.
  C. You are treating a patient with a deep laceration in his right forearm.
  D. Your patient loses consciousness while you are carrying her to the ambulance.

A 24. While in the living room of a private house treating a patient for nausea, headache, and general body weakness, your eyes begin to tear and three family members have the same symptoms. You should immediately
  A. evacuate all people from the building.
  B. call for three additional ambulances.
  C. notify the police department.
  D. begin to flush out everyone's eyes.

<u>B</u> **25.** If the number of patients is more than the responding units can effectively handle, the EMT-B should
   A. involve bystanders in care of the injured.
   B. call for additional EMS resources immediately.
   C. advise medical direction that assistance is needed.
   D. All of the above.

COMPLETE THE FOLLOWING

1. List the five parts of the scene size-up.

   Scene Safety
   BSI
   MOI or NOI
   # of Pt's
   Additional resources

2. List five signals of danger from violence that you may observe as you approach the scene.

   • Fighting or loud voices
   • Weapons visible, or in use
   • Signs of alcohol or drugs
   • Unusual silence
   • Knowledge of prior violence

3. List five types of motor vehicle collisions.

   • Head on
   • Rear-end
   • Side impact
   • Rollover
   • Rotational impact

CHAPTER

The Initial Assessment

MATCH TERMINOLOGY/DEFINITIONS

A. Steps taken by the EMT-B for the purpose of discovering and dealing with a patient's life-threatening problems

B. Level of a patient's responsiveness

C. Method of assessing circulation in a pediatric patient

D. Reason EMS was called by or for the patient

E. Part of the EMT-B's evaluation that includes assessment of the environment and the patient's chief complaint and appearance

F. Memory aid to keep the levels of responsiveness in mind

G. Actions taken to correct a patient's problems

H. Awake and oriented

I. Lack of response to any stimuli

J. Ability to respond to stimuli

H **1.** Alert

F **2.** AVPU

C **3.** Capillary refill

D **4.** Chief complaint

E **5.** General impression

A **6.** Initial assessment

G **7.** Interventions

B **8.** Mental status

J **9.** Responsive

I **10.** Unresponsive

MULTIPLE CHOICE REVIEW

D **1.** Which of the following steps is <u>not</u> a part of the initial assessment of a responsive patient with a medical problem?
 A. Assess the patient's mental status.
 B. Assess the adequacy of breathing.
 C. Determine the patient's priority.
 D. Obtain the blood pressure.

D **2.** The general impression is an evaluation of all of the following <u>except</u>
 A. chief complaint.   **C.** environment.
 B. appearance.   **D.** past medical history.

C **3.** An example of a patient's environment providing information about the patient's condition is
 A. a bruise on the patient's chest.   **C.** drug-use paraphernalia.
 B. an alleyway that is not well lit.   **D.** a medical history of asthma.

B **4.** Clinical judgment is also referred to as a(n)
 A. license to diagnose what is wrong with the patient.
 B. sixth sense that provides clues to the severity of a patient's condition.
 C. reliance on medical direction to recommend treatment.
 D. ability to judge the patient's mental status without using AVPU.

D   **5.** During the general impression, the EMT-B should
- **A.** look.
- **B.** listen.
- **C.** smell.
- **D.** All of the above.

B   **6.** One way to determine the patient's level of responsiveness is to
- **A.** put ammonia inhalants into each nostril.
- **B.** rub the patient's sternum briskly.
- **C.** place the patient's hands in water.
- **D.** press on the patient's nail beds.

D   **7.** The "A" in AVPU stands for
- **A.** action.
- **B.** airway.
- **C.** assess.
- **D.** alert.

C   **8.** The "V" in AVPU stands for
- **A.** violent.
- **B.** very painful.
- **C.** verbal.
- **D.** venous.

B   **9.** The "P" in AVPU stands for
- **A.** priority.
- **B.** painful.
- **C.** position.
- **D.** patient.

B   **10.** One major difference between the initial assessment of a responsive trauma patient and the initial assessment of an unresponsive trauma patient is
- **A.** the initial assessment is done more quickly on the responsive patient.
- **B.** the unresponsive patient is a higher priority for immediate transport.
- **C.** there is no difference between the two assessments.
- **D.** a jaw-thrust maneuver should always be used on the responsive patient.

D   **11.** If a patient is not alert and his breathing rate is slower than 8, the EMT-B should
- **A.** give high-concentration oxygen via nonrebreather mask.
- **B.** quickly evaluate the circulation and treat for shock.
- **C.** suction the patient and perform rescue breathing.
- **D.** provide positive pressure ventilations with 100% oxygen.

B   **12.** During the initial assessment, if the patient is alert and the breathing rate is faster than 24, provide the patient with
- **A.** positive pressure ventilations with 100% oxygen.
- **B.** high-concentration oxygen via nonrebreather.
- **C.** low-concentration oxygen via bag-valve mask.
- **D.** medium-concentration oxygen via nasal cannula.

_____ **13.** In the initial assessment, the circulation assessment includes evaluating all of the following except
- **A.** pulse.
- **B.** skin.
- **C.** severity of bleeding.
- **D.** blood pressure.

_____ **14.** If a patient's skin is warm, pink, and dry, it indicates
- **A.** a serious sunburn.
- **B.** heat exposure.
- **C.** alcohol abuse.
- **D.** good circulation.

_____ **15.** If a patient's skin is cool, pale, and moist, it indicates
- **A.** increased perfusion.
- **B.** high blood pressure.
- **C.** poor circulation.
- **D.** cold exposure.

_____ **16.** In order to evaluate skin color in a dark-skinned patient, the EMT-B should
- **A.** evaluate the tissues of the lips or nail beds.
- **B.** evaluate the tissues of the heels of the feet.
- **C.** check the pupils of the eyes.
- **D.** All of the above.

_____ **17.** When assessing the circulation, you should check for and control severe bleeding because
  A. open wounds can become infected.
  B. it may lead to long-term complications.
  C. a patient can bleed to death in minutes.
  D. the blood pressure may drop over time.

_____ **18.** When a life threat is observed in the initial assessment, the EMT-B should
  A. complete the assessment, then treat.
  B. treat it immediately.
  C. determine the patient's priority, then treat.
  D. package the patient for transport.

_____ **19.** High priority conditions include
  A. poor general impression.
  B. unresponsive.
  C. shock (hypoperfusion).
  D. All of the above.

_____ **20.** All of the following would be considered high priority conditions <u>except</u>
  A. difficulty breathing.
  B. responsive but not following commands.
  C. an uncomplicated childbirth.
  D. chest pain with systolic pressure less than 100.

COMPLETE THE FOLLOWING

1. List the six steps of the initial assessment.

_____

_____

_____

_____

_____

_____

2. State what the letters in AVPU stand for.

A _____

V _____

P _____

U _____

3. List five high priority conditions.

_____

_____

_____

_____

_____

EMT-BASIC SKILL PERFORMANCE CHECKLIST

▶ THE INITIAL ASSESSMENT

After taking body substance isolation precautions:

❑ Form a general impression based on assessment of the environment and the patient's chief complaint and appearance.

❑ Assess mental status (determine responsiveness/level of consciousness).

❑ Assess airway and breathing (assessment, initiate appropriate oxygen therapy, assure adequate ventilation).

❑ Assess circulation (assess/control major bleeding; assess pulse; assess skin color, temperature, and condition).

❑ Determine patient's priority/make transport decision.

Vital Signs and SAMPLE History

MATCH TERMINOLOGY/DEFINITIONS

▶ **PART A**

A. Pressure remaining in the arteries when the left ventricle of the heart relaxes and refills

B. Slow pulse; any pulse rate below 60 beats per minute

C. Force of blood against the walls of the blood vessels

D. Pulse felt along the large artery on either side of the neck

E. Feeling with the fingertips

F. Number of pulse beats per minute

G. Reacting to light by changing size such as occurs in the pupils of the eyes

H. Rhythmic beats felt as the heart pumps blood through the arteries

I. Rhythm (regular or irregular) and force (strong or weak) of the pulse

J. Major artery of the arm

K. Black center of the eye

L. When a stethoscope is used to listen for characteristic sounds

M. To get larger

N. To get smaller

O. Pulse felt at the wrist on the lateral (thumb) side

_____ **1.** Auscultation

_____ **2.** Blood pressure

_____ **3.** Brachial artery

_____ **4.** Bradycardia

_____ **5.** Carotid pulse

_____ **6.** Constrict

_____ **7.** Dilate

_____ **8.** Diastolic blood pressure

_____ **9.** Palpation

_____ **10.** Pulse

_____ **11.** Pulse quality

_____ **12.** Pulse rate

_____ **13.** Pupil

_____ **14.** Radial pulse

_____ **15.** Reactivity

▶ PART B

A. Normal or abnormal (shallow, labored, noisy) character of breathing

B. Number of breaths a person takes in one minute

C. Rapid pulse; any pulse rate above 100 beats per minute

D. Pressure created when the heart contracts and forces blood into the arteries

E. Regular or irregular spacing of breaths

F. Information about the present problem (signs and symptoms) and past medical history of the patient

G. An indication of a patient's condition that is objective—something you see, hear, feel, or smell

H. An indication of a patient's condition that cannot be observed by another person but rather is subjective—something felt and reported by the patient

I. Cuff and gauge used to measure blood pressure

J. Outward signs of what is going on inside the body, including respiration; pulse; skin color, temperature, and condition; pupils; and blood pressure

_____ 1. Respiratory quality

_____ 2. Respiratory rate

_____ 3. Respiratory rhythm

_____ 4. SAMPLE history

_____ 5. Sign

_____ 6. Sphygmomanometer

_____ 7. Symptom

_____ 8. Systolic pressure

_____ 9. Tachycardia

_____ 10. Vital signs

MULTIPLE CHOICE REVIEW

_____ 1. The assessed components of the vital signs include all of the following except
A. respiratory rate and quality.
B. skin color and condition.
C. pulse rate and quality.
D. pulse oximetry.

_____ 2. A sign that gives important information about the patient's condition but is not considered a "vital sign" is
A. blood pressure.
B. mental status.
C. pulse rate.
D. respiratory rhythm.

_____ 3. Why is it essential that vital signs be recorded as they are obtained?
A. to avoid having to take them more than once
B. to prevent forgetting them and to note the time they were taken
C. to give the patient a chance to calm down
D. because they will always change quickly

_____ 4. When a patient's pulse rate exceeds 100 beats per minute, this is called
A. normal.
B. regular.
C. bradycardia.
D. tachycardia.

_____ 5. Based upon the pulse alone, a sign that something may be seriously wrong with a patient could be
A. a sustained rate below 50 beats per minute.
B. a sustained rate above 120 beats per minute.
C. a rate above 150 beats per minute.
D. All of the above.

_____ 6. In addition to the answer to question number 5, another serious indicator found in the pulse may be a(n)
A. regular strong rhythm.
B. irregular rhythm.
C. athlete with a pulse of 50.
D. increase in rate after exercise.

_____ 7. The quality of the pulse includes determining the
   A. rhythm and rate.   C. rhythm and force.
   B. rate and force.   D. presence and balance.

_____ 8. A patient described as having a "thready" pulse has a
   A. strong pulse.   C. weak pulse.
   B. irregular pulse.   D. infrequent pulse.

_____ 9. The normal pulse rate for a school-age child (6–10 years) is
   A. 120 to 160.   C. 70 to 110.
   B. 60 to 100.   D. 80 to 120.

_____ 10. The normal pulse rate for an adult is
   A. 60 to 100.   C. 80 to 120.
   B. 70 to 110.   D. 90 to 140.

_____ 11. The pulse at the thumb side of the wrist is referred to as the _____ pulse.
   A. femoral   C. carotid
   B. radial   D. brachial

_____ 12. When assessing the carotid pulse, the EMT-Basic should
   A. palpate the artery as hard as he can.
   B. assess both sides at exactly the same time.
   C. be aware that excessive pressure can slow the heart.
   D. apply pressure until he feels the pulse rate rise.

_____ 13. The number of breaths a patient takes in one minute is called the
   A. minute volume.   C. respiratory rate.
   B. minute pressure.   D. quality of breathing.

_____ 14. The respiratory rate is classified as
   A. normal, slow, or rapid.   C. labored, quick, or noisy.
   B. noisy, shallow, or normal.   D. weak, thready, full.

_____ 15. If the EMT-B is treating a patient with a sustained respiratory rate above
   _____ or below _____ breaths per minute, high concentration oxygen must
   be administered.
   A. 20 : 10   C. 24 : 8
   B. 20 : 12   D. 24 : 10

_____ 16. The normal respiration rate for an adult at rest is
   A. 12 to 24.   C. 20 to 30.
   B. 12 to 20.   D. 20 to 40.

_____ 17. The normal respiration rate for a toddler (1–3 years) is
   A. 12 to 24.   C. 20 to 30.
   B. 12 to 20.   D. 20 to 40.

_____ 18. Shallow breathing occurs when
   A. there is only slight movement of the chest or abdomen.
   B. there is stridor or grunting on expiration.
   C. there is a complete obstruction.
   D. the chest muscles fully expand with each breath.

_____ 19. Many resting people breathe more with their _____ than with their _____
   muscles.
   A. diaphragm : pelvic   C. chest : abdominal
   B. diaphragm : chest   D. chest : pelvic

_____ 20. Signs of labored breathing include all of the following except:
   A. increase in the work of breathing.
   B. use of accessory muscles.
   C. retractions above the collarbones.
   D. delayed capillary refill.

_____ **21.** A harsh, high pitched sound heard on inspiration when a patient has labored breathing is called
    A. nasal flaring.
    B. grunting.
    C. stridor.
    D. gurgling.

_____ **22.** When the quality of a patient's respirations are abnormal due to something blocking the flow of air, this is referred to as _____ breathing.
    A. normal
    B. shallow
    C. noisy
    D. labored

_____ **23.** A sound made by the patient that usually indicates the need to suction the airway is called
    A. gurgling.
    B. crowing.
    C. stridor.
    D. wheezing.

_____ **24.** The best places to assess skin color in adults are the
    A. inside of the lower eyelids and the nostrils.
    B. inside of the cheek and the nail beds.
    C. nail beds and the upper chest.
    D. the toes and the lips.

_____ **25.** Blood loss, shock, hypotension, or emotional distress may result in skin that is
    A. flushed.
    B. gray.
    C. pale.
    D. jaundiced.

_____ **26.** A patient with a lack of oxygen in the red blood cells resulting from inadequate breathing or inadequate heart function will exhibit _____ skin.
    A. pink
    B. pale
    C. flushed
    D. cyanotic

_____ **27.** The skin of a patient who has liver abnormalities will appear
    A. flushed.
    B. mottled.
    C. pale.
    D. jaundiced.

_____ **28.** Cold, dry skin is frequently associated with
    A. high fever and/or heat exposure.
    B. exposure to cold.
    C. shock and anxiety.
    D. a body that is losing heat.

_____ **29.** Hot, dry skin is frequently associated with
    A. high fever, heat exposure.
    B. exposure to cold.
    C. shock and anxiety.
    D. heat loss.

_____ **30.** You notice that the patient's right arm is much cooler than the rest of the patient's body. This should lead you to consider a
    A. nervous system problem.
    B. respiratory system problem.
    C. circulatory system problem.
    D. endocrine system problem.

_____ **31.** If you press on a child's nail bed and watch how long it takes for the normal pink color to return, you are testing for
    A. reflexes.
    B. capillary refill.
    C. pain response.
    D. nail bed temperature.

_____ **32.** If a patient is in direct sunlight or very bright conditions, the EMT-B should test the pupils by
    A. using a very bright light that is similar to the environmental light.
    B. covering the patient's eyes for a few moments, then uncovering one eye at a time.
    C. applying a cold towel to the patient's eyelids for ten seconds.
    D. moving the patient indoors to an area that has dimmer light.

33. The pupils may be unequal due to any of the following conditions <u>except</u>
  A. stroke.   **C.** eye injury.
  B. head injury.   **D.** shock.

34. Fright, blood loss, drugs, and treatment with eye drops may cause the patient's pupils to become
  A. constricted.   **C.** unequal.
  B. dilated.   **D.** unreactive.

35. When the left ventricle of the heart relaxes and refills, the pressure in the arteries is called the
  A. diastolic pressure.   **C.** ventricular pressure.
  B. carotid pressure.   **D.** systolic pressure.

COMPLETE THE FOLLOWING

1. List five vital signs.

_____

_____

_____

_____

_____

2. List four types of noisy respiratory sounds.

_____

_____

_____

_____

3. List the six components of the SAMPLE History.

_____

_____

_____

_____

_____

_____

LABEL THE DIAGRAM

Fill in the name of the pulse that can be found at each numbered location on the line provided.

MAJOR ARTERIES

1.

Pulmonary artery

2.

Brachial

3.

4.

Posterior tibial

5.

MAJOR VEINS

Pulmonary vein

Superior vena cava

Inferior vena cava

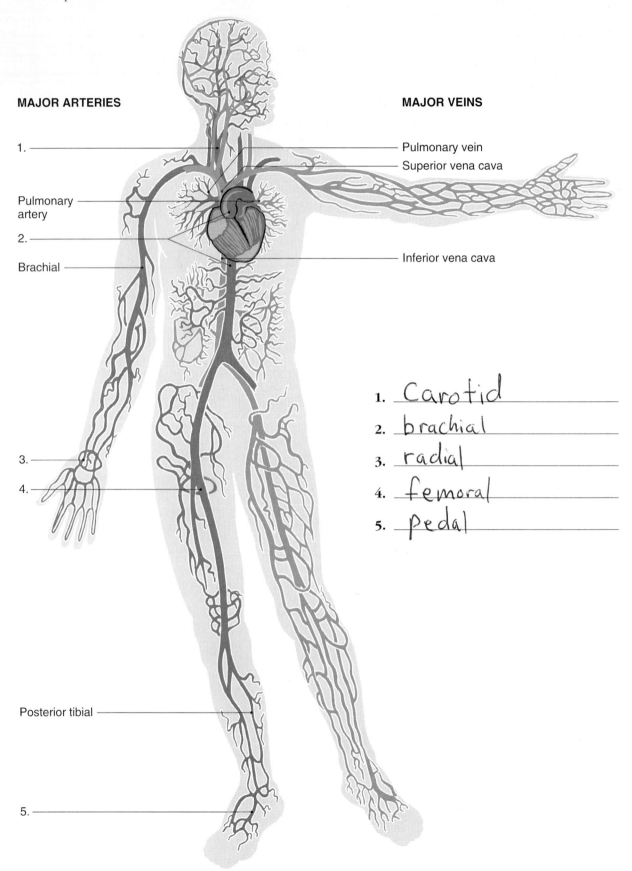

1. Carotid
2. brachial
3. radial
4. femoral
5. pedal

▶ DETERMINING THE BLOOD PRESSURE BY AUSCULTATION

❑ Place the stethoscope around your neck.

❑ The patient should be seated or lying down.

❑ If the patient has not been injured, support his arm at the level of his heart.

❑ Place the cuff snugly around the upper arm so that the bottom of the cuff is about one inch above the crease of the elbow.

❑ With your fingertips, palpate the brachial artery at the crease of the elbow.

❑ Place the tips of the stethoscope arms in your ears.

❑ Position the diaphragm of the stethoscope directly over the brachial pulse or over the medial anterior elbow (front of the elbow) if no brachial pulse can be felt.

❑ Inflate the cuff with the bulb valve (thumb valve) closed.

❑ Once you no longer hear the brachial pulse, continue to inflate the cuff until the gauge reads 30 mm Hg higher than the point where the sound pulse disappeared.

❑ Slowly release air from the cuff by opening the bulb valve, allowing the pressure to fall smoothly at the rate of approximately 10 mm per second.

❑ When you hear the first clicking or tapping sounds, note the reading on the gauge. This is the systolic pressure.

❑ Continue to deflate the cuff and listen for the point at which these distinctive sounds fade. When the sounds turn to dull, muffled thuds, the reading on the gauge is the diastolic pressure.

❑ After obtaining the diastolic pressure, let the cuff deflate rapidly.

▶ DETERMINING THE BLOOD PRESSURE BY PALPATION*

❑ Find the radial pulse on the limb to which the blood pressure cuff is applied.

❑ With the bulb valve closed, inflate the cuff to a point where you can no longer feel the radial pulse.

❑ Note this point on the gauge and continue to inflate the cuff until the gauge reads 30 mm Hg higher than the point where the pulse disappeared.

❑ Slowly deflate the cuff, noting the reading at which the radial pulse returns. This reading is the systolic pressure.

❑ After obtaining the systolic reading, let the cuff deflate.

*Note: You cannot determine a diastolic reading by palpation.

Assessment of the Trauma Patient

MATCH TERMINOLOGY/DEFINITIONS

A. When palpating a body part, the EMT-B elicits and locates a painful area

B. Movement of part of the chest in the opposite direction from the rest of the chest during respiration

C. Persistent erection of the penis that can result from spinal cord injury or certain medical problems

D. Quick assessment of the head, neck, chest, abdomen, pelvis, extremities, and posterior body on patients with significant mechanism of injury

E. Surgical opening in the wall of the abdomen with a bag in place to collect excretions from the digestive system; also called an ileostomy

F. Memory aid, the initials of which stand for deformities, contusions, abrasions, punctures/penetrations, burns, tenderness, lacerations, and swelling

G. Surgical incision in the neck held open by a metal or plastic tube

H. Bulging of the neck veins

I. Step of patient assessment that follows the initial assessment

J. Jagged cut, or open wound, that causes significant blood loss

K. Condition of being stretched, inflated, or larger than normal

L. To methodically visualize, palpate, and listen to each body part with a potential injury, including examination of the face, ears, eyes, nose, and mouth

M. Permanent surgical opening in the neck through which the patient breathes

N. Medical term for a bruise

O. Grating sensation or sound made when fractured bones rub against each other

_____ **1.** Colostomy

_____ **2.** Contusion

_____ **3.** Crepitation

_____ **4.** DCAP-BTLS

_____ **5.** Detailed physical exam

_____ **6.** Distention

_____ **7.** Focused history and physical exam

_____ **8.** Jugular vein distension

_____ **9.** Laceration

_____ **10.** Paradoxical motion

_____ **11.** Priapism

_____ **12.** Rapid trauma assessment

_____ **13.** Stoma

_____ **14.** Tenderness

_____ **15.** Tracheostomy

_____ **1.** When evaluating a patient during the focused physical exam, the EMT-B needs to _____ each body part.
    A. auscultate and visualize .
    B. percuss and palpate
    C. inspect and palpate
    D. visualize and percuss

_____ **2.** The memory aid for remembering what to look for when conducting a physical exam is
    A. AVPU.
    B. PULSE.
    C. SAMPLE.
    D. DCAP-BTLS.

_____ **3.** The "C" in DCAP-BTLS refers to
    A. compound.
    B. contusions.
    C. cardiac.
    D. circulation.

_____ **4.** The "A" in DCAP-BTLS refers to
    A. alert.
    B. appearance
    C. asthma.
    D. abrasions.

_____ **5.** The "P" in DCAP-BTLS refers to
    A. punctures/penetrations.
    B. palpation/pulse.
    C. priapism/penetrations.
    D. paradoxical motion/punctures.

_____ **6.** The "S" in DCAP-BTLS refers to
    A. soft tissue.
    B. stable.
    C. swelling.
    D. stomach.

_____ **7.** When a body part no longer has its normal shape, this is referred to as a
    A. hematoma.
    B. deformity.
    C. fracture.
    D. crepitation.

_____ **8.** Reddened, blistered, or charred-looking areas are called
    A. abrasions.
    B. burns.
    C. lacerations.
    D. contusions.

_____ **9.** The difference between pain and tenderness is
    A. pain only occurs when you squeeze an injury site, whereas tender areas hurt all the time.
    B. pain is considered unbearable, whereas tenderness is usually bearable.
    C. tenderness may not hurt unless the area is palpated, whereas pain is evident without palpation.
    D. pain only hurts for the first ten minutes whereas tenderness doesn't go away.

_____ **10.** A common result of injured capillaries bleeding under the skin is called
    A. swelling.
    B. puncture.
    C. laceration.
    D. abrasion.

_____ **11.** When is it appropriate to apply a cervical collar?
    A. if the mechanism of injury exerts great force on the upper body
    B. if there is any pain in the abdomen
    C. if there is any burn injury to the neck
    D. if the patient has experienced any trauma

_____ **12.** Any blow above the _____ may damage the cervical spine.
    A. clavicles
    B. diaphragm
    C. femur
    D. pelvis

_____ **13.** The experienced EMT-B may refer to a soft cervical collar as a
    A. device of choice for a neck injury.
    B. "neck warmer."
    C. requirement for all auto collision patients.
    D. preferred extrication collar.

_____ **14.** If a cervical collar is the wrong size, it may
    A. cause additional injury to the spine.
    B. make breathing more difficult or obstruct the airway.
    C. prevent the patient from moving his/her neck.
    D. take too much time to adjust and apply correctly.

_____ **15.** The need for a cervical immobilization should be based upon
    A. the trauma patient's level of consciousness.
    B. the location of injuries to the patient.
    C. the mechanism of injury.
    D. All of the above.

_____ **16.** Prior to applying the cervical collar, the EMT-B should
    A. complete the rapid trauma assessment.
    B. complete the detailed physical exam.
    C. assess the patient's neck.
    D. obtain the baseline vital signs.

_____ **17.** When reconsidering the mechanism of injury, which of the following would <u>not</u> be considered a significant mechanism of injury?
    A. a high speed motorcycle crash
    B. a vehicle-pedestrian collision
    C. an adult who fell 10 feet
    D. a roll-over vehicle collision

_____ **18.** You are treating a patient who was in the front seat of an automobile involved in a collision. You observe that there is a spider web cracked windshield and the patient has facial lacerations. Most likely the patient
    A. will have a life-threatening head injury.
    B. did not wear a seat belt or three-point harness.
    C. will also complain of leg injuries.
    D. was involved in a rollover collision.

_____ **19.** Why should the EMT-B "lift and look" under the airbag after the patient has been removed from the vehicle?
    A. to obtain the serial number of the airbag
    B. to see if a hazardous chemical has been released
    C. to note any visible damage to the steering wheel
    D. to determine if it deployed properly

_____ **20.** When assessing the head of a critical trauma patient, in addition to DCAP-BTLS, the EMT-B should inspect/palpate for
    A. hematoma.   **C.** crepitation.
    B. scalp lacerations.   **D.** abrasions.

_____ **21.** When assessing the neck of a critical trauma patient, in addition to DCAP-BTLS, the EMT-B should inspect/palpate for
    A. jugular vein distention.   **C.** lacerations.
    B. swelling.   **D.** burns.

_____ **22.** The neck veins are usually not visible when the patient is
    A. lying flat.   **C.** supine.
    B. sitting up.   **D.** prone.

_____ **23.** When assessing the chest of a critical trauma patient, in addition to DCAP-BTLS, the EMT-B should inspect/palpate for
    A. hematoma.   **C.** hemothorax.
    B. paradoxical motion.   **D.** jugular vein distention.

_____ **24.** When assessing the abdomen of a critical trauma patient, in addition to DCAP-BTLS, the EMT-B should inspect/palpate for
    A. distention of the kidneys.   **C.** crepitation.
    B. colostomy and/or ileostomy. **D.** paradoxical motion.

_____ 25. When assessing the pelvis of a critical trauma patient, in addition to DCAP-BTLS, the EMT-B should inspect/palpate for
A. paradoxical motion.　　　　C. priapism.
B. burns.　　　　　　　　　　D. bleeding.

_____ 26. The main difference between the rapid trauma assessment and the detailed physical exam is
A. the rapid trauma assessment is less detailed.
B. the detailed physical exam is only done on medical patients.
C. the rapid trauma exam is done in the ambulance.
D. the detailed physical exam is done more quickly.

_____ 27. If you are treating a severely injured patient, it may be appropriate to skip the
A. initial physical exam.　　　　C. vital signs.
B. detailed physical exam.　　　　D. initial assessment.

_____ 28. Areas you will assess in the detailed physical exam that were not assessed in the rapid trauma assessment are
A. face, ears, eyes, nose, and mouth.
B. head, neck, chest, and abdomen.
C. chest, abdomen, pelvis, and extremities.
D. extremities and posterior of the body.

_____ 29. The final step of the detailed physical exam is to
A. complete the head-to-toe exam.
B. reassess the vital signs.
C. conduct a rapid trauma assessment.
D. examine the posterior of the body.

_____ 30. A bruise behind the ear is called
A. raccoon's eyes.　　　　C. Battle's sign.
B. orbital hematoma.　　　　D. Cushing reflex.

_____ 31. When performing the detailed physical exam, you note blood in the anterior chamber of the eye. This tells you
A. the patient was wearing contact lenses.
B. the patient has a serious brain injury.
C. the patient's eye is bleeding inside.
D. All of the above.

_____ 32. Clear fluid that may be draining from the ears and nose is called _____ fluid.
A. lymphatic　　　　C. mucous
B. cerebrospinal　　　　D. synovial

_____ 33. In addition to looking for DCAP-BTLS when examining the mouth, you should look for all of the following except
A. possible airway obstructions.　　　　C. tongue lacerations or swelling.
B. loose or broken teeth.　　　　D. crepitation.

_____ 34. The detailed physical exam is not designed for the
A. trauma patient with a significant mechanism or injury.
B. patient with an unclear mechanism of injury.
C. medical patient with few signs and symptoms.
D. patient who could be either medical or trauma.

_____ 35. If you are treating a patient who could be either medical or trauma, it is always best to assess for
A. the medical problem first.　　　　C. the trauma problem first.
B. both problems at once.　　　　D. loss of consciousness.

COMPLETE THE FOLLOWING

1. List the eight components of the focused history and physical exam for a trauma patient who is found with significant mechanism of injury.

_____

_____

_____

_____

_____

_____

_____

_____

2. List the eight components of the rapid trauma assessment.

_____

_____

_____

_____

_____

_____

_____

_____

LABEL THE PHOTOGRAPHS

Fill in the name of each injury assessed for in the focused physical exam of the trauma patient.

1. _____

5. _____

2. _____

6. _____

3. _____

7. _____

4. _____

8. _____

COMPLETE THE CHART

Fill in the additional things to assess in each area of the body during rapid trauma assessment.

Body Part	DCAP-BTLS	Plus
Head	Yes	1.
Neck	Yes	2. 3.
Chest	Yes	4. 5. 6.
Abdomen	Yes	7. 8. 9.
Pelvis	Yes	10. 11. 12.
Extremities	Yes	13. 14. 15.
Posterior	Yes	—

▶ FOCUSED PHYSICAL EXAM AND HISTORY

❑ Take body substance isolation.

❑ Select appropriate assessment (focused or rapid assessment).

❑ Obtain baseline vital signs.

❑ Question patient about signs and symptoms (assess history of present illness).

❑ Question patient about allergies.

❑ Question patient about medications.

❑ Question patient about past medical history.

❑ Question patient about last meal.

❑ Question patient about events leading up to present illness (rule out trauma).

▶ LISTENING TO BREATH SOUNDS

❑ Take body substance isolation.

❑ Explain what a bronchial/tracheal sound is and where to listen for it.

❑ Explain what a vesicular sound is and where to listen for it.

❑ Demonstrate how to listen to the anterior chest.

❑ Explain the importance of listening by comparing the same location on the right side to the location on the left side.

❑ Demonstrate how to listen to the posterior chest.

❑ Explain what a rale, rhonchi, wheeze, and friction rub represent and how they sound.

▶ THE DETAILED PHYSICAL EXAM

❑ Take body substance isolation.

❑ Examine the head (inspect and palpate the scalp, cranium, face, ears, eyes, nose, and mouth).

❑ Examine the neck (inspect and palpate the neck, assess for JVD, and assess for tracheal deviation, crepitation).

❑ Examine the chest (inspect, palpate, and auscultate the chest).

❑ Examine the abdomen.

❑ Examine the pelvis (verbalize assessment of genitalia/perineum as needed).

❑ Examine the extremities (includes inspection, palpation, and assessment of distal pulses, sensation, and motor function).

❑ Examine the posterior body (assess thorax and lumbar).

❑ Manage secondary injuries and wounds appropriately.

❑ Verbalize reassessment of the vital signs.

CASE STUDY

▶ MOTORCYCLE MISHAP

You are dispatched to a motorcycle collision in an intersection in your community. Apparently a car made a right turn on the red without stopping and the motorcycle who had the green light collided with the left side of the car. On arrival, you conduct a quick scene size-up. What four things should you be concerned about in the scene size-up of this collision?

1. _____
   _____

2. _____

3. _____
   _____
   _____

4. _____

You find out from a witness who was standing on the corner at the bus stop that the vehicles were probably traveling 40 mph and the cyclist crashed into the rear left door of the car. He was thrown off the motorcycle onto the roof of the car and then landed on his back in the street. The witness immediately rushed to aid the cyclist and at the same time motioned people in another vehicle to stop traffic and to call 911. The witness stated that the patient was in a lot of pain but never hit his head or lost consciousness. The cyclist was wearing a helmet, which he removed after the collision.

Based on this information, what general impression of the patient can you form?

▶ GENERAL IMPRESSION

5. _____

6. _____

7. _____

8. _____

Your general impression reveals a 20-year-old responsive male trauma patient with severe external blood loss. The patient is able to talk with you, although he is experiencing considerable pain in both his thighs and lower back. He is able to describe what happened in the collision, knows the day of the week, and is concerned about his new Sportster! His name is Tony and he was on his way to the beach, which explains why he was wearing shorts and a tee shirt.

9. As you question Tony, what should one of your partners be doing?

10. What is Tony's mental status on the AVPU?

Although Tony keeps saying, "It's my legs!", which are obviously broken but no longer seriously bleeding, you proceed with the initial assessment beginning with an assessment of Tony's airway.

11. Explain why it would be wrong to be distracted by Tony and begin to treat his broken legs?

12. What should be checked in the **A)** third, **B)** fourth, and **C)** fifth steps of the initial assessment?

A) _____

B) _____

C) _____

Based upon your initial assessment of Tony, you have determined he is a high-priority patient, and an ALS unit should be requested if they are not en route already. You found his airway was open and clear, his breathing was present and adequate, he was moving air into both sides of his chest equally, but he has a weak, rapid radial pulse. One of your crew members has controlled the bleeding from Tony's thighs. His skin is pale, cool, and clammy to touch.

13. Why is Tony a high-priority patient?

14. How long should you wait for an ALS unit to arrive before transporting Tony?

As one of your crew members attends to Tony's injured legs and then places him onto a long backboard (you will learn this later in the course), you continue with the Focused History and Physical Exam. Since you have reconsidered the mechanism of injury, you have decided to provide early transport for Tony as soon as he is packaged.

15. What would you be looking for with DCAP-BTLS?

16. What would you be asking about with the SAMPLE?

17. What vitals should be assessed?

En route to the hospital you have time to conduct a detailed physical exam. Tony is immobilized, receiving oxygen via nonrebreather mask, the backboard is in the Trendelenburg position, and you are keeping him warm with a blanket. His vitals are a respiration rate of 20—good quality, a pulse rate of 120—weak and regular, a blood pressure of 110/70, and pale, cool, and clammy skin.

18. What would the detailed physical exam include?

You note that Tony's blood pressure is slowly dropping and his pulse rate is increasing. He is no longer alert but responds verbally.

19. What's happening to Tony?

CHAPTER 11

Assessment of the Medical Patient

MATCH TERMINOLOGY/DEFINITIONS

A. Description of where pain is located and where it spreads to

B. Description of the pain, such as stabbing, crampy, dull, or sharp

C. Description of what makes the pain worse, such as sitting, standing, eating certain foods

D. Description of how bad the pain is, often described on a scale of 1 to 10

E. Memory jogger designed to remind the EMT-B of what questions to ask the patient about his/her chief complaint

F. Necklace or bracelet designed to notify emergency personnel that a patient has a specific medical history or condition

G. Medicine-like bottle kept in the patient's refrigerator that contains a listing of his/her past medical history

H. Description of how fast or slow the pain came on and what the patient was doing when the pain started

I. The one thing that seems most seriously wrong with the patient

J. History relating to the patient's chief complaint

_____ **1.** Chief complaint

_____ **2.** Medic alert

_____ **3.** Onset of pain

_____ **4.** OPQRST

_____ **5.** Prior history

_____ **6.** Provocation of pain

_____ **7.** Quality of pain

_____ **8.** Radiation of pain

_____ **9.** Severity of pain

_____ **10.** Vial of life

_____ **1.** The components of the focused history and physical exam for a responsive medical patient include all of the following except
  A. history of the present illness.   **C.** baseline vital signs.
  B. SAMPLE history.   **D.** rapid trauma exam.

_____ **2.** OPQRST is a memory aid to help the EMT-B remember the
  A. questions that ask about the past medical history.
  B. questions that expand on the history of the present illness.
  C. status of the patient's condition.
  D. mental status.

_____ **3.** When you ask a patient "Can you think of anything that might have triggered this pain?", you are questioning about
  A. onset.   **C.** quality.
  B. provokes.   **D.** radiation.

_____ **4.** When you ask a patient "How bad is the pain?", you are questioning about
  A. quality.   **C.** time.
  B. severity.   **D.** radiation.

_____ **5.** The "T" in "OPQRST" stands for
  A. temperature.   **C.** time.
  B. tibia.   **D.** trembling.

_____ **6.** When you ask a patient "Have you vomited?", you are questioning about
  A. signs and symptoms.   **C.** medication.
  B. allergies.   **D.** pertinent past history.

_____ **7.** The "P" in "SAMPLE" stands for
  A. perforation.   **C.** puncture wound.
  B. pertinent past history.   **D.** prehospital care report.

_____ **8.** When you ask a patient "How have you felt today?", you are questioning about
  A. pertinent past history.   **C.** events leading to the illness.
  B. signs and symptoms.   **D.** last oral intake.

_____ **9.** A patient with a specific chief complaint and a known history may carry medication or other treatment with him. The EMT-B may need to request medical direction's permission to assist the patient with his
  A. inhaler.   **C.** epinephrine.
  B. nitroglycerin.   **D.** All of the above.

_____ **10.** When a medical patient complains of difficulty breathing, but does not take any prescribed medication for this condition, you should generally
  A. look for a Medic Alert tag.
  B. consult with the patient's personal physician.
  C. transport the patient to the hospital.
  D. All of the above.

_____ **11.** In terms of the initial approach to the focused history and physical exam, the biggest difference between a responsive and a unresponsive patient would be that
  A. the responsive patient gets the OPQRST questions last.
  B. the unresponsive patient will be given a rapid physical exam first.
  C. the bystanders and family become more important if the patient is responsive.
  D. a rapid trauma exam is not done on an unconscious patient.

_____ **12.** In addition to DCAP-BTLS in the rapid physical exam on an unresponsive
medical patient, you should also include all of the following except
  A. look for jugular vein distention.
  B. determine firmness or rigidity of abdomen.
  C. check for incontinence of urine or feces.
  D. ask the SAMPLE questions.

_____ **13.** When assessing a medical patient's extremities, be sure to check for
  A. central cyanosis.   **C.** pulmonary edema.
  B. sensation and motor function.   **D.** capillary refill.

_____ **14.** When conducting a physical exam, look for a necklace or bracelet. This is
important because it may
  A. reveal the patient's name.
  B. give clues to the patient's residence.
  C. be a medical identification device.
  D. be the cause of the emergency.

_____ **15.** Why might it be important to check the refrigerator of a patient who is
found unconscious at home?
  A. Last night's meal could be the cause.
  B. The patient may have a Vial-of-Life.
  C. Most medications are kept in the refrigerator.
  D. The person's diet could be the cause of the problem.

COMPLETE THE FOLLOWING

1. List five components of a focused history and physical exam for an
unresponsive medical patient.

_____

_____

_____

_____

_____

2. List four questions to ask bystanders who witness a patient's medical emergency.

_____

_____

_____

_____

COMPLETE THE CHART

Complete the chart by writing the remainder of the word that follows each letter in the acronyms.

1.	S
2.	A
3.	M
4.	P
5.	L
6.	E
7.	O
8.	P
9.	Q
10.	R
11.	S
12.	T

EMT-BASIC SKILLS PERFORMANCE CHECKLIST

▶ FOCUSED PHYSICAL EXAM AND HISTORY OF THE MEDICAL PATIENT

❏ Take body substance isolation.

❏ Determine if patient is responsive or unresponsive.*

❏ Question patient on signs and symptoms (assess history of present illness).

❏ Question patient on allergies.

❏ Question patient on medications.

❏ Question patient on pertinent past history.

❏ Question patient on last oral intake.

❏ Question patient on events leading up to present illness (rule out trauma).

❏ Conduct focused physical examination (assess affected body part/system or, if indicated, complete rapid assessment).

❏ Obtain baseline vitals.

❏ Interventions (obtain medical direction or verbalize standing order for medication interventions and verbalize proper additional intervention/treatment).

❏ Transport (re-evaluate transport decision).

❏ Complete detailed physical examination.

*If the patient is responsive, gather the history of the present illness (OPQRST) from the patient prior to a hands on physical exam. Likewise, if the patient is unresponsive, do a rapid physical exam assessing the head, chest, abdomen, pelvis, extremities, and posterior body before asking too many questions of bystanders.

CHAPTER 12

Ongoing Assessment

MATCH TERMINOLOGY/DEFINITIONS

A. Changes in a patient's condition over time, that may show improvement or deterioration, and that can be shown by documenting repeated assessments

B. Something that is done to a patient either physical or through the use of a medication that is expected to change the patient's condition

C. Four-step procedure for detecting changes in a patient's condition

_____ **1.** Intervention

_____ **2.** Ongoing assessment

_____ **3.** Trending

MULTIPLE CHOICE REVIEW

_____ **1.** Which of the following best describes the purpose of performing the ongoing assessment?
A. To detect changes in patient condition and to treat any life threats
B. To detect and treat life threats and to evaluate the EMS system's effectiveness
C. To evaluate the EMS system's effectiveness and to detect changes in patient condition
D. To repeat key elements of assessment procedures already performed and to detect changes in patient condition

_____ **2.** The ongoing assessment may be omitted if
A. the patient care report is not completed.
B. you do not want to interrupt patient conversation.
C. life-saving interventions prevent doing it.
D. a short transport time prevents completion.

_____ **3.** During the ongoing assessment of an infant or child patient,
A. avoid eye contact at all times.
B. stand above the patient.
C. speak in a loud voice.
D. use a reassuring voice.

_____ **4.** The ongoing assessment includes all the following steps <u>except</u>
A. reassess vital signs.
B. repeat the initial assessment for life-threats.
C. repeat the focused assessment.
D. repeat all interventions.

_____ **5.** Which of the following is the last step in the ongoing assessment?
A. Reassess the vital signs.
B. Check interventions.
C. Repeat the initial assessment.
D. Repeat the focused assessment.

_____ **6.** Which of the following is <u>not</u> a step when repeating the initial assessment?
   A. Reestablish patient priorities.
   B. Monitor skin color and temperature.
   C. Maintain an open airway.
   D. Apply a cervical collar.

_____ **7.** During your ongoing assessment, you note that the patient's pulse is rapid and his skin is cool and pale. This may indicate
   A. deterioration in mental status.   **C.** an occluded airway.
   B. heat exhaustion.   **D.** the onset of shock.

_____ **8.** The mental status of an unresponsive child or infant can be checked by
   A. a sternal rub.
   B. assessing the capillaries for refill.
   C. shouting or by flicking the feet.
   D. asking the parent to stick a pin in the child's foot.

_____ **9.** An example of checking interventions during the ongoing assessment of a medical patient is
   A. taking an initial blood pressure.
   B. tightening a bandage that was applied to a severe laceration.
   C. applying a tourniquet.
   D. assuring adequacy of oxygen delivery.

_____ **10.** Frequently reassessing a patient establishes
   A. a paper trail.   **C.** trends.
   B. legal evidence.   **D.** a reason for treating the patient.

_____ **11.** The best way to determine if the patient is improving or deteriorating is to
   A. ask the hospital.
   B. contact medical direction.
   C. do frequent ongoing assessments.
   D. keep repeating the initial assessment.

_____ **12.** If the patient is considered stable, the recommended interval for reassessment is every _____ minutes.
   A. 5   **C.** 15
   B. 10   **D.** 20

_____ **13.** You are treating a patient with a head injury who is breathing adequately, yet has an altered mental status. The recommended interval for reassessment is every _____ minutes.
   A. 5   **C.** 15
   B. 10   **D.** 20

_____ **14.** You should repeat at least the initial assessment
   A. after you have noticed and documented trends.
   B. whenever you or your partner have the time and opportunity to do so.
   C. whenever you believe there may have been a change in the patient's condition.
   D. when directed to do so by medical direction.

_____ **15.** During your ongoing assessment of an unresponsive patient, you hear gurgling sounds in her airway. What intervention should you take?
   A. Sit the patient up.   **C.** Check oxygen tubing.
   B. Suction the patient.   **D.** All of the above.

COMPLETE THE FOLLOWING

1. List the six steps involved in repeating the initial assessment.

_____

_____

_____

_____

_____

_____

_____

2. List the three steps for checking interventions.

_____

_____

_____

EMT-BASIC SKILLS PERFORMANCE CHECKLIST

▶ THE ONGOING ASSESSMENT

❑ Take body substance isolation.

❑ Repeat the initial assessment for life-threats.

    ❑ Reassess mental status.

    ❑ Maintain an open airway.

    ❑ Monitor breathing for rate and quality.

    ❑ Reassess pulse for rate and quality.

    ❑ Monitor skin color and temperature.

    ❑ Reestablish patient priorities.

❑ Reassess and record baseline vital signs.

❑ Repeat focused assessment regarding patient complaint or injuries.

❑ Check interventions performed for the patient.

    ❑ Assure adequacy of oxygen delivery and ventilation support.

    ❑ Assure management of bleeding.

    ❑ Assure adequacy of other interventions.

CHAPTER

Pediatric, Adolescent, and Geriatric Assessment

MATCH TERMINOLOGY/DEFINITIONS

A. Child from 1 to 3 years of age

B. Child from 3 to 6 years of age

C. Elderly person, generally considered over 65 years of age or older

D. Child less than 1 year of age

E. Child from 12 to 18 years of age

F. "Soft spot" on an infant's skull

G. Child from 6 to 12 years of age

H. Abnormally low body temperature

I. Chin thrust forward to maintain an open airway

J. Newborns and infants who do not know to open their mouths to breathe when the nose is obstructed

K. Tipping the head too far back

L. When under stress, a child acts like a younger child

M. Chronic disorder resulting in dementia

N. Abnormal heart rhythm

O. When an elderly person replaces lost circumstances with imaginary ones

_____ **1.** Adolescent

_____ **2.** Alzheimer's disease

_____ **3.** Arrhythmia

_____ **4.** Confabulation

_____ **5.** Fontanelle

_____ **6.** Geriatric

_____ **7.** Hyperextension

_____ **8.** Hypothermia

_____ **9.** Infant

_____ **10.** Obligate nose breathers

_____ **11.** Preschooler

_____ **12.** Regression

_____ **13.** School age

_____ **14.** Sniffing position

_____ **15.** Toddler

MULTIPLE CHOICE REVIEW

_____ **1.** For the purposes of the CPR standards, the American Heart Association defines a child as any patient between the ages of
   A. 5 and 12.
   B. 1 and 6.
   C. 1 and 8.
   D. 6 months and 16 years.

_____ **2.** In general emergency care, more useful age groupings for children would include
   A. newborns and infants.
   B. toddlers and preschoolers.
   C. school age and adolescents.
   D. All of the above.

_____ **3.** Infants up until about 18 months will have a soft spot called a
  A. bulging puncture.
  B. sunken suture.
  C. fontanelle.
  D. intracranial pressure.

_____ **4.** When an infant is crying, the fontanelle normally
  A. bulges out.
  B. sinks into the skull.
  C. remains the same in size.
  D. softens gradually.

_____ **5.** Newborns usually breathe
  A. through their noses.
  B. through their mouths.
  C. very slowly.
  D. through their mouths and noses.

_____ **6.** Hyperextension of the neck of an infant may result in
  A. swelling of the fontanelle.
  B. an airway obstruction.
  C. secretions that obstruct the airway.
  D. breathing from the diaphragm.

_____ **7.** "Blind" finger sweeps are not performed on infants or children to clear an airway obstruction because the
  A. finger might force an obstruction down and wedge it in the narrow trachea.
  B. finger could cause hyperextension of the neck.
  C. adult finger is too large to insert in an infant's mouth.
  D. tongue takes up too much space to allow for finger insertion.

_____ **8.** When faced with the stress of an emergency, some children will act like a younger child. This is called
  A. reflection.
  B. regression.
  C. transition.
  D. imitation.

_____ **9.** It is always a good idea to _____ when assessing a child.
  A. speak loudly and rapidly.
  B. stand and speak softly.
  C. kneel down and talk at eye level.
  D. stare directly into the child's eyes.

_____ **10.** If the parent is overreacting when you are caring for a child, you should
  A. ignore them.
  B. try to involve them in the child's care.
  C. let them help stabilize the child's head.
  D. ask the police to take them to the hospital in their vehicle.

_____ **11.** When forming a general impression of a child if the child talks in grunts only, you should consider that the child
  A. has a digestive condition.
  B. has significant respiratory distress.
  C. doesn't want to talk to you.
  D. has poor language skills.

_____ **12.** When forming a general impression, it is most likely that a withdrawn child or one who is emotionally flat is probably
  A. bored.
  B. sick.
  C. about to die.
  D. deaf.

_____ **13.** To assess a child's breathing, observe all of the following except
  A. skin color.
  B. chest expansion.
  C. capillary refill.
  D. effort of breathing.

_____ **14.** An infant's soft spot may bulge due to head trauma or
  A. meningitis.
  B. dehydration.
  C. excessive eating.
  D. anaphylaxis.

_____ **15.** Starting at age _____ , our organ systems lose about _____ percent function each year.

    A. 20 : 1   **C.** 30 : 1
    B. 20 : 2   **D.** 40 : 2

_____ **16.** Although older patients are at least twice as likely to use EMS as younger patients, they are less likely

    A. to accept care provided by EMS.
    B. to have medical problems, rather than injuries.
    C. to be involved in motor vehicle accidents.
    D. All of the above.

_____ **17.** Assessing the airway of an older patient is often difficult because of the patient's wearing dentures and because

    A. large, poorly chewed pieces of food are often found.
    B. arrhythmias occur frequently.
    C. an older person's trachea is usually narrower.
    D. of arthritic changes in the bones of the neck.

_____ **18.** Since older patients are less likely to show severe symptoms in certain conditions, it can be difficult to

    A. find a radial pulse.
    B. determine a patient's priority.
    C. assess for foreign body obstruction.
    D. note sudden onset of weakness.

_____ **19.** When interviewing an elderly patient, the family tells you the patient was wrong with some of her responses. This is sometimes the result of neurological problems as well as

    A. slurred speech.   **C.** medications.
    B. depression.   **D.** All of the above.

_____ **20.** When an elderly patient replaces lost circumstances with imaginary ones, this is known as

    A. depression.   **C.** flustering.
    B. confabulation.   **D.** arrythmia.

_____ **21.** Many older people have a _____ threshold for pain.

    A. high   **C.** zero
    B. low   **D.** None of the above.

_____ **22.** As a person ages, the systolic blood pressure has a tendency to

    A. decrease.   **C.** become erratic.
    B. increase.   **D.** stay constant.

_____ **23.** Hip fractures are common in elderly patients, especially women, due to

    A women's shorter legs   **C.** abnormal curvature of the hip
    B. motor vehicle accidents.   **D.** loss of calcium.

_____ **24.** An EMT-B should consider that any injury of an elderly person could be a sign of

    A. a severe fall.   **C.** abuse or neglect.
    B. Alzheimer's disease.   **D.** depression.

_____ **25.** The EMT-Basic can ease the fears of a geriatric patient by understanding the

    A. effect that loss of independence has on the patient.
    B. need to minimize the patient's fears.
    C. need to minimize the patient's concerns.
    D. proper treatment for all of the patient's diseases.

COMPLETE THE FOLLOWING

1. List six examples of patients who are high priority for immediate transport.

_____

_____

_____

_____

_____

_____

2. Explain how to deal with a geriatric patient's fears of loss of independence.

_____

_____

_____

_____

_____

EMT-BASIC SKILLS PERFORMANCE CHECKLIST

▶ DEALING WITH THE PEDIATRIC PATIENT

❑ Take body substance isolation.

❑ Identify yourself in a simple informal way.

❑ Let the child know someone will call his/her parents.

❑ Determine if there are life-threatening problems and treat them immediately.

❑ Let the child have a nearby toy that he/she may want.

❑ Kneel or sit at the child's eye level.

❑ Smile.

❑ Touch the child or hold his/her hand or foot if appropriate.

❑ Explain all equipment that you plan to use in simple terms to the child.

❑ Make eye contact without staring at the child.

❑ Stop occasionally to confirm that the child understands your actions.

❑ Never lie to a child.

CHAPTER 14

Communications

MATCH TERMINOLOGY/DEFINITIONS

A. Federal agency which regulates radio communications

B. Device that picks up signals from lower-power radio units such as mobile and portable radios and retransmits them at a higher power

C. Unit of measurement used in measuring output power of a radio

D. Hand-held two-way radio

E. Two-way radio at a fixed site such as a hospital or dispatch center

F. Update on the patient's condition given to hospital personnel either face-to-face or over a radio

G. Two-way radio that is used or affixed in a vehicle

H. Phone that transmits through the air instead of over wires so that the phone can be transported and used over a wide area

I. Equipment that permits transmission of standard messages in condensed form by punching a key

J. "Press to talk" button the EMS radio

_____ 1. Base station

_____ 2. Cellular phone

_____ 3. Digital radio equipment

_____ 4. FCC

_____ 5. Mobile radio

_____ 6. Portable radio

_____ 7. PTT

_____ 8. Repeater

_____ 9. Verbal report

_____ 10. Watt

MULTIPLE CHOICE REVIEW

_____ 1. The EMT-B's ability to communicate effectively is important because
A. all EMTs are expected to be a good public speakers.
B. little information about a patient's condition is obtained by talking to the patient, bystanders, or family members.
C. describing your assessment findings to the hospital may make a difference in the care the patient receives.
D. None of the above.

_____ 2. One of the key contributions to improvement in EMS over the years has been
A. the type II, van style ambulance vehicle.
B. development of radio links between dispatcher, mobile units, and hospitals.
C. the military anti-shock trousers.
D. air conditioning in the transport vehicles.

_____ 3. Components of a communications system include
A. base stations.
B. mobile units.
C. portable radios.
D. All of the above.

_____ **4.** A device which picks up radio signals from lower-powered units and retransmits them at a higher power is called a
    A. mobile.   **C.** repeater.
    B. cellular.   **D.** portable.

_____ **5.** The government agency that maintains order on the airwaves is called the
    A. FCC.   **C.** FEMA.
    B. FAA.   **D.** DOT.

_____ **6.** The purposes of always following the general principles of radio transmission is to allow all persons to use the frequencies and to
    A. avoid having to repeat orders from medical direction.
    B. enable the EMT-B to talk in code language.
    C. prevent delays.
    D. All of the above.

_____ **7.** Of the following components of a radio report, which is the correct order?
    1) Major past illness
    2) Chief complaint
    3) Unit identification and level of provider
    4) Emergency medical care given
    A. 4, 1, 2, 3   **C.** 3, 2, 1, 4
    B. 3, 4, 1, 2   **D.** 1, 2, 4, 3

_____ **8.** The reason why the ambulance was called is the
    A. major past illness.   **C.** presenting diagnosis.
    B. chief complaint.   **D.** call type.

_____ **9.** During a radio report when the EMT-B says "The patient's abdomen does not feel rigid," he/she is attempting to advise the hospital of
    A. the baseline vital signs.
    B. the emergency medical care given.
    C. response of patient to the emergency medical care.
    D. pertinent findings of the physical exam.

_____ **10.** During a radio report, when the EMT-B says "The patient's mental status has not changed during our care," he/she is attempting to advise the hospital of the
    A. baseline vital signs.
    B. emergency medical care given.
    C. response of patient to the emergency medical care.
    D. pertinent findings of the physical exam.

_____ **11.** Whenever the EMT-B is requesting an order for medical direction over the radio, it is a good practice to
    A. repeat the physician's order word for word back to the physician.
    B. question all verbal orders that are given.
    C. speak quickly because the physician is busy.
    D. call the physician back again to verify.

_____ **12.** If an order from the on-line physician appears to be inappropriate, then the EMT-B should
    A. switch to another frequency to find another physician.
    B. question the physician about the order.
    C. follow the physician's order as stated.
    D. ignore the order and do what he/she thinks is correct.

_____ **13.** When an EMT-B stands with arms crossed looking down at the patient, the non-verbal message is,
    A. "I am here to help you."
    B. "I am not really interested."
    C. "I can empathize with your problem."
    D. "I am afraid of catching your disease."

_____ **14.** If it is obvious that a patient has a broken leg with a bone protruding, and the patient asks, "Is my leg broken?", what would be the most appropriate response?

    A. Relax and stay calm, you will be all right.

    B. I am not qualified to make that determination.

    C. No, it's a bad cut, and I'll control the bleeding with a bandage.

    D. Yes it is, and I will be as gentle as possible splinting it.

_____ **15.** When treating a toddler, the best approach is to

    A. kneel down so you are at the child's level.

    B. speak louder so the child can hear you above all the crying.

    C. stare directly into the child's eyes.

    D. tell the child you are a friend of his parents.

COMPLETE THE FOLLOWING

1. List five examples of components of a communications system.

\
\
\
\
\

2. List six interpersonal communications guidelines to use when dealing with patients, families, friends, and bystanders.

\
\
\
\
\
\

▶ RADIO REPORT*

Pick an ambulance call on which you were recently an observer or a patient who you examined during the hospital observation portion of the EMT-Basic course. Without releasing any confidential information about the call, such as the patient's name and address, take a moment and organize your thoughts so you can provide a mock radio report to another crew member or your instructor.

The sample format offered in the *Emergency Care* 8th Edition text is as follows:

❑ Unit identification and level of provider.

❑ Estimated time of arrival.

❑ Patient's age and sex.

❑ Chief complaint.

❑ Brief, pertinent history of the present illness or injury.

❑ Major past illnesses.

❑ Mental status.

❑ Baseline vital signs.

❑ Pertinent findings of the physical exam.

❑ Emergency medical care given.

❑ Response to emergency medical care.

❑ Does medical direction have any questions or orders?

*There are a number of local formats for radio reports that may differ somewhat, yet they all adhere to the same principles. They should follow a logical order, be concise, and paint a picture of the patient's problem and the priorities for the hospital personnel.

CHAPTER 15

Documentation

MATCH TERMINOLOGY/DEFINITIONS

A. Information from an individual point of view

B. Standardized report form used by EMS agencies to document prehospital assessment and care

C. Inaccurate entry or misrepresentation on a prehospital care report usually intended to cover up serious flaws in assessment or in care

D. Observable, measurable, and verifiable information

E. Exam finding that is not present or not true but is important to note (i.e., patient denies any shortness of breath)

F. Report on unusual, complex, or involved situations that is completed according to your service's standard operating procedures

G. Each individual box on a prehospital care report

H. Minimum elements that are recommended by the U.S. Department of Transportation be included in all prehospital care reports nationwide

I. Clipboard-format device that is able to recognize handwriting and convert it to computer text

J. Item affixed to a patient at an MCI used to record chief complaint and injuries, vital signs, and treatment given

_____ **1.** Data element

_____ **2.** Falsification

_____ **3.** Minimum data set

_____ **4.** Objective information

_____ **5.** PCR

_____ **6.** Pen-based computer

_____ **7.** Pertinent negative

_____ **8.** Special situation report

_____ **9.** Subjective information

_____ **10.** Triage tag

MULTIPLE CHOICE REVIEW

_____ **1.** The prehospital care report serves as a legal document as well as
   A. a press release form for your EMS agency.
   B. a receipt for the patient.
   C. an aid to research, education, and administrative efforts.
   D. a form to report all calls to the local police department.

_____ **2.** Why is it necessary to complete a prehospital care report if on each call you give the emergency department staff a good oral report?
   A. The QI committee needs something to hold you to.
   B. It provides a means for the emergency department staff to review the patient's prehospital care.
   C. They usually do not listen to oral reports.
   D. Duplication is helpful in emergency call documentation.

_____ **3.** The copy of the prehospital care report left at the hospital
    A. is returned to the state for quality review and follow-up.
    B. is thrown out once it is key punched and added to computer file.
    C. should become part of the patient's permanent hospital record.
    D. is sent to the regional Emergency Medical Services agency.

_____ **4.** You are called to court to testify about a civil matter when a patient sues the city for an injury that occurred in a public place. Which of the following will best help you recall the events of the call?
    A. the questioning by the defense's attorney
    B. the questioning by the plaintiff's attorney
    C. a complete and accurate prehospital care report
    D. your tape recording of the call dispatch

_____ **5.** The person who completed a prehospital care report may be called to court to testify about the
    A. call in a criminal proceeding.   **C.** call in a civil proceeding.
    B. care provided to the patient.   **D.** All of the above.

_____ **6.** The routine review of prehospital care reports for conformity to current medical and organizational standards is a process called
    A. initial feedback.   **C.** stress debriefing.
    B. quality improvement.   **D.** system research.

_____ **7.** Each individual box on a prehospital care report is called a(n)
    A. narrative.   **C.** key punch.
    B. data element.   **D.** assessment.

_____ **8.** According to the U.S. Department of Transportation, in addition to other data elements, the minimum data set on a prehospital care report should include all of the following except
    A. respiratory rate and effort and skin color and temperature.
    B. times of incident, dispatch, and arrival at the patient.
    C. patient's social security number.
    D. capillary refill for patients less than 6 years old.

_____ **9.** The minimum data set includes all of the following except
    A. vital signs.   **C.** chief complaint.
    B. vehicle mileage.   **D.** times of the call.

_____ **10.** The time of dispatch is an example of _____ data on the prehospital care report.
    A. assessment   **C.** patient
    B. run   **D.** narrative

_____ **11.** Examples of patient data on a prehospital care report would be
    A. date of birth and age.
    B. time of arrival at the hospital.
    C. ambulance identification number.
    D. the hospital transported to.

_____ **12.** Experienced EMT-Bs consider a good prehospital care report as one that
    A. protects them against a QA review.
    B. is vague enough to prevent lawsuits.
    C. paints a picture of the patient.
    D. identifies symptoms overlooked by the patient.

_____ **13.** A statement such as "The patient has a swollen, deformed extremity" on the narrative portion of the prehospital care report is an example of
    A. subjective information.   **C.** pertinent negative information.
    B. objective information.   **D.** non-standard abbreviations.

_____ **14.** Each of the following are examples of information that should be put in quotation marks on the prehospital care report <u>except</u>
  A. bystander information.   **C.** objective information.
  B. chief complaint information.   **D.** police officer's information.

_____ **15.** In the narrative section of a prehospital care report, the EMT-B should
  A. list his/her conclusions about the situation.
  B. include pertinent negatives.
  C. use the radio codes for each treatment.
  D. list the vital signs and times obtained.

_____ **16.** Medical abbreviations should be used on a prehospital care report
  A. to save space in the narrative section.
  B. to replace all words you cannot spell.
  C. only if they are standardized.
  D. to ensure correct interpretation by physicians.

_____ **17.** The prehospital care report form itself and the information on it should be considered
  A. the property of the ambulance service.
  B. confidential information.
  C. privileged information.
  D. the patient's property.

_____ **18.** When a patient refuses transport, before the EMT-B leaves the scene, he/she should
  A. document assessment findings and care given.
  B. try again to persuade the patient to go to a hospital.
  C. ensure the patient is able to make a rational, informed decision.
  D. All of the above.

_____ **19.** When completing a prehospital care report on a patient refusal, the EMT-B should document all of the following <u>except</u>
  A. that he/she was willing to return if the patient changed his/her mind.
  B. the complete patient assessment.
  C. that alternative methods of care were offered.
  D. the patient's diagnosis.

_____ **20.** If the EMT-B forgot to administer a treatment that is required by a state protocol, he/she should
  A. document on the prehospital care report only what treatment was actually given.
  B. be sure to document an excuse why the treatment was skipped.
  C. record that the patient was given the forgotten treatment.
  D. None of the above.

_____ **21.** Falsification of information on a prehospital care report may lead to
  A. suspension or revocation of your license or certification.
  B. better EMT-B education.
  C. longer response times.
  D. None of the above.

_____ **22.** To correct an error discovered while writing the prehospital care report, the EMT-B should
  A. scribble out the error so it cannot be seen.
  B. draw a single horizontal line through the error, initial it, and write the correct information.
  C. place his/her initials over the error.
  D. erase the error, then write the correction.

_____ **23.** If information was omitted on a prehospital care report, the EMT-B should
  A. prepare another report and substitute that for the earlier one.
  B. notify the service medical director immediately.
  C. add a note with the correct information, the date, and initial it.
  D. do nothing, as information should never be added after the call.

_____ **24.** An example of an instance in which it would <u>not</u> be unusual for the EMT-B to obtain only a limited amount of information is
  A. during a mass casualty incident.
  B. during an interhospital transfer.
  C. while performing a non-emergency run.
  D. when you encounter a child abuse case.

_____ **25.** Special situation reports
  A. are used to document events that should be reported to local regulatory authorities.
  B. can be submitted at any time after the call.
  C. need not be accurate and/or objective.
  D. are required on each call.

COMPLETE THE FOLLOWING

List ten examples of patient data on a prehospital care report.

_____

_____

_____

_____

_____

_____

_____

_____

_____

_____

16

General Pharmacology

MATCH TERMINOLOGY/DEFINITIONS

A. Specific signs, symptoms, or circumstances under which it is appropriate to administer a drug to a patient

B. Spray device with a mouthpiece that contains an aerosol form of a medication that a patient can spray directly into his airway

C. Semi-solid paste form of a drug

D. Medication given by mouth to treat a conscious patient with an altered mental status and a history of diabetes

E. Brand name of a medication

F. Drug that helps to constrict the blood vessels and relax airway passages; it may be used to counter a severe allergic reaction.

G. Solid form of a drug; compressed powder

H. Powder, usually pre-mixed with water, that will absorb some poisons and help prevent them from being absorbed by the body

I. This gas, in its pure form, is used as a drug to treat any patient whose medical or traumatic condition causes them to be hypoxic, or in danger of becoming hypoxic.

J. Liquid form of a drug in which a powder is mixed with a slurry or water

_____ 1. Activated charcoal

_____ 2. Epinephrine

_____ 3. Gel

_____ 4. Indications

_____ 5. Inhaler

_____ 6. Oral glucose

_____ 7. Oxygen

_____ 8. Suspension

_____ 9. Tablet

_____ 10. Trade name

MULTIPLE CHOICE REVIEW

_____ 1. The study of drugs and their effects is called
   A. anatomy.
   B. physiology.
   C. medicinology.
   D. pharmacology.

_____ 2. Medications that are routinely carried on the EMS unit are
   A. activated charcoal, oral glucose, and oxygen.
   B. oxygen and nitroglycerin.
   C. epinephrine and prescribed inhalers.
   D. All of the above.

_____ 3. Activated charcoal is an example of a
   A. powder, usually pre-mixed with water.
   B. prescribed inhaler.
   C. liquid for injection.
   D. fine powder for inhalation.

_____ **4.** Activated charcoal is given to a patient because it
   A. displaces poisons by surface tension.
   B. will bind some poisons to its surface.
   C. prevents the patient from vomiting.
   D. can be used in a patient without a gag reflex.

_____ **5.** Poorly managed diabetes can cause
   A. hypoxia, or low oxygen.   **C.** dilation of the coronary arteries.
   B. altered mental status.   **D.** absorption of poisons.

_____ **6.** Oral glucose is given between the patient's cheek and gum because
   A. this area contains blood vessels that allow easy absorption into
       the bloodstream.
   B. it will not be aspirated if the patient suddenly becomes unconscious.
   C. it will cause the patient to regurgitate the stomach's contents.
   D. it will assist in dilating the coronary vessels as much as possible.

_____ **7.** Examples of medications that the patient may have in his possession that
   the EMT-B may assist the patient in taking under the appropriate
   circumstances are
   A. activated charcoal, glucose injections, and anticonvulsants.
   B. home oxygen, antihypertensives, and anti-inflammatories.
   C. epinephrine auto-injector, a prescribed inhaler, nitroglycerin.
   D. insulin, antihypertensives, and anticonvulsants.

_____ **8.** Patients who have a medical history of asthma, emphysema, and chronic
   bronchitis may carry a(n) _____ .
   A. nitroglycerin   **C.** bronchodilator.
   B. epinephrine auto-injector   **D.** bronchoconstrictor.

_____ **9.** The drug nitroglycerin is used to
   A. dilate the peripheral vessels.   **C.** dilate the coronary vessels.
   B. constrict the peripheral vessels. **D.** constrict the coronary vessels.

_____ **10.** The government publication listing all drugs in the U.S. is called the
   A. _Physician's Desk Reference._   **C.** _U.S. Pharmacopoeia._
   B. _Hazmat Guidebook._   **D.** _National Medicine Guidebook._

_____ **11.** The name that the manufacturer uses in marketing a drug is called
   the _____ name.
   A. generic   **C.** official
   B. trade   **D.** original

_____ **12.** A circumstance in which a drug should not be used because it may cause
   harm to the patient or offer no effect in improving the patient's condition
   or illness is called a(n)
   A. indication.   **C.** adverse reaction.
   B. side effect.   **D.** contraindication.

_____ **13.** An action of a drug that is other than the desired action is called a(n)
   A. side effect.   **C.** contraindication.
   B. overdose.   **D.** systemic effect.

_____ **14.** Prior to administering a medication to a patient, you must know all of the
   following except
   A. the route of administration.
   B. the proper dose to administer.
   C. the actions the medication will take.
   D. both the generic and chemical names.

_____ **15.** Drugs prescribed for pain relief are called
   A. antiarrhythmics.   **C.** anticonvulsants.
   B. analgesics.   **D.** antihypertensives.

_____ **16.** Drugs prescribed to reduce high blood pressure are called
  A. antiarrhythmics.   **C.** anticonvulsants.
  B. analgesics.   **D.** antihypertensives.

_____ **17.** Drugs prescribed for heart rhythm disorders are called
  A. antidiabetics.   **C.** antiarrhythmics.
  B. bronchodilators.   **D.** anticonvulsants.

_____ **18.** Drugs prescribed to relax the smooth muscles of the bronchial tubes
  are called
  A. bronchospasms.   **C.** anticonvulsants.
  B. bronchodilators.   **D.** bronchoconstrictors.

_____ **19.** Drugs prescribed for prevention and control of seizures are called
  A. antidiabetics.   **C.** anticonvulsants.
  B. antihypertensives.   **D.** antidepressants.

_____ **20.** Drugs prescribed to help regulate the emotional activity of the patient to
  minimize the peaks and valleys in their psychological and emotional state
  are called
  A. antidepressants.   **C.** antiarrhythmics.
  B. analgesics.   **D.** anticonvulsants.

COMPLETE THE FOLLOWING

1. List six medications an EMT-Basic can administer or assist a patient
in taking.

_____

_____

_____

_____

_____

_____

2. List the four "rights" to adhere to when administering a medication.

_____

_____

_____

_____

Respiratory Emergencies

17

MATCH TERMINOLOGY/DEFINITIONS

A. Active process in which the intercostal muscles and the diaphragm contract, expanding the size of the chest cavity and causing air to flow into the lungs; also called inhalation

B. Sporadic, irregular breaths that are usually seen just before respiratory arrest

C. Blockage of the bronchi that lead from the trachea to the lungs

D. Pulling in of the accessory muscles to breathe

E. Passive process in which the intercostal muscles and the diaphragm relax, causing the chest cavity to decrease in size and forcing air from the lungs; also called exhalation

_____ **1.** Agonal respirations

_____ **2.** Bronchoconstriction

_____ **3.** Expiration

_____ **4.** Inspiration

_____ **5.** Retractions

MULTIPLE CHOICE REVIEW

_____ **1.** The muscular structure that divides the chest cavity from the abdominal cavity is called the
　A. intercostal muscle.　　　**C.** diaphragm.
　B. sternocleidomastoid muscle.　　　**D.** inguinal muscle.

_____ **2.** Expiration is a(n)
　A. active process that involves the relaxation of the intercostal muscles and the diaphragm.
　B. passive process that involves the relaxation of the intercostal muscles and the diaphragm.
　C. active process that involves the contraction of the intercostal muscles and the diaphragm.
　D. passive process that involves the contraction of the intercostal muscles and the diaphragm.

_____ **3.** To determine the quality of breathing, check for all of the following except
　A. presence of breath sounds.　　　**C.** breathing rhythm.
　B. chest expansion.　　　**D.** depth of respirations.

_____ **4.** An unconscious patient with shallow, gasping breaths with only a few breaths per minute requires
　A. oxygen given via nasal cannula.
　B. immediate transport to a medical facility.
　C. immediate artificial ventilation with supplemental oxygen.
　D. oxygen given via nonrebreather mask.

_____ **5.** The muscles in the neck and abdomen which sometimes assist in breathing are called _____ muscles.
    A. extra
    B. accessory
    C. sub-diaphragmatic
    D. smooth

_____ **6.** Since oxygenation of the body's tissue is reduced in a patient with inadequate breathing, the skin may be _____ in color, and feel _____ .
    A. pale : dry and cool
    B. red : clammy and hot
    C. yellow : dry and warm
    D. blue : clammy and cool

_____ **7.** If an unresponsive adult patient makes _____ sounds, he may have a serious airway problem requiring immediate intervention.
    A. snoring or gurgling
    B. slight wheezing
    C. sniffling
    D. whistling or grunting

_____ **8.** Statistically, a leading killer of infants and children is
    A. motor vehicle collisions.
    B. heart attacks.
    C. respiratory conditions.
    D. infection.

_____ **9.** The structure of infant's and children's airway is different from an adult's in each of the following ways except
    A. all airway structures are smaller and are more easily obstructed.
    B. their tongues are proportionately larger than an adult's.
    C. the trachea is softer and more flexible.
    D. the cricoid cartilage is more rigid.

_____ **10.** Because the chest wall is softer in infants and children, they
    A. must inhale twice the amount of air to breathe.
    B. depend more heavily on the diaphragm for breathing.
    C. grunt and gurgle whenever they breathe.
    D. expend less energy than adults do when breathing.

_____ **11.** The signs of inadequate breathing in infants and children include all of the following except
    A. nasal flaring.
    B. grunting.
    C. "seesaw breathing."
    D. quivering jaw.

_____ **12.** Which of the following would be most important to observe related to a patient's breathing?
    A. presence of breathing and pulse rate
    B. breathing pattern and adequacy of breathing
    C. presence of breathing and adequacy of breathing
    D. patient position and adequacy of breathing

_____ **13.** The first preference for providing artificial ventilation is the
    A. pocket face mask with supplemental oxygen.
    B. two-person bag-valve mask with supplemental oxygen.
    C. flow-restricted, oxygen-powered ventilator.
    D. one-person bag-valve mask with supplemental oxygen.

_____ **14.** If you are unsure if a patient requires artificial ventilation, you should
    A. contact medical direction immediately.
    B. move to the ambulance and transport rapidly.
    C. increase the liter flow rate to the nonrebreather mask.
    D. provide artificial ventilation.

_____ **15.** The adequate rate of artificial ventilations for a non-breathing adult patient is _____ breaths per minute.
    A. 8
    B. 12
    C. 16
    D. 20

_____ **16.** The adequate rate of artificial ventilations for a non-breathing infant or child patient is _____ breaths per minute.
    A. 10   **C.** 20
    B. 15   **D.** 25

_____ **17.** If an infant or child has _____ in the setting of a respiratory emergency, this usually indicates trouble.
    A. a fever   **C.** a low pulse
    B. cold skin   **D.** a rapid pulse

_____ **18.** You are artificially ventilating an adult patient in respiratory arrest. The chest does not rise and fall with each ventilation. The <u>first</u> action to take is to
    A. increase the oxygen flow rate.
    B. increase the force of ventilations.
    C. change the ventilatory device.
    D. recheck the airway.

_____ **19.** Why is it important to try to distinguish between a lower airway and an upper airway problem in an infant and child?
    A. Suctioning can cause spasms with some lower respiratory diseases.
    B. You will need to give this information to the emergency department.
    C. Finger sweeps will not help to clear an upper airway obstruction.
    D. The lower airway may wheeze when treated with oxygen.

_____ **20.** The sign(s) of a lower respiratory problem include all of the following <u>except</u>
    A. wheezing.
    B. increased breathing effort upon exhalation.
    C. rapid breathing without stridor.
    D. yellow skin color.

_____ **21.** If your patient is able to speak only in short choppy sentences, this may mean he/she
    A. may have a language problem.
    B. is unable to hear you clearly.
    C. is experiencing breathing difficulty.
    D. is afraid of you.

_____ **22.** When an EMT-B states that the patient was in the tripod position due to respiratory distress, this means the patient was
    A. holding self up by two legs and one arm.
    B. leaning forward with hands resting on knees.
    C. in the recovery position.
    D. supine with knees flexed against the chest.

_____ **23.** Which pair of signs/symptoms is <u>not</u> commonly associated with breathing difficulty?
    A. crowing/restlessness
    B. retractions/shortness of breath
    C. increased pulse/tightness in chest
    D. vomiting/headache

_____ **24.** If a patient is suffering from breathing difficulty and is breathing adequately, administer oxygen via
    A. nasal cannula.
    B. nonrebreather mask.
    C. pocket face mask.
    D. bag-valve mask with supplemental oxygen.

_____ **25.** If a patient is experiencing breathing difficulty and is breathing adequately, it is usually best to place him in the _____ position.
    A. tripod   **C.** sitting-up
    B. supine   **D.** None of the above.

_____ **26.** A patient with respiratory problems that causes bronchoconstriction may carry a(n)
   A. bronchoconstrictor.
   B. metered dose aspirator.
   C. inhaler or puffer.
   D. antihypertensive medication.

_____ **27.** Once you receive permission from medical direction to assist a patient with an inhaler, make sure you have all of the following except
   A. the right dose.
   B. an inhaler that is not expired.
   C. a large enough syringe.
   D. a patient who is alert enough to cooperate.

_____ **28.** Prior to coaching the patient in the use of an inhaler, the EMT-B should
   A. shake the inhaler vigorously.
   B. test the unit by spraying into the air.
   C. ensure that the patient is no longer alert.
   D. call the patient's personal physician.

_____ **29.** To ensure that the most medication is absorbed when using an inhaler, you should try to
   A. encourage the patient to take short shallow breaths.
   B. encourage the patient to hold the breath as long as possible.
   C. discourage the patient from breath holding.
   D. encourage the patient to hyperventilate.

_____ **30.** The best way to document that a patient has a respiratory complaint is to
   A. describe your opinion of the patient's problem in detail.
   B. see if the patient can answer all the SAMPLE and OPQRST questions.
   C. ask the patient to describe the difficulty in his own words.
   D. carefully count the patient's breathing rate for at least two minutes.

COMPLETE THE FOLLOWING

1. List nine conditions of inadequate breathing.

_____

_____

_____

_____

_____

_____

_____

_____

_____

2. List four signs of inadequate breathing in infants and children.

_____

_____

_____

_____

3. List ten signs of breathing difficulty.

_____

_____

_____

_____

_____

_____

_____

_____

_____

_____

_____

LABEL THE DIAGRAMS

Fill in each phase of respiration on the line provided.

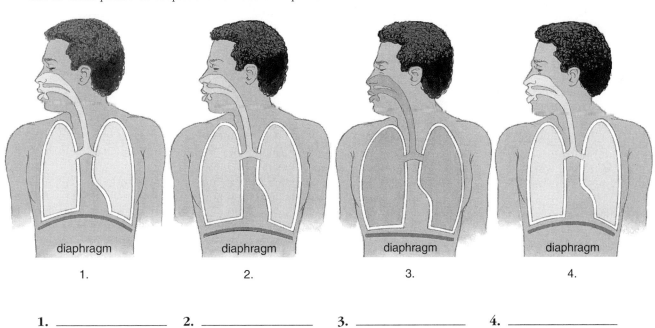

diaphragm   diaphragm   diaphragm   diaphragm

1.   2.   3.   4.

1. _____ **2.** _____ **3.** _____ **4.** _____

EMT-BASIC SKILLS PERFORMANCE CHECKLIST

▶ **THE PRESCRIBED INHALER**

❑ Conduct a scene size-up.

❑ Take body substance isolation.

❑ Perform initial assessment.

❑ Perform focused history and physical exam.

❑ Confirm indications for inhaler use.

❑ Obtain medical direction for prescribed patient assisted inhaler.
(generics: albuterol, isoetharine, metaproteranol, etc.)

❑ Check contraindications for inhaler use.

❑ Assure right patient, right medication, right dose, right route.

❑ Check expiration date of inhaler.

❑ Check if patient has already taken any doses.

❑ Make sure inhaler is at room temperature or warmer.

❑ Shake inhaler vigorously several times.

❑ Make sure the patient is alert enough to use the inhaler properly.

❑ Make sure the patient first exhales deeply.

❑ Have the patient put the lips around the opening and press the inhaler to
activate the spray as he/she inhales deeply.

❑ After the patient inhales, make sure he/she holds his/her breath as long as
possible so the medication can be absorbed into the bronchial tree.

❑ Put oxygen back on patient.

❑ Reassess patient.

CHAPTER 18

Cardiac Emergencies

MATCH TERMINOLOGY/DEFINITIONS

▶ PART A

A. Buildup of fatty deposits on the inner walls of arteries

B. Dilation, or ballooning, of a weakened section in the wall of an artery

C. Condition of excessive fluid buildup in the lungs and/or other organs and body parts because of the inadequate pumping of the heart

D. Condition in which artery walls become hard and stiff due to calcium deposits

E. When the heart has ceased generating electrical impulses

F. Blanket term for any kind of heart problem

G. Irregular, or absent, heart rhythm

H. Diseases that affect the arteries of the heart

I. Condition in which a portion of the myocardium dies as a result of oxygen starvation; often called a heart attack by lay persons

J. Pain in the chest that occurs when the blood supply to the heart is reduced and a portion of the heart muscle is not receiving enough oxygen

_____ 1. Acute myocardial infarction

_____ 2. Aneurysm

_____ 3. Angina pectoris

_____ 4. Arrhythmia

_____ 5. Arteriosclerosis

_____ 6. Asystole

_____ 7. Atherosclerosis

_____ 8. Cardiac compromise

_____ 9. Congestive heart failure

_____ 10. Coronary artery disease

PART B

A. Condition in which the heart's electrical impulses are disorganized, preventing the heart muscle from contracting normally

B. Blockage of an artery that cuts off blood flow

C. Accumulation of fluid in the feet or ankles

D. Cardiac arrest that occurs within two hours of the onset of symptoms

E. Accumulation of fluid in the lungs

F. Condition in which the heartbeat is quite rapid; if rapid enough, it will not allow the heart's chambers to fill with enough blood between beats to produce blood flow sufficient to meet the body's needs

G. Clot of blood and debris from plaque that has broken loose from the wall of an artery and then moves to smaller arteries and blocks blood flow

H. Clot formed of blood and plaque attached to the inner wall of an artery

I. Condition in which the heart's electrical rhythm remains relatively normal, yet the mechanical pumping activity fails to follow the electrical activity, causing cardiac arrest

J. Swelling resulting from a buildup of fluid in tissues

_____ **1.** Edema

_____ **2.** Embolism

_____ **3.** Occlusion

_____ **4.** Pedal edema

_____ **5.** Pulmonary edema

_____ **6.** Pulseless electrical activity

_____ **7.** Sudden death

_____ **8.** Thrombus

_____ **9.** Ventricular fibrillation

_____ **10.** Ventricular tachycardia

MULTIPLE CHOICE REVIEW

_____ **1.** Cardiac compromise is a term that refers to
   A. a heart attack.
   B. sudden death.
   C. any kind of problem with the heart.
   D. a period of time when the heart stops.

_____ **2.** Chest pain from the heart is typically described by the patient as any of the following except
   A. dull.   **C.** tearing.
   B. squeezing.   **D.** crushing.

_____ **3.** The pain or discomfort from a heart problem commonly radiates to the
   A. arms and jaw.   **C.** stomach and lower abdomen.
   B. feet and head.   **D.** right arm and lower abdomen.

_____ **4.** In addition to chest pain or discomfort, the patient with cardiac compromise will also complain of
   A. diarrhea.   **C.** dyspnea.
   B. shivering.   **D.** headache.

_____ **5.** Patients with heart problems may complain of any of the following except
   A. pain in the center of the chest.
   B. mild chest discomfort.
   C. sudden onset of sharp abdominal pain.
   D. difficulty breathing.

_____ 6. If the heart is beating too fast or too slow, the patient with cardiac compromise may also
   A. have stomach pain.
   B. lose consciousness.
   C. have a seizure or convulsion.
   D. have right-side weakness.

_____ 7. The signs and symptoms of cardiac compromise include all of the following except
   A. difficulty breathing and abnormal pulse rate.
   B. sudden onset of sweating with nausea or vomiting.
   C. sharp lower abdominal pain and a fever.
   D. pain in the chest or upper abdomen.

_____ 8. The emergency medical care of the patient with cardiac compromise should include all of the following except
   A. placing the patient in the position of comfort.
   B. administering high concentration oxygen by nonrebreather mask.
   C. administering high flow oxygen by a nasal cannula.
   D. assisting the patient with nitroglycerin administration if medical direction authorizes.

_____ 9. What is the typical "position of comfort" for a conscious patient who is having chest pain and difficulty breathing?
   A. Fowler's
   B. supine
   C. sitting up
   D. lying down with knees bent

_____ 10. All of the following cardiac compromise patients are candidates for immediate transport except
   A. a patient with no history of cardiac problems.
   B. a patient with a history of cardiac problems, who does not have nitroglycerin.
   C. a patient with prescribed nitroglycerin.
   D. a patient with a systolic blood pressure of less than 100.

_____ 11. You should consider using nitroglycerin when the patient
   A. is hypertensive and has a headache.
   B. has his own nitroglycerin and has crushing chest pain.
   C. loses consciousness after feeling dizzy.
   D. has chest pain for over five minutes and is hypotensive.

_____ 12. Which of the following is the best description of the role of medical direction in the treatment of a cardiac compromise patient?
   A. authorizing the EMT-B to administer oxygen via nonrebreather mask
   B. prescribing nitroglycerin that the EMT-B can then assist the patient in taking
   C. authorizing the EMT-B to assist the patient in taking his prescribed nitroglycerin
   D. contacting the patient's physician to ensure the patient's nitroglycerin prescription is not out of date

_____ 13. A patient is complaining of chest pain. In order for the EMT-B to administer nitroglycerin, all of the following conditions must be met except
   A. medical direction should authorize its administration.
   B. the patient's physician should have prescribed the medication.
   C. the patient's blood pressure is lower than 100 systolic.
   D. the patient's blood pressure is greater than 100 systolic.

_____ 14. The maximum number of doses of nitroglycerin routinely given in the field is
   A. one.
   B. two.
   C. three.
   D. four.

_____ 15. After administering three doses of nitroglycerin, if the patient's blood pressure falls below 100 systolic, you should
A. administer another dose of nitroglycerin.
B. reassess the patient's vital signs.
C. treat for shock and transport promptly.
D. All of the above.

_____ 16. Nitroglycerin is contraindicated for the patient who has
A. a head injury.
B. a systolic blood pressure of 110.
C. not yet taken the maximum dose.
D. been complaining of the pain for at least twenty minutes.

_____ 17. Which of the following is not a common side effect to nitroglycerin?
A. hypotension   C. pulse rate changes
B. headache   D. palpitations

_____ 18. After administering nitroglycerin, it is important to
A. immediately administer the next dose.
B. discontinue the oxygen therapy.
C. reassess the vital signs.
D. lay the patient down.

_____ 19. Cardiovascular emergencies are caused, directly or indirectly, by all of the following except
A. changes in the inner walls of arteries.
B. problems with the heart's electrical function.
C. problems with the heart's mechanical function.
D. complications resulting from cardiovascular surgery.

_____ 20. When the body is subjected to exertion or stress, the heart rate will normally
A. increase.   C. become irregular.
B. decrease.   D. stop temporarily.

_____ 21. Two conditions commonly cause narrowing or blocking of the arteries. One condition is atherosclerosis, and the other is
A. aneurysm.   C. arteriosclerosis.
B. arrhythmia.   D. congestive heart failure.

_____ 22. Factor(s) that put a person at risk for developing coronary artery disease include
A. lack of exercise. C. obesity.
B. cigarette smoking. D. All of the above.

_____ 23. Which of the following risk factors can be modified to reduce the risk of coronary artery disease?
A. age   C. hypertension
B. heredity   D. None of the above.

_____ 24. The reason an emergency occurs in most cardiac-related medical emergencies is due to
A. reduced blood flow to the myocardium.
B. cardiac arrest.
C. loss of consciousness.
D. breathing difficulty.

_____ 25. Angina pectoris means, literally,
A. a small heart attack.   C. paralyzed chest muscles.
B. a pain in the chest.   D. breathing difficulty.

_____ 26. Why is nitroglycerin administered to the patient with chest pain?
   A. It increases blood flow to the brain.
   B. It dilates the blood vessels and decreases the work of the heart.
   C. It constricts the blood vessels and raises the blood pressure.
   D. It is easy to administer in unconscious patients.

_____ 27. A condition in which a portion of the myocardium dies as a result of oxygen starvation is known as
   A. coronary occlusion.
   B. acute myocardial infarction.
   C. myocardial starvation.
   D. acute angina attack.

_____ 28. When a cardiac arrest occurs within two hours of the onset of cardiac symptoms, this is referred to as
   A. prehospital death.
   B. prehospital arrest.
   C. sudden death.
   D. ventricular tachycardia.

_____ 29. Unfortunately, nearly _____ of the patients who experience a cardiac arrest within two hours of the onset of symptoms have no previous history of cardiac problems.
   A. 10%   C. 60%
   B. 25%   D. 80%

_____ 30. Changes in the field care of the acute myocardial infarction (AMI) have made _____ and _____ two of the most important treatment methods.
   A. oxygen : PASG   C. thrombolytics : defibrillation
   B. rapid transport : surgery   D. None of the above.

_____ 31. Congestive heart failure is a(n)
   A. clotting of the coronary artery.
   B. condition in which excessive fluids buildup in the lungs and/or other organs.
   C. infection in the heart that makes it difficult to oxygenate the blood.
   D. chronic lung condition that requires a low concentration of oxygen administration.

_____ 32. When there is damage to the left ventricle and blood backs up into the lungs, this usually presents in the form of
   A. pedal edema.   C. thrombolytics.
   B. pulmonary edema.   D. diaphoresis.

_____ 33. The elements of the chain of survival include early access and all of the following except
   A. early CPR.   C. early advanced care.
   B. early defibrillation.   D. early diagnosis.

_____ 34. Ways to decrease the EMS access time include
   A. installing a 911 system.
   B. placing 911 stickers on telephones.
   C. providing public information workshops.
   D. All of the above.

_____ 35. Which of the following steps is unnecessary in order to ensure CPR can be delivered earlier to cardiac arrest victims?
   A. Send CPR trained professionals to patients faster.
   B. Ensure that heart specialists are involved in CPR training.
   C. Train lay people in CPR.
   D. Have dispatchers instruct callers in how to perform CPR.

_____ **36.** Who is the typical cardiac arrest victim?
  A. a male in his sixties
  B. a female in her forties
  C. a male in his seventies
  D. There is no pattern to cardiac arrests.

_____ **37.** The most common witness to a cardiac arrest is a
  A. male in his forties.   **C.** man in his sixties.
  B. female in her forties.   **D.** female in her sixties.

_____ **38.** The single most important factor in determining survival from cardiac arrest is
  A. nitroglycerin administration.
  B. training middle-aged and older people in CPR.
  C. early CPR.
  D. early defibrillation.

_____ **39.** If the response time from the time a call is received to arrival of the defibrillator is longer than _____ minutes, virtually no one survives a cardiac arrest.
  A. 6   **C.** 10
  B. 8   **D.** 12

_____ **40.** When treating a cardiac arrest patient and there is no ACLS unit in the community, the EMT-B should
  A. discontinue resuscitative efforts and pronounce the patient.
  B. package quickly and transport to the closest medical facility.
  C. call for ACLS from another town and wait for their arrival.
  D. continue to provide CPR at the scene until the patient regains a pulse.

_____ **41.** In order to manage a patient in cardiac arrest, in addition to the skills taught in the CPR course, the EMT-B should be able to do all of the following except
  A. use a bag-valve-mask device with oxygen.
  B. use an automated external defibrillator.
  C. request advanced life support backup (when available).
  D. administer epinephrine via IV or ET tube.

_____ **42.** Which of the following is an unnecessary step for the EMT-B to take when using a fully automated defibrillator?
  A. Assess the patient.
  B. Turn on the power.
  C. Put the pads on the patient's chest.
  D. Press the button to deliver the shock.

_____ **43.** The primary electrical disturbance resulting in cardiac arrest is
  A. asystole.   **C.** ventricular tachycardia.
  B. ventricular fibrillation.   **D.** pulseless electrical activity.

_____ **44.** The shockable rhythms include all of the following except
  A. asystole and PEA.   **C.** pulseless ventricular tachycardia.
  B. ventricular fibrillation.   **D.** ventricular tachycardia.

_____ **45.** A nonshockable rhythm which can be the result of a terminally sick heart or severe blood loss is called
  A. pulseless electrical activity. **C.** pulseless ventricular tachycardia.
  B. ventricular tachycardia.   **D.** ventricular fibrillation.

_____ **46.** A nonshockable rhythm that is commonly called "flatline" is named
  A. pulseless electrical activity. **C.** asystole.
  B. ventricular tachycardia.   **D.** ventricular fibrillation.

_____ 47. When the AED is analyzing the patient's heart rhythm, the EMT-B must
   A. continue the CPR compressions.
   B. avoid touching the patient.
   C. hyperventilate the patient.
   D. reassess for a carotid pulse.

_____ 48. The AED should routinely be used on
   A. trauma victims.
   B. patients under 90 pounds.
   C. patients under 12 years of age.
   D. patients with a shockable rhythm.

_____ 49. The AED pads are first attached to the cables. Then the pad attached to the
   A. white cable goes on the left lower ribs.
   B. white cable goes on the right lower ribs.
   C. red cable goes on the left lower ribs.
   D. red cable goes on the right lower ribs.

_____ 50. After the first set of three stacked shocks, you check the patient's carotid pulse. The patient has a pulse and is breathing adequately. You should then _____ and transport.
   A. give high-concentration oxygen via bag-valve-mask
   B. provide artificial ventilations with high-concentration oxygen
   C. give high-concentration oxygen via nonrebreather mask
   D. repeat the cycle of three stacked shocks

_____ 51. After six shocks, the EMT-B should _____ unless their local protocol says otherwise.
   A. give two more in a row
   B. transport the patient
   C. terminate the arrest
   D. increase the rate of ventilation

_____ 52. Which of the following is not a general principle of AED use?
   A. Hook up oxygen before beginning defibrillation.
   B. Avoid contact with patient during rhythm analysis.
   C. Be sure everyone is "clear" before delivering each shock.
   D. Avoid defibrillation in a moving ambulance.

_____ 53. Of the cardiac arrest patients listed below, which is the one that can be defibrillated immediately?
   A. a soaking wet patient lying in the rain
   B. a trauma patient with severe blood loss
   C. a patient on a metal deck being cradled by another person
   D. a patient with an implanted defibrillator

_____ 54. If it is necessary to remove a nitroglycerin patch to defibrillate a patient, you should
   A. wear gloves.
   B. wear goggles.
   C. ensure you have a replacement patch.
   D. cleanse the patient's skin with alcohol.

_____ 55. If a patient has a cardiac pacemaker and needs to be defibrillated, the EMT-B should
   A. perform the procedure as she would for other cardiac patients.
   B. remove the pacemaker before defibrillation.
   C. place the pad several inches away from the pacemaker battery.
   D. double the power setting on the AED.

COMPLETE THE FOLLOWING

1. List five signs and symptoms of congestive heart failure.

_____

_____

_____

_____

_____

2. List the four elements of the chain of survival.

_____

_____

_____

_____

LABEL THE DIAGRAM

Fill in the name of each component of the cardiovascular system on the line provided.

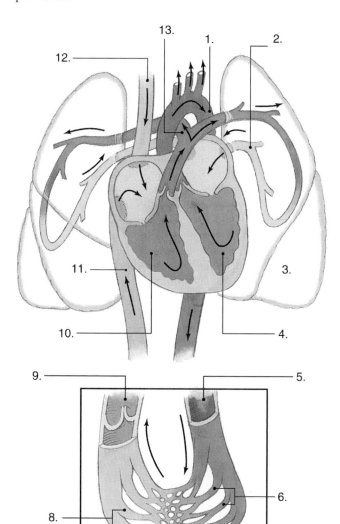

1. _____

2. _____

3. _____

4. _____

5. _____

6. _____

7. _____

8. _____

9. _____

10. _____

11. _____

12. _____

13. _____

► NITROGLYCERIN ASSIST

❏ Take body substance isolation.

❏ Scene size-up.

❏ Perform initial assessment.

❏ Perform focused history and physical exam.

❏ Contact medical direction for authorization to administer.

❏ Assure baseline vital signs.

❏ Assure right patient, right medication, right dose, right route.

❏ Assist patient with nitroglycerin administration.

❏ Reassess vital signs and chest pain after each dose.* Document findings.

*If the blood pressure falls below 100 systolic, treat the patient for shock (hypoperfusion). Transport promptly.

► CARDIAC ARREST MANAGEMENT/AUTOMATED EXTERNAL DEFIBRILLATION

❏ Take body substance isolation.

❏ Briefly question rescuer about arrest events.

❏ Direct rescuer to stop CPR.

❏ Verify absence of spontaneous pulse.

❏ Turn on defibrillator power.

❏ Attach automated defibrillator to patient.

❏ Ensure all individuals are standing clear of the patient.

❏ Initiate analysis of rhythm.

❏ Deliver shock (up to three successive shocks).

❏ Verify presence or absence of spontaneous pulse.

❏ If pulse absent, direct resumption of CPR.

❏ Gather additional information on arrest event.

❏ Confirm effectiveness of CPR (ventilation and compressions).

❏ Direct insertion of a simple airway adjunct (oropharyngeal/nasopharyngeal).

❏ Direct ventilation of patient.

❏ Assure high concentration of supplemental oxygen connected to the ventilatory adjunct.

❏ Assure CPR continues without unnecessary/prolonged interruption.

❏ In approximately one minute, re-evaluate patient/CPR.

❏ Repeat defibrillator sequence.

❏ Check carotid pulse.

❏ If there is a spontaneous pulse, check patient's breathing.

❏ If breathing is adequate, provide high-concentration oxygen by nonrebreather mask. If breathing is inadequate, ventilate patient with high-concentration oxygen.

❏ Transport patient without delay.

Diabetic Emergencies and Altered Mental Status

MATCH TERMINOLOGY/DEFINITIONS

A. Form of sugar that provides the body's basic source of energy

B. Condition brought about by decreased insulin production; also called "sugar diabetes" or simply "diabetes"

C. Hormone produced by the pancreas or taken as a medication by many diabetics that aids cells in utilizing glucose

D. Uncontrolled muscular movements

E. Prolonged seizure, or when a person suffers two or more convulsive seizures without regaining full consciousness

F. Low blood sugar

G. Medical condition that sometimes causes seizures

H. High blood sugar

I. Sudden change in sensation, behavior, or movement that can, in its most severe form, produce convulsions

J. Blockage or bursting of a major blood vessel supplying the brain; also called a cerebrovascular accident (CVA)

_____ **1.** Convulsions

_____ **2.** Diabetes mellitus

_____ **3.** Epilepsy

_____ **4.** Glucose

_____ **5.** Hyperglycemia

_____ **6.** Hypoglycemia

_____ **7.** Insulin

_____ **8.** Seizure

_____ **9.** Status epilepticus

_____ **10.** Stroke

MULTIPLE CHOICE REVIEW

_____ **1.** The relationship of glucose to insulin is often described as
    A. oppositional.
    B. synergistic.
    C. a lock and key mechanism.
    D. antagonistic.

_____ **2.** The condition brought about by decreased insulin production is known as
    A. diabetes mellitus.
    B. hypotension.
    C. hypoglycemia.
    D. cerebrovascular accident.

_____ **3.** The most common medical emergency for the diabetic patient is called
    A. diabetes mellitus.
    B. hypotension.
    C. hypoglycemia.
    D. cerebroascular accident.

_____ **4.** When a diabetic overexercises or overexerts, a medical condition called _____ can develop.
    A. hypoglycemia
    B. hyperglycemia
    C. diabetes mellitus
    D. acute pulmonary edema.

5. Of the potential causes of hypoglycemia listed below, which is <u>not</u> a cause?
    A. The patient may have taken too much insulin by mistake.
    B. The patient ate a box of candy too fast.
    C. The patient has been vomiting.
    D. The patient has been fasting.

6. If sugar is not replenished quickly for the hypoglycemic patient, the
    A. patient may have permanent brain damage.
    B. patient may go into pulmonary edema.
    C. patient will have chest pain.
    D. body can live off its internal sugar supply for up to two weeks.

7. The clues that a patient is a diabetic include all of the following <u>except</u>
    A. a medical identification bracelet.
    B. the presence of insulin in the refrigerator.
    C. low fat food in the freezer.
    D. information provided by family members.

8. Of the following, which is <u>not</u> a common oral medication used to treat diabetes?
    A. Diabinese.   **C.** Micronase.
    B. Sugunoil.   **D.** Orinase.

9. An intoxicated appearance and uncharacteristic behavior are typical of
    A. shock.   **C.** cardiac arrest.
    B. dehydration.   **D.** diabetic emergency.

10. Diabetics often present the EMT-B with all of the following signs and symptoms <u>except</u>
    A. cold, clammy skin.   **C.** anxiety.
    B. decreased heart rate.   **D.** combativeness.

11. In order for the EMT-B to consider administering oral glucose, the patient must have altered mental status and meet which other criteria?
    A. have a history of diabetes and be awake enough to swallow
    B. have prescribed medication and an absent gag reflex
    C. have a history of seizures and be awake
    D. have a Medic Alert tag that says "diabetic" and a head injury

12. When reassessing a patient to whom you have administered oral glucose, you note the patient's condition has not improved. What action should you take?
    A. Call the patient's personal physician.
    B. Give glucose in orange juice.
    C. Consult medical direction about whether to administer more glucose.
    D. Administer oxygen by nasal cannula.

13. Which position is most appropriate for transport of the diabetic patient who is not awake enough to swallow and does not need ventilation?
    A. supine   **C.** recovery
    B. prone   **D.** Fowler's

14. Which statement is most correct related to children with diabetes?
    A. Children are more likely than adults to eat correctly.
    B. Children are less likely than adults to exhaust blood sugar levels.
    C. Children are more at risk than adults for developing hypoglycemia.
    D. Children have a greater risk for medical emergencies than adults.

15. Which of the following would <u>most</u> likely indicate an alteration in the patient's blood sugar level?
    A. right lower abdominal pain   **C.** change in mental status
    B. nausea and vomiting   **D.** rigid abdomen on palpation

_____ **16.** Before and after administering oral glucose, make sure you
  A. check for distal pulses in both arms.
  B. document the mental status of the patient.
  C. increase the oxygen flow rate by 5 liters per minute.
  D. have the patient drink a glass of water.

_____ **17.** A trade name for oral glucose is
  A. D$_5$W.
  B. Lactose.
  C. Insulin.
  D. Insta-glucose.

_____ **18.** A patient is very confused and disoriented. Before deciding the patient has a behavioral problem, the EMT-B should consider all of the following except
  A. a potential head injury.
  B. brain tumor.
  C. hypoxia.
  D. glucose allergy.

_____ **19.** The most common cause of seizures in adults is
  A. taking a double dose of anti-seizure medication.
  B. taking a small dose of anti-seizure medication.
  C. not taking anti-seizure medication.
  D. use of illicit street drugs.

_____ **20.** Seizures are commonly caused by all of the following except
  A. cold exposure.
  B. high fever.
  C. brain tumor.
  D. infection.

_____ **21.** Which of the following is not a characteristic of idiopathic seizures?
  A. They last longer than 5 to 10 minutes.
  B. They occur spontaneously.
  C. They have an unknown cause.
  D. They often start in childhood.

_____ **22.** Convulsive seizures may be seen with
  A. epilepsy or hypoglycemia.
  B. hyperventilation or AMI.
  C. anaphylaxis or pulmonary embolism.
  D. hyperglycemia or asthma.

_____ **23.** The best-known condition that results in seizures is
  A. a stroke.
  B. epilepsy.
  C. measles.
  D. eclampsia.

_____ **24.** The type of seizure that most people associate with epilepsy and seizure disorders is called
  A. generalized tonic-clonic seizure.
  B. complex partial seizure.
  C. simple partial seizure.
  D. idiopathic seizure.

_____ **25.** When obtaining the medical history of a seizure patient find out from bystanders all of the following except
  A. how long the seizure lasted.
  B. what the patient did after the seizure.
  C. what the patient was doing prior to the seizure.
  D. what was the family's reaction to the seizure.

_____ **26.** A seizure patient becomes cyanotic. After convulsions have ended, what action should you take?
  A. Wait for patient's color to return to normal.
  B. Place a nonrebreather mask with oxygen on the patient.
  C. Provide artificial ventilations with supplemental oxygen.
  D. Monitor the pulse closely for 2 minutes.

_____ **27.** When you arrive on the scene of a seizure patient, you notice that a
bystander has placed a tongue blade in the corner of the patient's mouth.
What should you do?
  A. Begin oxygen therapy with a nonrebreather mask.
  B. Carefully remove the object from his mouth.
  C. Immobilize the patient on a long spine board.
  D. Immediately transport to the hospital.

_____ **28.** A seizure will normally last about _____ minutes.
  A. 1 to 3   **C.** 7 to 10
  B. 4 to 6   **D.** 30

_____ **29.** A patient has two or more back to back seizures without regaining full
consciousness. This is called
  A. repeating seizure.   **C.** status asthmaticus.
  B. status epilepticus.   **D.** convulsions.

_____ **30.** If you suspect a conscious patient has had a stroke, you should transport
him in the _____ position.
  A. recovery   **C.** prone
  B. supine   **D.** semi-sitting

COMPLETE THE FOLLOWING

1. List six of the signs and symptoms associated with a diabetic emergency.

_____

_____

_____

_____

_____

_____

_____

_____

2. Give four reasons a diabetic may develop hyperglycemia.

_____

_____

_____

_____

_____

_____

_____

EMT-BASIC SKILLS PERFORMANCE CHECKLIST

▶ **ORAL GLUCOSE ADMINISTRATION**

❑ Conduct a scene size-up.

❑ Take body substance isolation.

❑ Perform initial assessment.

❑ Obtain patient's history.

❑ Perform focused history and physical exam and take vital signs.

❑ Consult medical direction.

❑ Assure signs and symptoms of altered mental status are consistent with a history of diabetes.

❑ Assure patient is awake enough to swallow.

❑ Administer oral glucose.

❑ Perform on-going assessment.

CHAPTER 20

Allergies

MATCH TERMINOLOGY/DEFINITIONS

A. Red, itchy raised blotches on the skin that often result from an allergic reaction

B. Severe or life-threatening allergic reaction in which the blood vessels dilate, causing a drop in blood pressure, and the tissues lining the respiratory system swell, interfering with the airway

C. Something that causes an allergic reaction

D. Hormone produced by the body; as a medication it constricts blood vessels and dilates respiratory passages and is used to relieve severe allergic reactions.

E. Syringe pre-loaded with medication that has a spring-loaded device that pushes the needle through the skin when the tip of the device is pressed firmly against the body

_____ **1.** Allergen

_____ **2.** Anaphylaxis

_____ **3.** Auto-injector

_____ **4.** Epinephrine

_____ **5.** Hives

MULTIPLE CHOICE REVIEW

_____ **1.** An exaggerated response of the body's immune system to any substance is called a(n) _____ reaction.
  A. vasoconstricting
  B. immune
  C. allergic
  D. syncopal

_____ **2.** Why are allergic reactions sometimes treated as a high priority?
  A. The patient can vomit.
  B. The patient can become covered with hives.
  C. They can speed up the heart rate.
  D. They can cause airway obstruction.

_____ **3.** The first time a patient is exposed to an allergen, the person's immune system
  A. reacts violently.
  B. shuts down.
  C. forms antibodies.
  D. ignores the allergen.

_____ **4.** The second time a patient is exposed to an allergen, the body reactions include all of the following except
  A. destruction of antibodies.
  B. difficulty breathing.
  C. massive swelling.
  D. dilation of the blood vessels.

_____ **5.** Common causes of allergic reactions include all of the following except
  A. hornet stings.
  B. eggs and milk.
  C. poison ivy and penicillin.
  D. red fruits and vegetables.

_____ **6.** Why is it important to find out if a patient is allergic to latex?
  A. So you do not wear gloves that could cause an allergic reaction.
  B. Because the patient will also be allergic to milk.
  C. Because latex allergy can produce antitoxins.
  D. Because a latex allergy causes immediate cardiac arrest.

_____ **7.** The respiratory signs and symptoms of anaphylactic shock include all of the following except
  A. rapid breathing.   **C.** cough.
  B. hives.   **D.** stridor.

_____ **8.** The effects on the cardiac system of an allergic reaction could include _____ blood pressure.
  A. decreased heart rate and decreased
  B. increased heart rate and increased
  C. decreased heart rate and increased
  D. increased heart rate and decreased

_____ **9.** To be considered a severe allergic reaction, a patient must have signs and symptoms of shock or
  A. a history of allergies.   **C.** respiratory distress.
  B. massive swelling.   **D.** increased blood pressure.

_____ **10.** After administering epinephrine, the EMT-B should
  A. prepare another dose.
  B. reassess the patient after 2 minutes.
  C. decrease the oxygen being administered.
  D. allow the patient to remain at home.

_____ **11.** If you see a patient who has no history of allergies and is having her first allergic reaction, you should
  A. consult with medical direction.
  B. treat for shock and transport immediately.
  C. administer epinephrine via auto-injector.
  D. attempt to determine the cause immediately.

_____ **12.** If a patient has an epinephrine auto-injector, besides helping him/her take the medication, you should always
  A. ask if the patient has any spare auto-injectors for the trip to the hospital.
  B. call the patient's physician and request another dosage of the medication.
  C. determine if other family members have a history of allergic reactions.
  D. take the insect or substance that caused the reaction to the hospital.

_____ **13.** The recommended location for injection with the auto-injector is the
  A. center of the back.   **C.** buttocks.
  B. lateral mid thigh.   **D.** biceps.

_____ **14.** Epinephrine auto-injectors come in two different sizes. The child size contains
  A. 0.05 mg.   **C.** 0.5 mg.
  B. 0.15 mg.   **D.** 1.0 mg.

_____ **15.** Which statement is true related to anaphylactic reactions in infants and children?
  A. Infants frequently experience anaphylactic reactions.
  B. Children "outgrow" allergies as they mature.
  C. Anaphylactic reactions are common in younger children.
  D. Parents seldom can provide useful information about the child's medical history.

COMPLETE THE FOLLOWING

1. List ten signs and symptoms of allergic reaction or anaphylactic shock.

_____

_____

_____

_____

_____

_____

_____

_____

_____

_____

2. For a patient to be considered in anaphylaxis, list two signs either of which must be evident.

_____

_____

LABEL THE DIAGRAMS

Fill in the name of each substance which may cause an allergic reaction on the line provided.

1. _____

2. _____

3. _____

4. _____

EMT-BASIC SKILLS PERFORMANCE CHECKLIST

► EPINEPHRINE AUTO-INJECTOR ASSIST

❑ Take body substance isolation.

❑ Perform an initial assessment. Provide high concentration oxygen by nonrebreather mask.

❑ Obtain SAMPLE history.

❑ Take the patient's vital signs.

❑ Contact medical direction for authorization.

❑ Obtain patient's auto-injector.

❑ Check medication for expiration date.

❑ Check medication for cloudiness or discoloration.

❑ Remove safety cap from the injector.

❑ Assure injector is prescribed for the patient.

❑ Select appropriate injection site (mid lateral thigh).

❑ Push injector firmly against site.

❑ Hold injector against site for a minimum of ten (10) seconds.

❑ Properly discard auto-injector.

❑ Document patient's response to the medication.

❑ Perform ongoing assessment, paying special attention to the patient's ABCs and vital signs, while transporting.

CASE STUDY ━━━━━━━━━━━━━━━━━━━━━━━━━━━━━━━━━━━

▶ **THE LAKEFRONT EMERGENCY**

You respond to a camp on the lake for a call from a woman having difficulty breathing. Upon your arrival, after ensuring the scene is safe, you find a woman in her forties who is clutching her chest and is having obvious breathing difficulty.

1. Is there a need for another ambulance?

2. Should you call for an ALS unit to respond?

After donning body substance isolation, you begin your initial assessment. There is no reason to suspect trauma, and the patient has an open airway. She is responsive, although she talks in short, choppy sentences. She knows her name, where she is, and the day of the week.

3. Why is she talking in short, choppy sentences?

4. What would be your assessment of her level of consciousness?

A high-pitched musical tone is heard as she breathes. She shows other signs of respiratory distress.

5. What is the name of her breathing sound and what are some of the potential causes of this sound?

6. What are some additional signs of breathing difficulty that you may observe in this patient?

You decide that beginning oxygen administration is an appropriate thing to do at this time.

7. How would you deliver the oxygen and how many liters per minute would you administer?

You note the patient has a weak and rapid radial pulse. There is no reason to suspect any life-threatening external bleeding in this instance. The patient is very pale and is sweating profusely. She also complains of chest tightness and dizziness, which she denies she has ever had before.

8. Would you prioritize this patient low or high priority? Why?

9. What would be the best position to transport the patient in and why?

As you begin to prepare the patient for transport, you start the focused history and physical exam. The patient has chest tightness and breathing difficulty which came on suddenly. The pain is across the upper chest, doesn't radiate, and is constant. Nothing the patient does makes the pain go away; she states it is a 7 on a scale of 1 to 10 with 10 being the worst pain she ever had. The pain has been present for approximately 15 minutes. You assign a crew member to obtain a complete set of vital signs as you quickly listen to her lungs. She has a weak and rapid pulse at 110, respirations are labored at 26 per minute, and her blood pressure is 88/50.

10. As you load the patient into the ambulance, what additional history should you obtain?

Your patient states she was cleaning out the gutter and may have been stung by a bee. She previously reacted severely to a bee sting and carries a "bee-sting kit."

11. A) What medicine is usually in these kits? **B)** Should you help her take the medicine?

12. A) Is it necessary to call a doctor? **B)** What must be checked prior to administering the medicine?

As you leave the scene, the driver arranges for an ALS intercept on the way to the hospital. Other than reassessing the patient after administering the medication, you continue to monitor the patient. About five minutes en route, your driver pulls the ambulance to the side of the road momentarily as the ALS paramedic jumps in with his equipment. Then you proceed to the hospital.

13. What would be your quick report to the paramedic on **A)** the patient's chief complaint, **B)** your assessment of the situation, and **C)** the treatment you have given?

14. What care would you expect to see the paramedic give en route to the hospital?

CHAPTER 21

Poisoning and Overdose Emergencies

MATCH TERMINOLOGY/DEFINITIONS

A. Any substance that can harm the body by altering cell structure or functions

B. Stimulants, such as amphetamines, that affect the central nervous system to excite the user

C. When a patient's body reacts severely when deprived of an abused substance

D. Poisons that are taken into the body through unbroken skin

E. Depressants, such as barbiturates, that depress the central nervous system, often used to bring a more relaxed state of mind

F. Poisons that are swallowed

G. Class of drugs that affects the nervous system and changes many normal body activities; their legal use is for relief of pain. Illicit use is to produce an intense state of relaxation.

H. Substance that absorbs many poisons and prevents them from being absorbed by the body

I. Thinning down or weakening by mixing with something else

J. Severe reaction that can be part of alcohol withdrawal, characterized by sweating, trembling, anxiety, and hallucinations

K. Poisons that are breathed in

L. Mind-affecting or -altering drugs that act on the central nervous system to produce excitement and distortion of perceptions

M. Poisonous substance secreted by bacteria, plants, or animals

N. Vaporizing compounds, such as cleaning fluid, that are breathed in by an abuser to produce a "high"

O. Substance that will neutralize a poison or its effects

_____ 1. Absorbed poisons

_____ 2. Activated charcoal

_____ 3. Antidote

_____ 4. Delirium tremens

_____ 5. Dilution

_____ 6. Downers

_____ 7. Hallucinogens

_____ 8. Ingested poisons

_____ 9. Inhaled poisons

_____ 10. Narcotics

_____ 11. Poison

_____ 12. Toxin

_____ 13. Uppers

_____ 14. Volatile chemicals

_____ 15. Withdrawal

_____ 1. Which of the following is an environmental clue at the scene that can be used to help you determine that your patient may have been poisoned?
   A. The patient appears to have been vomiting.
   B. There is an empty pill bottle on the night table.
   C. The patient has an altered level of consciousness.
   D. The patient states he has a headache.

_____ 2. Which of the following is the most accurate definition of a poison?
   A. any substance that can harm the body, sometimes seriously enough to create a medical emergency
   B. any foreign substance swallowed by the patient
   C. any substance that could kill the patient if it is injected into the body
   D. any substance labeled with a hazardous material placard or label

_____ 3. Most of the over one million poisonings in the U.S. yearly are due to
   A. suicide attempts by adults.
   B. attempts to murder someone.
   C. accidents involving young children.
   D. teenagers on illicit drugs.

_____ 4. A substance secreted by plants, animals, or bacteria that is poisonous to humans is called a
   A. chemical.   C. narcotic.
   B. toxin.   D. drug.

_____ 5. Due to the poisons they produce, plants such as _____ can be dangerous to humans or pets.
   A. mistletoe   C. rubber plants
   B. mushrooms   D. All of the above.

_____ 6. Bacteria may produce toxins that cause deadly diseases such as
   A. HIV.   C. penicillin.
   B. botulism.   D. steroids.

_____ 7. For most poisonous substances, the reaction is more serious in
   A. the evening hours.   C. smaller concentrations.
   B. the elderly and the ill.   D. Spring time.

_____ 8. Which of the following is not a way that poisons damage the body?
   A. destroying skin and other tissues
   B. enhancing normal biochemical processes
   C. overstimulating the central nervous system
   D. displacing oxygen on the hemoglobin

_____ 9. Poisons may enter the body through any of the following routes except
   A. inhalation.   C. injection.
   B. ingestion.   D. excretion.

_____ 10. Carbon monoxide, chlorine, and ammonia are examples of _____ poisons.
   A. ingested   C. inhaled
   B. injected   D. swallowed

_____ 11. Examples of absorbed poisons include
   A. insecticides and agricultural chemicals.
   B. carbon monoxide and ammonia.
   C. insect stings and snake bites.
   D. aspirin and LSD.

_____ 12. The venom of a snake bite is an example of an _____ poison.
   A. ingested   C. inhaled
   B. injected   D. absorbed

_____ 13. Why is it important to determine when the ingestion of a poison occurred?
  A. Different poisons act on the body at different rates.
  B. Those who ingest poison in the evening tend to vomit more.
  C. Dilution of the poison is not effective after ten minutes.
  D. The antidote will work more effectively once the poison is in the intestines.

_____ 14. If you suspect poisoning by ingestion, after assuring a child has a patent airway, ask the parent for the child's
  A. name.   C. last visit to a physician.
  B. weight.   D. favorite drink.

_____ 15. The most common results of poison ingestion are
  A. altered mental status and diarrhea.
  B. nausea and vomiting.
  C. abdominal pain and diarrhea.
  D. chemical burns around the mouth and stomach pain.

_____ 16. Activated charcoal is used to
  A. act as an antidote.
  B. dilute the poisonous substance.
  C. reduce the amount of poison absorbed by the body.
  D. speed up the digestion of most chemicals in the body.

_____ 17. The difference between activated charcoal and regular charcoal is that
  A. activated charcoal is manufactured to have many cracks and crevices.
  B. regular charcoal is too large to swallow.
  C. activated charcoal is mixed with a substance to cause vomiting.
  D. regular charcoal is not diluted when used.

_____ 18. The decision on when to use activated charcoal is best made
  A. en route to the hospital.
  B. upon arrival at the emergency department.
  C. with medical direction or poison-control center consultation.
  D. in consultation with the patient's family physician.

_____ 19. Activated charcoal is not routinely used with ingestion of
  A. caustic substances.   C. strong alkalis.
  B. strong acids.   D. All of the above.

_____ 20. Examples of caustic substances include all of the following except
  A. lye.   C. toilet bowl cleaner.
  B. venom.   D. oven cleaner.

_____ 21. A patient who continues to cough violently after a gasoline ingestion should
  A. not be given activated charcoal.
  B. not be given oxygen.
  C. be transported immediately.
  D. be treated like a patient with an airway obstruction.

_____ 22. When a physician orders dilution of an ingested substance, you can use either water or
  A. a cola drink.   C. milk.
  B. coffee.   D. apple juice.

_____ 23. The most common inhaled poison is
  A. carbon dioxide.   C. carbon monoxide.
  B. nitrogen.   D. phosgene.

_____ 24. As you approach a patient who has passed out while cleaning a large tank, you smell an unusual odor. What should you do?
  A. Stand back and attempt to learn more about the chemical involved.
  B. Rapidly remove the patient from the area using a drag maneuver.
  C. Ignore the smell; it is probably a normal odor around industrial sites.
  D. Ask his coworkers to bring the patient to your ambulance.

_____ 25. The principal prehospital treatment of a patient who has inhaled poison is
   A. administering activated charcoal to the patient.
   B. administering high concentration oxygen.
   C. providing full spinal immobilization.
   D. administering an antidote.

_____ 26. Besides motor-vehicle exhaust, where else might you find carbon monoxide?
   A. in the patient compartment of your ambulance
   B. wherever you can smell its odor
   C. around an improperly vented wood-burning stove
   D. around the foundation of a house

_____ 27. How does carbon monoxide affect the body?
   A. It causes severe respiratory burns.
   B. It prevents the normal carrying of oxygen by the red blood cells.
   C. It causes the tissues in the airway to swell, making breathing difficult.
   D. It stimulates the central nervous system to decrease oxygen consumption.

_____ 28. A conscious patient who you suspect has carbon monoxide poisoning may exhibit any of the following except
   A. cyanosis.   **C.** dizziness.
   B. altered mental status.   **D.** cherry red lips.

_____ 29. If a patient has been contaminated by a poisonous powder, how should she be treated?
   A. Brush off as much powder as possible, then irrigate.
   B. Immediately start irrigation with very cold water.
   C. Leave the powder in place and transport immediately.
   D. Irrigate with water for 20 minutes.

_____ 30. If you smell alcohol on the breath or clothes of a patient, you should
   A. call for police immediately.
   B. not let this sidetrack you from doing a complete assessment.
   C. ask the patient how much he/she has had to drink today.
   D. assume that the patient will not give you the entire truth about his/her condition.

_____ 31. Of the following signs and symptoms, which is not seen with alcohol abuse but is with a diabetic emergency?
   A. acetone breath
   B. hallucinations
   C. slurred speech
   D. swaying and unsteadiness of movement

_____ 32. The sweating, trembling, anxiety, and hallucinations found in the alcohol withdrawal patient are called
   A. withdrawal signs.   **C.** delirium tremens.
   B. seizures.   **D.** Parkinson's tremors.

_____ 33. A patient who has mixed alcohol and drugs will exhibit with
   A. uncontrolled shivering.   **C.** extreme calmness.
   B. depressed vital signs.   **D.** All of the above.

_____ 34. When interviewing an intoxicated patient, do not begin by asking if he has taken any drugs. The reason for this statement is that
   A. the presence of drugs will negate the presence of the alcohol.
   B. the patient may feel you are accusing him of a crime.
   C. alcoholics generally do not take drugs.
   D. the patient would probably not tell the truth.

_____ 35. Drugs that stimulate the nervous system to excite the user are called
   A. uppers.   **C.** narcotics.
   B. downers.   **D.** antihypertensives.

_____ **36.** Tranquilizers or sleeping pills are examples of
    A. uppers.   **C.** narcotics.
    B. downers.   **D.** hallucinogens.

_____ **37.** Drugs that have a depressant effect on the central nervous system are called
    A. uppers.   **C.** narcotics.
    B. downers.   **D.** hallucinogens.

_____ **38.** Drugs capable of producing stupor or sleep that are often used to relieve pain are called
    A. uppers.   **C.** narcotics.
    B. downers.   **D.** hallucinogens.

_____ **39.** Mind-altering drugs that act on the nervous system to produce an intense state of excitement or distortion of the user's perceptions are called
    A. uppers.   **C.** narcotics.
    B. downers.   **D.** hallucinogens.

_____ **40.** A class of drugs which have few legal uses and are dissolved in the mouth are called
    A. narcotics.   **C.** hallucinogens.
    B. uppers.   **D.** downers.

_____ **41.** Cleaning fluid, glue, and model cement are examples of
    A. hallucinogens.   **C.** diuretics.
    B. volatile chemicals. **D.** narcotics.

_____ **42.** A patient who has overdosed on an upper may have signs and symptoms such as
    A. excitement, increased pulse and breathing rates, dilated pupils, and rapid speech.
    B. sluggishness, sleepiness, lack of coordination of body and speech.
    C. fast pulse rate, dilated pupils, flushed face, and "see" or "hear" things.
    D. reduced pulse rate and rate and depth of breathing, constricted pupils, and sweating.

_____ **43.** A patient who has overdosed on a downer may have signs and symptoms such as
    A. excitement, increased pulse and breathing rates, dilated pupils, and rapid speech.
    B. sluggishness, sleepiness, lack of coordination of body and speech.
    C. fast pulse rate, dilated pupils, flushed face, and "see" or "hear" things.
    D. reduced pulse rate and rate and depth of breathing, constricted pupils, and sweating.

_____ **44.** A patient who has overdosed on a hallucinogen may have signs and symptoms such as
    A. excitement, increased pulse and breathing rates, dilated pupils, and rapid speech.
    B. sluggishness, sleepiness, lack of coordination of body and speech.
    C. fast pulse rate, dilated pupils, flushed face, and "see" or "hear" things.
    D. reduced pulse rate and rate and depth of breathing, constricted pupils, and sweating.

_____ **45.** A patient who has overdosed on a narcotic may have signs and symptoms such as
    A. excitement, increased pulse and breathing rates, dilated pupils, and rapid speech.
    B. sluggishness, sleepiness, lack of coordination of body and speech.
    C. fast pulse rate, dilated pupils, flushed face, and "see" or "hear" things.
    D. reduced pulse rate and rate and depth of breathing, constricted pupils, and sweating.

COMPLETE THE FOLLOWING

1. What information should the EMT-Basic document for medical direction when treating a patient you suspect was poisoned?

_____   _____

_____   _____

_____   _____

_____   _____

2. List at least six signs and symptoms of alcohol abuse.

_____

_____

_____

_____

_____

_____

_____

LABEL THE DIAGRAMS

Fill in the way that each type of poison enters the body.

1. _____

2. _____

3. _____

4. _____

1.

Cleaning Fluid

Sprays

2.

Drugs

3.

Lye

Rat poison   Drain cleaners

4.

Household
cleaners

Insecticides

COMPLETE THE CHART

Fill in the type of commonly abused drug on the line provided. Indicate on the chart whether each drug is an upper, downer, narcotic, mind-altering, or volatile chemical.

AMPHETAMINE   **1.** _____

CODEINE   **2.** _____

LSD   **3.** _____

PSILOCYBIN   **4.** _____

GASOLINE   **5.** _____

SECOBARBITAL   **6.** _____

METHAQUALONE   **7.** _____

COCAINE   **8.** _____

DEXTROAMPHETAMINE   **9.** _____

CHLORAL HYDRATE   **10.** _____

MESCALINE   **11.** _____

MORNING GLORY SEEDS   **12.** _____

STP   **13.** _____

HEROIN   **14.** _____

BUTYL NITRATE   **15.** _____

PCP   **16.** _____

PRELUDIN   **17.** _____

METHADONE   **18.** _____

BARBITURATES   **19.** _____

DEMEROL   **20.** _____

▶ MANAGEMENT OF INGESTED POISONS

❑ Take body substance isolation.

❑ Maintain an open airway.

❑ Conduct initial assessment.

❑ Perform a focused history and physical exam.

❑ Assess baseline vital signs.

❑ Quickly gather information about the substance.

❑ Call medical direction on the scene or en route.

❑ If directed, administer activated charcoal.

❑ Position patient for vomiting and save all vomitus. Have suction ready.

❑ Perform ongoing assessment.

❑ Transport as soon as possible.

▶ MANAGEMENT OF INHALED POISONS

❑ Size-up the situation to prevent injury to yourself and your crew.

❑ Take body substance isolation. Remove patient from the source.*

❑ Avoid touching contaminated clothing and jewelry.

❑ Maintain an open airway. Stay alert for vomiting. Properly position patient and have suction equipment ready.

❑ Conduct initial assessment.

❑ Administer a high concentration of oxygen.

❑ Perform a focused history and physical exam.

❑ Remove contaminated clothing and jewelry.

❑ Assess baseline vital signs.

❑ Quickly gather information about the substance.

❑ Call medical direction on the scene or en route.

❑ Perform ongoing assessment.

❑ Transport as soon as possible.

*Safety Note: In the presence of hazardous fumes or gases, wear protective clothing and self-contained breathing apparatus or wait for those who are properly trained and equipped to enter the scene and bring the patient out.

▶ MANAGEMENT OF ABSORBED POISONS

❑ Size-up the situation to prevent injury to yourself and your crew.

❑ Take body substance isolation.

❑ Remove the patient from the source. Avoid contaminating yourself with the poison.

❑ Maintain an open airway.

❑ Conduct initial assessment.

❑ Administer a high concentration of oxygen.

❑ Perform a focused history and physical exam.

❑ Brush powders from the patient. Be careful not to abrade the patient's skin.

❑ Remove contaminated clothing and other articles.

❑ Assess baseline vital signs.

❑ Quickly gather information about the substance.

❑ If appropriate, wash with clear water. Call medical direction. Follow directions.

❑ Perform ongoing assessment.

❑ Be alert for shock and transport as soon as possible.

CHAPTER 22

Environmental Emergencies

MATCH TERMINOLOGY/DEFINITIONS

▶ **PART A**

A. Change from liquid to gas; as perspiration on the skin vaporizes, the body experiences a cooling effect.

B. Abbreviation that stands for arterial gas embolism

C. Application of an external heat source to rewarm the body of a hypothermic patient

D. Carrying away of heat by currents of air or water or other gases or liquids

E. Death caused by changes in the lungs resulting from immersion in water

F. Direct transfer of heat from one material to another through direct contact

G. Condition resulting from nitrogen trapped in the body's tissues caused by coming up too quickly from a deep, prolonged dive

H. Application of heat to the lateral chest, neck, armpits, and groin of a hypothermic patient

I. Increase in body temperature above normal; life-threatening in its extreme

J. Gas bubble in the bloodstream; more accurately called an arterial gas embolism

_____ **1.** Active rewarming

_____ **2.** AGE

_____ **3.** Air embolism

_____ **4.** Central rewarming

_____ **5.** Conduction

_____ **6.** Convection

_____ **7.** Decompression sickness

_____ **8.** Drowning

_____ **9.** Evaporation

_____ **10.** Hyperthermia

A. Condition of having begun to drown; the patient may be conscious, unconscious with heartbeat and pulse, or with no heartbeat or pulse but still able to be resuscitated.

B. Covering a hypothermic patient and taking other steps to prevent further heat loss and help the body rewarm itself

C. Sending out energy, such as heat, in waves into space

D. Breathing; during this process, the body loses heat as warm air is exhaled from the body.

E. Cooling or freezing of particular parts of the body

F. Generalized cooling that reduces body temperature below normal; life-threatening in its extreme

G. Substances produced by animals or plants that are poisonous to humans

H. Chilling caused by conduction of heat from the body when the body or clothing is wet

I. Toxin produced by certain animals such as snakes, spiders, and some marine life forms

J. Chilling caused by convection of heat from the body in the presence of air currents

_____ 1. Hypothermia

_____ 2. Local cooling

_____ 3. Near-drowning

_____ 4. Passive rewarming

_____ 5. Radiation

_____ 6. Respiration

_____ 7. Toxins

_____ 8. Venom

_____ 9. Water chill

_____ 10. Wind chill

MULTIPLE CHOICE REVIEW

_____ 1. Water conducts heat away from the body _____ than still air.
   A. 25 times faster
   B. 25 times slower
   C. 50 times faster
   D. 50 times slower

_____ 2. The body loses heat from respiration, radiation, conduction, convection, and
   A. excretion.
   B. induction.
   C. evaporation.
   D. condensation.

_____ 3. When there is _____ wind, there is _____ heat loss.
   A. more : less
   B. less : greater
   C. more : greater
   D. no : maximum

_____ 4. Most radiant heat loss occurs from a person's
   A. arms and legs.
   B. chest and back.
   C. head and neck.
   D. feet and hands.

_____ 5. Predisposing factors to hypothermia include all of the following except
   A. burns.
   B. diabetes.
   C. spinal cord injuries.
   D. headache.

_____ 6. Which of the following is not a reason infants and children are more prone to hypothermia?
   A. They have small muscle mass.
   B. They have large skin surface in relation to their total body mass.
   C. They are unable to shiver effectively.
   D. They have more body fat than do adults.

_____ 7. You are treating an elderly patient with a possible leg fracture who was found lying on his cold garage floor where he had been all night. You should also consider
   A. a cerebrovascular accident.
   B. hypothermia.
   C. pulmonary edema.
   D. hypoperfusion.

_____ 8. When a patient's core body temperature drops below 90°F, the patient
   A. may be shivering uncontrollably.
   B. may no longer be shivering.
   C. will be pulseless.
   D. will suddenly become alert.

_____ 9. All of the following are signs and symptoms of hypothermia except
   A. high blood pressure and low pulse.
   B. stiff or rigid posture.
   C. cool abdominal skin temperature.
   D. loss of motor coordination.

_____ 10. Passive rewarming involves
   A. applying heat packs to the patient.
   B. covering the patient.
   C. administering heated oxygen to the patient.
   D. massaging the patient's limbs.

_____ 11. The treatment of the hypothermic patient who is alert and responding
   includes all of the following except
   A. removal of all of the patient's wet clothing.
   B. actively rewarming the patient during transport.
   C. rapidly giving the patient plenty of hot liquids.
   D. providing care for shock and providing oxygen.

_____ 12. When actively rewarming a patient,
   A. apply heat to the chest, neck, armpits, and groin.
   B. quickly rewarm the patient.
   C. give the patient stimulants to drink.
   D. immerse the arms and feet in hot water.

_____ 13. The reason why you should rewarm the body's core first is to
   A. prevent blood from collecting in the extremities due to vasodilation.
   B. quickly circulate cold blood throughout the body.
   C. speed up the blood flow to the extremities.
   D. increase blood flow to the brain to prevent unconsciousness.

_____ 14. When transporting an alert patient with mild hypothermia, it is recommended
   that you
   A. transport in Fowler's position.
   B. massage the legs so the patient can walk.
   C. keep the patient at rest.
   D. leave the wet clothes in place.

_____ 15. When treating the unresponsive patient with severe hypothermia,
   A. keep the patient's head raised above the feet for the transport to the
      hospital.
   B. place the patient in a warm bath tub for at least twenty minutes.
   C. provide high concentration oxygen that has been passed through a
      warm humidifier.
   D. massage the extremities for 35–45 seconds.

_____ 16. Because patients with extreme hypothermia may not reach biological death
   for over 30 minutes, the medical philosophy is
   A. if there is a pulse, start CPR.
   B. they are not dead until they're warm and dead.
   C. resuscitate for no longer than 30 minutes.
   D. always resuscitate very aggressively.

_____ 17. A cold injury usually occurring to exposed areas of the body that is brought about by direct contact with a cold object or exposure to cold air is called a(n)
A. early local cold injury.   C. frostbite.
B. superficial late cold injury.   D. deep local cold injury.

_____ 18. The skin color of a patient with a superficial local cold injury will change from _____ to _____ .
A. red : white   C. red : blue
B. white : red   D. white : blue

_____ 19. If a superficial local cold injury is on an extremity, the EMT-B should
A. splint and leave uncovered.
B. rub the extremity briskly.
C. not re-expose the injury to cold.
D. immerse the extremity in hot water.

_____ 20. When muscles, bones, deep blood vessels, and organ membranes become frozen, this type of injury is called
A. a superficial local cold injury.   C. a deep local cold injury.
B. frostnip.   D. local cooling.

_____ 21. In frostbite, the affected area first appears
A. black and stiff.   C. red and blotchy.
B. white and waxy.   D. blue and abraded.

_____ 22. Do not allow the frostbite patient to drink alcohol or smoke because
A. the patient may suffer altered mental status or fall asleep.
B. these would stimulate the patient to move, which could cause further injury.
C. constriction of blood vessels and decreased circulation to the injured tissues may result.
D. either could contaminate the frostbitten area.

_____ 23. Active rewarming of a frozen part
A. is seldom recommended in the field.
B. includes using very hot water.
C. is performed without removing the patient's clothing.
D. includes covering the patient's face.

_____ 24. The environment associated with hyperthermia includes
A. heat and high winds.   C. heat and high humidity.
B. heat and light rain.   D. heat and low humidity.

_____ 25. The higher the humidity the
A. less you perspire.
B. less your perspiration evaporates.
C. less you radiate heat.
D. more you lose heat from your body.

_____ 26. The medical problems resulting from dry heat are often worse than those from moist heat because
A. dry heat is more common.
B. moist heat tires people quickly.
C. dry heat causes more sunburn.
D. dry heat affects the respiratory system more quickly.

_____ 27. When salts are lost by the body through sweating, the patient may have all of the following except
A. muscle cramps.   C. dizziness or periods of faintness.
B. weakness or exhaustion.   D. fluid buildup in the lungs.

_____ 28. A patient with heat exhaustion will present with
A. dry, hot skin.
B. moist, pale, normal to cool skin.
C. a lack of sweating.
D. rapid strong pulse.

_____ 29. The signs and symptoms of a heat emergency in patients who have hot, dry or moist skin include
A. slow and shallow breathing.
B. seizures.
C. constricted pupils.
D. muscle cramps.

_____ 30. The signs and symptoms of a heat emergency in patients who have hot, dry or moist skin include all of the following except
A. generalized weakness.
B. loss of consciousness or altered mental status.
C. profuse perspiration.
D. full and rapid pulse.

_____ 31. Which of the following is a large contributor to adolescent and adult drownings?
A. inexperience with equipment
B. substance abuse
C. stomach cramps
D. car accident immersions

_____ 32. During a drowning incident, water flowing past the epiglottis causes
A. a reflex to close the mouth.
B. the victim to gasp for more air.
C. a reflex spasm of the larynx.
D. the victim to begin hyperventilating.

_____ 33. About 10 percent of the drowning victims die from
A. too much fluid in their lungs.
B. lack of air.
C. cervical spine injuries.
D. crushing chest injury.

_____ 34. If you are not an experienced swimmer, you should
A. never attempt to go into the water to do a rescue.
B. don a floatation device prior to going into the water.
C. use a boat as your first approach to conduct the rescue.
D. coach the patient in floating techniques.

_____ 35. If you suspect that a patient still in the pool has a possible spine injury,
A. spineboard the patient as you pull him from the water.
B. immobilize and spineboard him while still in the water.
C. quickly remove him from the water to prevent hypothermia.
D. encourage the patient to swim to the side of the pool.

_____ 36. A toxin produced by some animals that is harmful to humans is called
A. poison.
B. lymph.
C. venom.
D. allergen.

_____ 37. Typical sources of injected poisons include _____ bites and stings.
A. spider
B. scorpion
C. snake
D. All of the above.

_____ 38. While cleaning out the crawl space below the house you experience blotchy skin, redness in your arm, weakness, and nausea. It is possible that you
A. are developing heat stroke.
B. were bitten by a poisonous spider.
C. are having a diabetic reaction.
D. are allergic to something in the air.

_____ 39. Signs and symptoms of injected poisoning include all of the following except
A. lack of sensation in one side of the body.
B. puncture marks.
C. muscle cramps, chest tightening, and joint pains.
D. excessive saliva formation and profuse sweating.

_____ **40.** If you suspect that your patient has been bitten by a snake, you should do all of the following except
  A. call for medical direction.
  B. clean the injection site with soap and water.
  C. remove rings, bracelets, or other constricting items on the bitten limb.
  D. capture the live snake and bring it in the ambulance to the emergency department.

COMPLETE THE FOLLOWING

1. List six of the signs and symptoms of heat exhaustion.

_____

_____

_____

_____

_____

_____

2. List six of the signs and symptoms of heat stroke (hot, dry or moist skin).

_____

_____

_____

_____

_____

_____

3. List ten of the signs and symptoms of an insect bite or sting.

_____

_____

_____

_____

_____

_____

_____

_____

_____

_____

▶ **ACTIVE RAPID REWARMING OF FROZEN PARTS**

❑ Take body substance isolation.

❑ Conduct initial assessment.

❑ Obtain baseline vital signs.

❑ Conduct focused history and physical exam.

❑ Consider administering oxygen by nonrebreather mask.

❑ Heat water to a temperature between 100° and 105°F.

❑ Fill the container with the heated water and prepare the injured part by removing clothing, jewelry, bands, or straps.

❑ Fully immerse the injured part. Do not allow the injured area to touch the sides or bottom of the container. Do not place any pressure on the affected part. Continuously stir the water. When the water cools below 100°F, remove the affected part and add more warm water. The patient may complain of moderate pain as the affected area rewarms or may experience some period of intense pain.

❑ If you complete rewarming of the part, gently dry the affected area and apply a dry sterile dressing. Place dry sterile dressings between fingers and toes before dressing hands and feet.

❑ Cover the site with blankets or whatever is available to keep the affected area warm. Do not allow these coverings to come in contact with the injured area or to put pressure on the site.

❑ Keep the patient at rest. Do not allow the patient to walk if a lower extremity has been frostbitten or frozen.

❑ Keep the entire patient warm.

❑ Continue to monitor the patient.

❑ Assist circulation according to local protocol. (Some systems recommend rhythmically and carefully raising and lowering the affected limb.)

❑ Do not allow the limb to refreeze.

❑ Transport patient as soon as possible with the affected limb slightly elevated.

❑ Take body substance isolation.

❑ Conduct initial assessment.

❑ Splint head and neck with arms.

❑ Roll patient over into supine position.

❑ Ensure airway and breathing. (Note: If patient is not breathing, remove him/her from the water on a backboard as soon as possible.)

❑ Provide manual stabilization of the head and neck.

❑ Assess sensory and motor function in all four extremities.

❑ Slide backboard under the patient.

❑ Apply rigid extrication collar.

❑ Tie down torso, then the head and neck with straps.

❑ Float board to the edge of the water.

❑ Remove patient from water with as much assistance as needed.

❑ Obtain baseline vital signs.

❑ Conduct focused history and physical exam.

❑ Reassess sensory and motor function in all four extremities.

❑ Apply oxygen and prepare to transport patient.

CHAPTER

Behavioral Emergencies

23

MATCH TERMINOLOGY/DEFINITIONS

A. Humane device made of leather used to hold a patient still to prevent the patient from injuring himself or others

B. Display of emotions, such as fear, grief, or anger, in response to an accident, serious illness, or death

C. Death of a person due to a body position that restricts breathing for a prolonged time

D. When a patient's behavior is not typical for the situation; when the patient's behavior is unacceptable or intolerable to the patient, his family, or the community; or when the patient may harm himself or others

E. Manner in which a person acts

_____ **1.** Behavioral emergency

_____ **2.** Behavior

_____ **3.** Positional asphyxia

_____ **4.** Soft restraint

_____ **5.** Stress reaction

MULTIPLE CHOICE REVIEW

_____ **1.** Physical causes of altered behavior include all of the following except
   A. inadequate blood flow to the brain.
   B. mind-altering substances.
   C. excessive heat or cold.
   D. differing lifestyles.

_____ **2.** Altered behavior ranging from irritability to altered mental status can be due to any of the following except
   A. lack of oxygen.
   B. head trauma.
   C. hypoactivity.
   D. hypoglycemia.

_____ **3.** To calm a patient who is experiencing a stress reaction, you should
   A. complete your assessment as quickly as possible.
   B. allow the patient to control the situation.
   C. explain things to the patient honestly.
   D. restrain the patient quickly.

_____ **4.** Which of the following is not usually a common presentation of a patient experiencing a behavioral emergency?
   A. panic or anxiety
   B. neat appearance
   C. repetitive motions
   D. pressured-sounding speech

_____ **5.** When you are called to care for a patient who has attempted suicide or is about to attempt suicide, your first concern should be
   A. how you will restrain the patient.
   B. your personal safety.
   C. determining the patient's method for suicide.
   D. the patient's and family's safety.

_____ **6.** High suicide rates occur at ages
    A. 15–25.   **C.** 30–35.
    B. 25–30.   **D.** 35–40.

_____ **7.** Which of the following is <u>not</u> an example of a self-destructive activity?
    A. a defined lethal plan of action which has been verbalized
    B. giving away personal possessions
    C. denial of suicidal thoughts
    D. previous suicide threats

_____ **8.** When a suicidal patient exhibits sudden improvement from depression, the EMT-B should consider that the patient is
    A. no longer suicidal.   **C.** still at risk for suicide.
    B. is now ready to accept care.   **D.** None of the above.

_____ **9.** When assessing an aggressive patient for a possible threat to you or your crew, take all of the following actions <u>except</u>
    A. try to determine the patient's history of aggressive behavior.
    B. pay attention to the patient's vocal activity.
    C. take note of the patient's posturing.
    D. assess the patient in the kitchen.

_____ **10.** If a patient stands in a corner of the room with fists clenched and screaming obscenities, you should
    A. request police backup and keep the doorway in sight.
    B. raise your voice to a higher level than the patient's.
    C. challenge the patient in an attempt to calm him.
    D. explain that you would respond in the same way.

_____ **11.** Use of reasonable force to restrain a patient should involve an evaluation of all of the following <u>except</u>
    A. the patient's size and strength.
    B. the family's ability to pay for your services.
    C. the patient's mental status.
    D. the available methods of restraint.

_____ **12.** The use of force by an EMT-B is allowed
    A. to defend against an attack by an emotionally disturbed patient.
    B. only when the police are present.
    C. whenever a patient refuses any of your treatments.
    D. whenever you suspect the patient has been drinking.

_____ **13.** Once the decision has been made to restrain a patient, which of the following steps should be avoided?
    A. Use multiple straps to restrain the patient.
    B. Reassure the patient throughout the procedure.
    C. Reassess the patient's distal circulation frequently.
    D. Use two rescuers to secure the patient.

_____ **14.** A restrained patient who is spitting on rescuers can best be managed by
    A. placing in a prone position on the stretcher.
    B. wrapping the patient's mouth with roller gauze.
    C. placing 3-inch tape across the patient's mouth.
    D. placing a surgical mask on the patient's face.

_____ **15.** When a patient is a danger to himself or others and needs to be transported against his will, the EMT-B should
    A. restrain the patient immediately.
    B. transport the patient with the family's assistance.
    C. contact the police for assistance.
    D. contact the patient's physician.

COMPLETE THE FOLLOWING

1. List nine potential risk factors for suicide.

_____

_____

_____

_____

_____

_____

_____

_____

_____

2. List four precautions for your safety and that of your crew when you feel your patient may hurt himself or others.

_____

_____

_____

_____

CHAPTER

Obstetrics and Gynecological Emergencies

MATCH TERMINOLOGY/DEFINITIONS

▶ **PART A**

A. Normal head-first birth

B. Neck of the uterus at the entrance to the birth canal

C. Implantation of the fertilized egg in an oviduct, the cervix of the uterus, or in the abdominopelvic cavity

D. Placenta, umbilical cord, and some tissues from the amniotic sac and lining of the uterus that are delivered after the birth of the baby

E. Baby developing in the womb

F. Condition in which the placenta separates from the uterine wall

G. Deliberate actions taken to stop a pregnancy

H. When more than one baby is born during a single delivery

I. Spontaneous (miscarriage) or induced termination of pregnancy

J. Three stages of the delivery of a baby that begin with the contractions of the uterus and end with the expulsion of the placenta

K. Thin, membranous "bag of waters" that surrounds the developing fetus

L. Amniotic fluid that is greenish or brownish-yellow rather than clear; an indication of possible maternal or fetal distress during labor

M. When the buttocks or both legs of a baby delivers first during birth

N. Skin between the vagina and the anus

O. When the presenting part of the baby first appears through the vaginal opening

_____ **1.** Abortion

_____ **2.** Abruptio placentae

_____ **3.** Afterbirth

_____ **4.** Amniotic sac

_____ **5.** Breech presentation

_____ **6.** Cephalic presentation

_____ **7.** Cervix

_____ **8.** Crowning

_____ **9.** Ectopic pregnancy

_____ **10.** Fetus

_____ **11.** Induced abortion

_____ **12.** Labor

_____ **13.** Meconium staining

_____ **14.** Multiple birth

_____ **15.** Perineum

CHAPTER 24 Obstetrics and Gynecological Emergencies

▶ **PART B**

A. When the umbilical cord presents first and is squeezed between the vaginal wall and the baby's head

B. Dizziness and a drop in blood pressure caused when the mother is in a supine position and the weight of the uterus, infant, placenta, and amniotic fluid compress the inferior vena cava, reducing return of blood to the heart and cardiac output

C. When the fetus and placenta deliver before the 28th week of pregnancy, commonly called a miscarriage

D. Muscular abdominal organ where the fetus develops; also called the womb

E. Born dead

F. Any newborn weighing less than 5½ pounds or one that is born before the 37th week of pregnancy

G. Fetal structure containing the blood vessels that carry blood to and from the placenta

H. Organ of pregnancy where exchange of oxygen, foods, and wastes occurs between a mother and fetus

I. Condition in which the placenta is formed in an abnormal location (usually low in the uterus and close to or over the cervical opening) that will not allow for a normal delivery of the fetus

J. Birth canal

_____ 1. Placenta

_____ 2. Placenta previa

_____ 3. Premature infant

_____ 4. Prolapsed umbilical cord

_____ 5. Spontaneous abortion

_____ 6. Stillborn

_____ 7. Supine hypotensive syndrome

_____ 8. Umbilical cord

_____ 9. Uterus

_____ 10. Vagina

MULTIPLE CHOICE REVIEW

_____ 1. The nine months of pregnancy are divided into three-month trimesters. During the second trimester, the
   A. fetus is being formed and there is little uterine growth during this period.
   B. uterus grows very rapidly while the woman's blood volume, cardiac output, and heart rate increase.
   C. uterus is often seen reaching up to the epigastrium by this time.
   D. uterus develops to full size.

_____ 2. The normal birth position is _____ and is called a _____ birth.
   A. head first : breech   C. feet first : breech
   B. head first : cephalic   D. feet first : cephalic

_____ 3. The first stage of labor starts
   A. with conception.
   B. at the nine-month point.
   C. with regular contractions of the uterus.
   D. when the cervix is dilated.

_____ 4. The second stage of labor starts with
   A. the birth of the baby.
   B. regular contractions of the uterus.
   C. the delivery of the afterbirth.
   D. the entry of the baby into the birth canal.

_____ 5. The third stage of labor begins with
   A. the birth of the baby.   C. dilation of the cervix.
   B. delivery of the afterbirth.   D. full growth of the uterus.

_____ **6.** The third stage of labor is complete when
   A. the baby is born.
   B. the afterbirth is expelled.
   C. twenty minutes have passed since the delivery.
   D. the uterus is firm again.

_____ **7.** The process by which the cervix gradually widens and thins out is called
   A. delivery.   **C.** staining.
   B. dilation.   **D.** contraction.

_____ **8.** As the fetus moves downward and the cervix dilates, normally the amniotic sac breaks and fluid leaks out. If this fluid is greenish or brownish-yellow in color this may indicate
   A. fetal or maternal distress.
   B. the fetus is dead.
   C. the mother is pushing too hard.
   D. the amniotic sac broke too early.

_____ **9.** The greenish or brownish-yellow fluid expelled from the amniotic sac is called
   A. a bloody show.   **C.** meconium staining.
   B. vena cava syndrome.   **D.** amniotic bile.

_____ **10.** When a mother in labor states she feels the need to move her bowels, this means the
   A. birth will be delayed.   **C.** birth moment is nearing.
   B. uterus is almost dilated.   **D.** baby is in distress.

_____ **11.** The contraction duration is timed from the
   A. start of the pain till the delivery of the infant.
   B. beginning of contraction to when the uterus relaxes.
   C. end of a contraction to the beginning of the next one.
   D. peak of the contraction to the end of the contraction.

_____ **12.** The contraction interval, or frequency, is timed from the
   A. start of one contraction to the start of the next.
   B. beginning of contraction to when the uterus relaxes.
   C. peak of the contraction to the end of the contraction.
   D. start of the pain until the delivery of the infant.

_____ **13.** Delivery is imminent when the contractions last
   A. 15 seconds and are 5 to 8 minutes apart.
   B. 30 seconds and are 2 to 3 minutes apart.
   C. 45 seconds or more and are 8 to 10 minutes apart.
   D. 90 seconds or more and are 5 to 8 minutes apart.

_____ **14.** The EMT-B's primary roles at a normal childbirth scene are to determine whether the delivery will occur at the scene and, if so, to
   A. determine if the delivery can be delayed.
   B. assist the mother as she delivers the child.
   C. carefully deliver the infant.
   D. immobilize the patient.

_____ **15.** The sterile obstetrical kit does <u>not</u> contain
   A. a rubber bulb syringe for suctioning.
   B. several individually wrapped sanitary napkins.
   C. heavy flat twine to tie the cord.
   D. cord clamps or hemostats.

_____ **16.** When evaluating the mother for a possible home delivery, the EMT-B should ask
   A. if pregnancy problems run in the family.
   B. the frequency and duration of contractions.
   C. if the mother feels she needs to urinate.
   D. the father's blood type and medical history.

_____ **17.** When is it important to ask the mother if you can examine for crowning?
   A. if the mother is straining during contractions
   B. if the mother is in her ninth month of pregnancy
   C. if the mother is pregnant for the first time
   D. it is not important to ask permission to examine the mother.

_____ **18.** You are treating a 25-year-old female who is 8 months pregnant. She states she has contractions every fifteen minutes or so which last for about twenty seconds. She is not exactly sure what labor pain is like because this is her first pregnancy. Her vitals are pulse of 96, blood pressure of 130/70, and respirations of 22. What should you do next?
   A. Administer oxygen and transport immediately.
   B. Prepare for a home delivery immediately.
   C. Ask if her water broke and prepare for a quiet ride to the hospital.
   D. Tell her to call you back when the contractions are more frequent.

_____ **19.** If you determine that the delivery is imminent based on the presence of crowning and other signs, you should
   A. contact medical direction.
   B. transport as quickly as possible.
   C. ask the mother to go the bathroom first.
   D. ask the mother to hold her legs closed.

_____ **20.** When a full-term pregnant woman in a supine position complains of dizziness and you note a drop in blood pressure, this could be due to a condition called _____ syndrome.
   A. diabetes mellitus   **C.** Cushing's reflex
   B. supine hypotension   **D.** fluid retention

_____ **21.** To counteract the pressure of the uterus on the inferior vena cava, you should
   A. raise the patient's legs.
   B. transport the patient on her left side.
   C. raise the patient's head.
   D. apply the PASG (MAST).

_____ **22.** During a delivery, the EMT-B will need all of the following infection control gear except
   A. surgical gloves.   **C.** eye protection.
   B. a mask.   **D.** a Tyvek suit.

_____ **23.** During delivery, encourage the mother to
   A. breathe rapidly and deeply.
   B. hold her breath every 2 minutes.
   C. close her mouth and breathe through her nose.
   D. breathe deeply through her mouth.

_____ **24.** When supporting the baby's head during a delivery, the EMT-B should do all of the following except
   A. pull on the baby's shoulders when they appear.
   B. apply gentle pressure to control the delivery.
   C. place one hand below the baby's head.
   D. spread fingers evenly around the baby's head.

_____ **25.** If the amniotic sac has not broken by the time the baby's head is delivered, you should
   A. stop the delivery and transport immediately.
   B. use your finger to puncture the membrane.
   C. contact medical control immediately.
   D. delay the delivery until it breaks.

_____ **26.** If you cannot loosen or unwrap the umbilical cord from around the infant's neck, you should
   A. stop the delivery and transport immediately.
   B. tell the mother to push more forcefully.
   C. clamp the cord in two places and cut between the clamps.
   D. contact medical direction for advice.

_____ **27.** Most babies are born
   A. face down and then rotate to either side.
   B. face up and then rotate to either side.
   C. feet and buttocks first and do not rotate.
   D. face up and do not rotate.

_____ **28.** When suctioning a newborn,
   A. compress the bulb syringe when inside the baby's mouth.
   B. compress the syringe before placing it in the baby's mouth.
   C. suction the nose and then the mouth.
   D. insert the syringe about 22 inches into the baby's mouth.

_____ **29.** Once the baby's feet are delivered,
   A. pick the baby up by the feet using a firm grasp.
   B. lay the baby on its side with head slightly lower than its torso.
   C. lay the baby on its side and massage its back.
   D. pick the baby up by the feet and massage its back.

_____ **30.** To assess the newborn, the EMT-B should do all of the following except
   A. note ease of breathing.
   B. check movement in the extremities.
   C. note skin coloration.
   D. check the response to a sternal rub.

_____ **31.** Why is it necessary to suction the baby's mouth before the nose?
   A. so the baby can gasp and begin breathing
   B. so the baby is stimulated to cry
   C. to prevent aspiration of materials from its mouth
   D. because this will open the nasopharynx passageway.

_____ **32.** If assessment of the infant's breathing reveals shallow, slow, or absent respirations, the EMT-B should
   A. provide oxygen by nonrebreather mask.
   B. use a gentle but vigorous rubbing of the infant's back.
   C. provide artificial ventilations at 40 to 60 per minute.
   D. provide artificial ventilations at 20 to 30 per minute.

_____ **33.** In a normal birth, the infant must be breathing on its own
   A. before you clamp and cut the cord.
   B. prior to transportation to the hospital.
   C. prior to considering ventilation.
   D. in order to use an oral airway.

_____ **34.** The first umbilical cord clamp should be placed about _____ inches from the baby.
   A. 4   **C.** 8
   B. 6   **D.** 10

_____ **35.** The second umbilical cord clamp should be placed about _____ inches from the baby.
  A. 3
  B. 5
  C. 7
  D. 9

_____ **36.** If the placenta does not deliver within _____ minutes of the baby's birth, transport the mother and baby to a medical facility without delay.
  A. 5
  B. 10
  C. 15
  D. 20

_____ **37.** It is not uncommon for the mother to tear part of the perineum during a delivery. If this occurs
  A. massage the uterus for at least fifteen minutes.
  B. apply a sanitary napkin and gentle pressure.
  C. transport the patient on her left side immediately.
  D. contact medical direction immediately.

_____ **38.** Which of the following is an appropriate action to take for a breech presentation?
  A. Place the mother on her left side.
  B. Provide low-concentration oxygen.
  C. Pull on the baby's legs to deliver.
  D. Initiate rapid transport upon recognition.

_____ **39.** If you see the umbilical cord presenting first,
  A. gently push up on the baby's head or buttocks to take pressure off of the cord.
  B. use two gloved fingers to check the cord for a pulse and keep the cord cool.
  C. raise the mother's head and lower buttocks to lessen pressure on the birth canal.
  D. attempt to push the cord back if it is not wrapped around the baby's neck.

_____ **40.** When a baby's limb presents first, the EMT-B should
  A. push gently on the extremity to prevent it from advancing.
  B. pull gently on the limb to encourage delivery.
  C. administer low-concentration oxygen to the mother.
  D. begin rapid transport of the patient immediately.

_____ **41.** When assisting with the delivery of twins,
  A. the afterbirth will be delivered after each individual infant.
  B. clamp the cord of the first baby before the second baby is born.
  C. labor contractions will stop after the first delivery.
  D. transport the mother immediately.

_____ **42.** Premature infants are at high risk for hypothermia because
  A. they are smaller than most babies.
  B. their brains are less developed than full-term baby.
  C. they lack fat deposits that would normally keep them warm.
  D. their temperature-regulating structures are not fully developed.

_____ **43.** When oxygen is administered to an infant, it should be given by
  A. a nonrebreather mask.
  B. flowing it past the baby's face.
  C. a pediatric nasal cannula.
  D. a demand valve unit.

_____ **44.** If you suspect meconium staining when the infant is born,
  A. contact medical control for advice.
  B. avoid stimulating the infant before suctioning the oropharynx.
  C. suction the nose, then the mouth.
  D. provide oxygen to the mother.

_____ **45.** A condition in which the placenta is formed low in the uterus and close to the cervical opening preventing the normal delivery of the fetus is called
    A. abruptio placentae.   **C.** placenta toxemia.
    B. stillborn birth.   **D.** placenta previa.

_____ **46.** Which of the following is true of seizures in pregnancy?
    A. They are usually associated with low blood pressure.
    B. They tend to occur early in pregnancy.
    C. They pose a threat to the mother but not the unborn baby.
    D. They are usually associated with extreme swelling of the extremities.

_____ **47.** The greatest danger associated with blunt trauma to the pregnant woman's abdomen and pelvis is
    A. cramping abdominal pains.
    B. spontaneous abortion.
    C. massive bleeding and shock.
    D. elevated blood pressure.

_____ **48.** Which of the following is true about the physiology of a pregnant woman?
    A. Vital signs may be interpreted as suggestive of shock when they are actually normal.
    B. The pregnant woman has a pulse rate that is 10-15 beats per minute slower than the nonpregnant female.
    C. A woman in later pregnancy may have a blood volume that is up to 48% lower than her nonpregnant state.
    D. Assessing for shock is easier in the pregnant patient than for a nonpregnant patient.

_____ **49.** Unless a back or neck injury is suspected, all pregnant women who have suffered blunt trauma injury should be transported in the _____ position.
    A. supine   **C.** Trendelenburg
    B. left lateral recumbent   **D.** Fowler's

_____ **50.** Which of the following is true of the treatment necessary for a woman with vaginal bleeding associated with abdominal pain?
    A. Massage the abdomen vigorously.
    B. Assume the woman is pregnant and transport.
    C. Treat as if she has potentially life-threatening injury.
    D. Determine the cause before treatment is begun.

COMPLETE THE FOLLOWING

1. List seven things you should do when evaluating the expectant mother.

_____

_____

_____

_____

_____

_____

_____

2. List eight steps you should take when providing care for the premature infant.

_____

_____

_____

_____

_____

_____

_____

_____

LABEL THE DIAGRAMS

Fill in the name of each structure of pregnancy on the line provided.

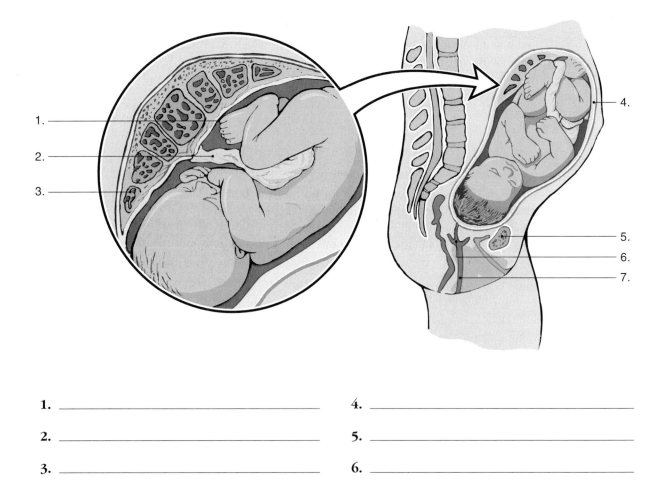

1. _____   4. _____

2. _____   5. _____

3. _____   6. _____

                           7. _____

EMT-BASIC SKILLS PERFORMANCE CHECKLIST

▶ **EVALUATING THE MOTHER FOR IMMINENT DELIVERY**

❑ Take body substance isolation.

❑ Conduct scene size-up.

❑ Conduct initial assessment.

❑ Ask name, age, and expected due date.

❑ Ask which pregnancy this is and the number of children she has given birth to.

❑ Ask how long labor pain has been present and the duration.

❑ Ask if the "bag of waters" has broken.

❑ Time the frequency and length of contractions.

❑ Ask if she is straining or feels the urge to move her bowels.

❑ With mother's permission, examine the mother for crowning.

❑ Feel for uterine contractions when she says she is having a contraction.

❑ Take another set of vitals and make the decision to prepare for a delivery or to begin transport to the hospital.

INTERIM EXAM 2

Use the answer sheet on pages 185–186 to complete this exam. It is perforated so it can be easily removed from this book.

1. During the initial assessment, all of the following are assessed except
   A. airway.
   B. mental status.
   C. circulation.
   D. blood pressure.

2. Which is not a component of the initial assessment?
   A. determining patient priority
   B. evaluating extremity mobility
   C. forming a general impression
   D. assessing breathing

3. When forming your general impression of a child's condition, the environment can provide clues. An example would be a child
   A. complaining of nausea or vomiting.
   B. holding pieces of a toy in his hand.
   C. with a blood pressure of 120/80.
   D. with a rapid heart beat.

4. When forming a general impression, the EMT-B takes into consideration all of the following except
   A. patient's position.
   B. patient's age and sex.
   C. patient's blood pressure.
   D. patient's sounds.

5. After forming a general impression, the next step of the initial assessment is
   A. assessing breathing.
   B. assessing mental status.
   C. determining the priority of the patient.
   D. assessing airway.

6. The "V" in "AVPU" stands for
   A. virtual.
   B. visible.
   C. verbal.
   D. vertex.

7. The "P" in "AVPU" stands for
   A. pulse.
   B. painful.
   C. paralysis.
   D. paraesthesia.

8. The lowest and the most serious mental status is
   A. A.
   B. V.
   C. P.
   D. U.

9. If a patient's level of responsiveness is lower than Alert, you should
   A. apply a cervical collar.
   B. administer high-concentration oxygen.
   C. place him in a recovery position.
   D. bandage all bleeding wounds.

10. If a patient is talking or crying, assume the patient
    A. is in little pain.
    B. has no life-threatening bleeding.
    C. has an open airway.
    D. has an "A" mental status.

11. If the patient is not alert and his breathing rate is slower than 8 breaths per minute, the EMT-B should
    A. insert an oral airway.
    B. place the patient in a prone position.
    C. provide ventilations with a bag-valve mask.
    D. apply the PASG.

12. If the skin is pale and clammy, this indicates
    A. nervous system damage.
    B. poor circulation.
    C. extremely high temperature.
    D. an airway problem.

13. A patient who gives a poor general impression should be considered a _____ priority.
    A. high
    B. low
    C. delayed
    D. stable

14. Which of the following is not an example of a high-priority condition?
    A. difficulty breathing
    B. nausea and vomiting
    C. a severed artery
    D. a mental status of "U"

15. The initial assessment takes different forms, which depend on the age of the patient and whether she
    A. has a medical problem or a trauma problem.
    B. is alert or conscious.
    C. has a history of diabetes.
    D. has a history of head injury.

16. When evaluating the circulation in infants, the EMT-B should use
    A. the femoral pulse.
    B. the distal pulse check.
    C. capillary refill.
    D. the radial pulse.

17. The mental status of an unconscious infant is typically checked by
   A. shouting at the infant while applying cold water.
   B. shouting at the infant and flicking the infant's feet.
   C. performing a pin prick on the bottom of the feet.
   D. applying a sternal rub.

18. Which is <u>not</u> a high-priority condition?
   A. shock
   B. a fever and rash
   C. a complicated childbirth
   D. severe pain anywhere

19. The difference between the general impression steps for a medical patient and those for a trauma patient is
   A. manual stabilization of the head for a trauma patient.
   B. no SAMPLE is taken for a trauma patient.
   C. the medical patient is treated faster.
   D. the AVPU is not used for a medical patient.

20. When the EMT-B documents that the chest pain patient denies shortness of breath, this is most appropriately termed
   A. objective information.
   B. advisory information.
   C. a pertinent negative.
   D. run data information.

21. When writing the narrative section of a prehospital care report, the EMT-B should do all of the following <u>except</u>
   A. use medical terminology correctly.
   B. avoid non-standard abbreviations.
   C. write legibly and use correct spelling.
   D. state one's personal opinion of the patient's condition.

22. Which statement best describes an important concept of documentation?
   A. Always fill out a continuation sheet.
   B. If its not written down, you didn't do it.
   C. It should include plenty of medical terms.
   D. Document everything you see at the scene.

23. If the patient does not wish to go to the hospital, you should
   A. document with a refusal-of-care form.
   B. take the patient to the hospital anyway.
   C. end your assessment immediately.
   D. call for another crew to help subdue the patient.

24. When an important part of the assessment or care was not performed, this is called
   A. malpractice.   C. libel.
   B. omission.   D. commission.

25. When an EMT-B makes up a set of vitals for inclusion on the prehospital care report, this is called
   A. malpractice.   C. falsification.
   B. libel.   D. omission.

26. An objective statement is
   A. one that is made from a particular point of view.
   B. one that is made by the patient or a family member.
   C. one that describes observable or measurable information.
   D. one's own assessment of what is wrong with the patient.

27. When the EMT-B writes "The patient is agitated and hostile towards us" on the prehospital care report, this is an example of
   A. objective information.
   B. a statement beyond his/her training.
   C. subjective information.
   D. non-factual information.

28. When you are documenting exactly what a patient told you on the prehospital care report, you should
   A. paraphrase for brevity.
   B. summarize the key points.
   C. use medical terminology.
   D. use quotes around the statement.

29. Writing a statement such as "The patient's daughter was rude to us" on a prehospital care report is
   A. not relevant.
   B. objective information.
   C. run data information.
   D. an example of what should be included in quotes.

30. The next step in the initial assessment after establishing unresponsiveness is to
   A. ensure an open airway.
   B. check for adequate breathing.
   C. check for circulation.
   D. look for profuse bleeding.

31. The term "sixth sense" is used to describe
   A. an EMT-B's clinical judgment.
   B. the six steps in an initial assessment.
   C. a patient's sensory functions.
   D. the ability to hear.

32. Which of the following is a true vital sign?
   A. nausea
   B. skin temperature

C. level of consciousness
D. age

33. The normal pulse rate for an adult at rest is between _____ beats per minute.
A. 50 and 70   C. 65 and 95
B. 60 and 100   D. 80 and 100

34. During the determination of vital signs, the initial pulse rate for patients 1 year and older is normally taken at the _____ pulse.
A. carotid   C. pedal
B. femoral   D. radial

35. When the pulse force is weak and thin, it is described as
A. shallow.   C. partial.
B. full.   D. thready.

36. Normal at rest respiration rates for adults vary from _____ breaths per minute.
A. 5 to 10   C. 15 to 30
B. 12 to 20   D. 20 to 32

37. A noisy harsh sound heard during inhalation that is an indication the patient needs prompt transport is
A. gurgling.
B. snorting.
C. stertorous respirations.
D. crowing.

38. Systolic blood pressure indicates the arterial pressure created as the
A. artery contracts.   C. heart contracts.
B. artery relaxes.   D. heart relaxes.

39. Diastolic blood pressure indicates the arterial pressure created as the
A. heart contracts.   C. artery contracts.
B. heart refills.   D. artery relaxes.

40. The technique of measuring blood pressure with a sphygmomanometer and a stethoscope is called
A. palpation.   C. oscillation.
B. auscultation.   D. priapism.

41. Determining blood pressure by palpation is
A. not as accurate as the auscultation method.
B. used when there is no noise around a patient.
C. is documented as the "palp/diastolic"
D. used whenever the patient is hypertensive.

42. Information that you can see, hear, feel, and smell are called
A. signs.   C. symptoms.
B. sensations.   D. assessments.

43. When the EMT-B asks the patient "Have you recently had any surgery or injuries?", he/she is inquiring about the
A. patient's medications.
B. patient's pertinent past history.
C. events leading up to the illness.
D. allergies that the patient may have.

44. When the EMT-Basic asks the patient "Are you on birth control pills?", he/she is inquiring about the
A. patient's medications.
B. patient's pertinent past history.
C. events leading up to the illness.
D. allergies that the patient may have.

45. An acronym used to remember what questions to ask about the patient's present problem and past history is
A. AVPU.   C. SAMPLE.
B. CUPS.   D. PEARL.

46. When conducting a patient interview on an adult patient, the EMT-B should do all of the following except
A. position oneself close to the patient.
B. identify oneself and reassure the patient.
C. gently touch the patient's shoulder or rest a hand over the patient's.
D. avoid asking the patient's age.

47. Normal diastolic pressures range from _____ mm Hg.
A. 50 to 80   C. 60 to 80
B. 50 to 90   D. 60 to 90

48. Using the formula presented in the text, a 36-year-old man would have an estimated systolic blood pressure of
A. 116 mm Hg.   C. 136 mm Hg.
B. 126 mm Hg.   D. 146 mm Hg.

49. Using the formula presented in the text, a 26-year-old woman would have an estimated systolic blood pressure of
A. 106 mm Hg   C. 126 mm Hg.
B. 116 mm Hg.   D. 136 mm Hg.

50. Why should the stethoscope not be placed under the cuff and then inflated when evaluating the blood pressure?
A. It may give a false reading.
B. It can dent the stethoscope.
C. The patient will not like the feeling.
D. It will prevent pumping the cuff to the proper pressure.

51. When taking a patient's blood pressure, the stethoscope is placed over the _____ artery.
A. carotid   C. brachial
B. radial   D. femoral

52. The best indication of potential injury is the
    A. type of accident.
    B. type of injury.
    C. mechanism of injury.
    D. position of the patient.

53. When there are no apparent hazards at the scene of a collision, the danger zone should extend _____ feet in all directions from the wreckage.
    A. 25   C. 75
    B. 50   D. 100

54. In the up-and-over injury pattern, the patient is most likely to sustain _____ injuries.
    A. knee   C. head
    B. hip   D. leg

55. A keen awareness that there may be injuries based on the mechanism of injury is called
    A. sixth sense.
    B. general impression.
    C. index of suspicion.
    D. kinesthetic sense.

56. The purpose of the initial assessment is to
    A. take the patient's vital signs.
    B. gather information about the accident.
    C. discover and treat life-threatening conditions.
    D. obtain the patient's history.

57. The first step in the focused history and physical exam for any trauma patient is to
    A. make a status decision.
    B. check for an open airway.
    C. reconsider the mechanism of injury.
    D. treat life-threatening conditions.

58. The "A" in DCAP-BTLS stands for
    A. allergies.   C. abrasions.
    B. alert.   D. arrhythmia.

59. All of the following are clues that help an EMT-B determine the need for cervical immobilization except
    A. mechanism of injury.
    B. level of consciousness.
    C. location of injuries.
    D. breathing rate.

60. Which of the following is true of the rapid trauma assessment?
    A. It begins with examination of the posterior body and ends with examination of the head.
    B. It evaluates areas of the body where the greatest threats to the patient may be.
    C. It is performed on a trauma patient without significant mechanism of injury.
    D. It includes careful examination of the face, eyes, ears, nose, and mouth.

61. On which type of patient is the detailed physical exam most often performed?
    A. trauma patient with a significant mechanism of injury
    B. trauma patient with no significant mechanism of injury
    C. a responsive medical patient
    D. an unresponsive medical patient

62. To obtain a history of a patient's present illness,
    A. ask the OPQRST questions.
    B. conduct the subjective interview.
    C. ask the SAMPLE questions.
    D. use the look, listen, feel, and smell method.

63. The "P" in OPQRST stands for
    A. punctures.   C. provokes.
    B. penetrations.   D. pulses.

64. The steps in the focused history and physical exam of the unresponsive medical patient include the following:
    1. Obtain baseline vital signs.
    2. Gather the history of the present illness from bystanders and family.
    3. Conduct a rapid physical exam.
    4. Gather a SAMPLE history from bystanders and family.

    Which is the correct order in which the above steps should be performed?
    A. 3, 1, 2, 4   C. 3, 2, 4, 1
    B. 2, 3, 4, 1   D. 1, 2, 3, 4

65. For a stable patient, the EMT-B should perform the ongoing assessment every _____ minutes.
    A. 5   C. 15
    B. 10   D. 20

66. During the ongoing assessment, whenever you believe there may have been a change in the patient's condition, you should immediately
    A. repeat the initial assessment.
    B. transport the patient immediately.
    C. document trends in vital signs.
    D. repeat the rapid trauma assessment.

67. Cool, clammy skin most likely indicates
    A. high fever.
    B. exposure to cold.
    C. mild fever.
    D. hypoperfusion (shock).

68. As an EMT-B, your overriding concern at all times is
    A. the patient's safety.
    B. the safety of patients and bystanders.
    C. the patient's life.
    D. your own safety.

69. During the detailed physical exam of the head of a trauma patient, inspect the
   A. ears and nose for blood or clear fluids.
   B. inner surface of the eyelids.
   C. skin color of the cheeks.
   D. mouth for blood and clear fluids.

70. Meningitis and _____ trauma can cause the fontanelle to bulge in an infant.
   A. multiple   C. extremity
   B. head   D. abdominal

71. Infants and young children under the age of _____ are abdominal breathers.
   A. 2   C. 8
   B. 4   D. 16

72. This age group generally feel that they are indestructible but may have fears of permanent injury or disfigurement.
   A. toddlers   C. adolescent
   B. preschool   D. school age

73. Geriatric patients usually have decreased elasticity of the lungs and decreased activity of cilia that results in
   A. increased risk of heart attack.
   B. diminished activity and tolerance of physical stress.
   C. decreased ability to clear foreign substances from the lungs.
   D. decreased energy and tolerance of hot and cold.

74. Loss of skin elasticity and shrinking of sweat glands in a geriatric patient causes
   A. diminished activity and tolerance of physical stress.
   B. decreased ability to clear foreign substances from the lungs.
   C. decreased energy and tolerance of hot and cold.
   D. thin, dry, wrinkled skin.

75. Diminished function of the thyroid gland is one of the effects of aging. This results in
   A. thin, dry, wrinkled skin.
   B. decreased energy and tolerance of heat and cold.
   C. depression and loss of social support.
   D. decreased strength.

76. When an elderly patient falls, this may be an indication of a more serious problem such as
   A. viral pneumonia.
   B. acute alcoholism.
   C. abnormal heart rhythm.
   D. severe depression.

77. Repeaters are
   A. phones that transmit radio signals over air waves instead of wires.
   B. devices used to transmit radio signals over long distances.
   C. patients who consistently call 911.
   D. a type of cellular phone used in EMS.

78. Which of the following is an appropriate interpersonal communication technique?
   A. standing above a patient
   B. avoiding eye contact
   C. directly facing a patient
   D. standing, arms crossed

79. What is the first item given to the hospital in your medical radio report to the receiving facility?
   A. the patient's age and sex
   B. unit identification/level of provider
   C. estimated time of arrival
   D. emergency medical care given

80. Which of the following is not considered an essential component of the verbal report to the receiving facility?
   A. patient's chief complaint
   B. additional treatment given en route
   C. additional vital signs taken en route
   D. patient's mental attitude.

81. Which of the following is true of the medical radio report?
   A. Use codes to communicate patient information.
   B. Ensure that you give the hospital your patient diagnosis.
   C. Paint a picture of the patient's problem in words.
   D. Speak rapidly to limit transmission time.

82. To avoid misunderstanding and miscommunication when speaking with medical direction, you should do all of the following except
   A. Give information clearly and accurately.
   B. Repeat back the order you are given word for word.
   C. Ask the physician to repeat the order if it is unclear.
   D. Avoid questioning the physician about the order.

83. Medications that are carried on the ambulance and that EMT-Bs can administer include activated charcoal, oxygen, and
   A. oral glucose.   C. epinephrine.
   B. nitroglycerin.   D. All of the above.

84. Any action of a drug other than the desired action is called a
   A. contraindication. C. reflex.
   B. indication.   D. side effect.

85. When a drug is administered subcutaneously, this means the drug is
    A. dissolved under the tongue.
    B. injected into a vein.
    C. injected into a muscle.
    D. injected under the skin.

86. Which of the following is true of the structure of infants' and children's airways?
    A. The trachea is more rigid and less flexible than adults'.
    B. Their tongues are proportionately smaller than an adults'.
    C. The cricoid cartilage is more rigid than an adults'.
    D. They depend more on the diaphragm for respiration than adults.

87. The means of providing artificial ventilation are
    1. Pocket face mask with supplemental oxygen.
    2. Two-person bag-valve mask with supplemental oxygen.
    3. Flow-restricted, oxygen-powered ventilator
    4. One-person bag-valve mask with supplemental oxygen

    What is the order of preference?
    A. 1, 2, 3, 4   C. 2, 3, 4, 1
    B. 1, 3, 4, 2   D. 3, 4, 2, 1

88. The adequate rate of artificial ventilations for a non-breathing adult patient is _____ breaths per minute.
    A. 8   C. 16
    B. 12   D. 20

89. The adequate rate of artificial ventilations for a non-breathing infant or child patient is _____ breaths per minute.
    A. 10   C. 20
    B. 15   D. 25

90. Which of the following respiratory sounds made by an unresponsive adult most likely indicates a serious airway problem requiring immediate intervention?
    A. snoring or gurgling
    B. slight wheezing
    C. sniffling
    D. whistling or grunting

91. The skin of a patient with inadequate breathing will most likely be _____ in color and feel _____ .
    A. pale: cool and dry.
    B. red: hot and clammy.
    C. yellow: warm and dry.
    D. blue: cool and clammy.

92. If a patient is experiencing breathing difficulty, but is breathing adequately, it is usually best to place him in the _____ position.
    A. tripod   C. sitting-up
    B. supine   D. recovery

93. Which of the following is a cause of adult chest pain due to a decreased blood supply to the heart muscle?
    A. cerebral vascular accident
    B. arrhythmia
    C. congestive heart failure
    D. angina pectoris

94. Most heart attacks are caused by the narrowing or occlusion of a _____ artery.
    A. cephalic   C. coronary
    B. brachial   D. carotid

95. Which of the following is the condition in which a portion of the myocardium dies because of oxygen starvation?
    A. angina pectoris
    B. mechanical pump failure
    C. cardiogenic shock
    D. acute myocardial infarction

96. An irregular, or absent heart rhythm is called
    A. mechanical pump failure.
    B. arrhythmia.
    C. cardiogenic shock.
    D. congestive heart failure.

97. Which term applies to a pulse slower than 60 beats per minute?
    A. bradycardia
    B. ventricular fibrillation
    C. tachycardia
    D. atrial fibrillation

98. An at-rest heart beat faster than 100 beats per minute is referred to as
    A. bradycardia.
    B. ventricular fibrillation.
    C. tachycardia.
    D. atrial fibrillation.

99. Which of the following is the condition caused by excessive fluid buildup in the lungs and/or other organs and body parts because of the inadequate pumping of the heart?
    A. congestive heart failure
    B. acute heart failure
    C. acute myocardial infarction
    D. chronic myocardial infarction

100. The conscious AMI patient is best transported in the
    A. recovery position.
    B. medical coma position.

C. traumatic coma position.
D. position of comfort.

101. A diabetic found with a weak, rapid pulse and cold, clammy skin who complains of hunger pangs suffers from
A. hypoglycemia.
B. cardiogenic shock.
C. hyperglycemia.
D. ulcers.

102. Which of the following conditions frequently results in an acetone smell on the patient's breath?
A. stroke
B. hyperglycemia
C. ulcers
D. hypoglycemia

103. A conscious hypoglycemic patient who is able to swallow is frequently administered
A. oral glucose.
B. insulin.
C. nitroglycerin.
D. epinephrine.

104. If you cannot administer glucose to the diabetic patient because he is not alert enough to swallow, you should
A. wait until his mental status improves.
B. contact medical direction immediately.
C. treat him like any other patient with altered mental status.
D. place him in a position of comfort.

105. The first time a person is exposed to an allergen, the immune system
A. reacts violently.
B. shuts down.
C. forms antibodies.
D. ignores the allergen.

106. To be considered a severe allergic reaction, a patient must have signs and symptoms of shock and/or
A. a history of allergies.
B. massive swelling.
C. respiratory distress.
D. increased blood pressure.

107. A patient has no history of allergies and is having his first allergic reaction. What action should you take?
A. Consult with medical direction.
B. Treat for shock and transport immediately.
C. Administer epinephrine via auto-injector.
D. Attempt to determine the cause immediately.

108. Carbon monoxide, chlorine, and ammonia are examples of _____ poisons.
A. ingested
B. injected
C. inhaled
D. absorbed

109. It is important for the EMT-B to determine when the ingestion of a poison occurred because
A. different poisons act on the body at different rates.
B. those who ingest poison in the evening tend to vomit frequently.
C. dilution of the poison is never effective after ten minutes.
D. the antidote is more effective once the poison reaches the stomach.

110. The principal prehospital treatment of a patient who has inhaled poisonous gas is
A. administering activated charcoal.
B. administering high concentration oxygen.
C. rapidly administering an antidote.
D. irrigating the respiratory tract with water.

111. Drinking alcohol along with taking other drugs frequently results in
A. uncontrolled shivering.
B. depressed vital signs.
C. extreme agitation.
D. All of the above.

112. Activated charcoal is contraindicated for patients who have ingested
A. alkalis.
B. gasoline.
C. acids.
D. All of the above.

113. Most cases of poisoning
A. are intentional in nature.
B. involve elderly patients.
C. involve young children.
D. lead to disability or death.

114. Poisons that are swallowed are _____ poisons.
A. absorbed
B. inhaled
C. ingested
D. injected

115. Which of the following is a true emergency that requires rapid cooling and immediate transport?
A. heat cramps
B. heat stroke
C. heat exhaustion
D. heat prostration

116. As frostbite progresses and exposure continues, the skin will turn from white and waxy to
A. blotchy and grayish yellow.
B. pale and pinkish red.
C. deep blue at the nose and cheeks.
D. cherry red, except for the extremities.

117. To treat a patient with deep frostbite,
A. immerse the limb in 100–105°F water and transport the patient.
B. rub snow on the frozen area or apply cold packs if available.

C. cover the frostbitten area, handle it as gently as possible, and transport patient.
D. protect the frostbitten area by keeping it cold and transport the patient.

118. With frostbite, the
A. underlying tissues feel frozen to the touch.
B. skin is commonly mottled and grayish blue.
C. skin blisters and swells.
D. affected area feels frozen, but only on the surface.

119. The initial sign of hypothermia is
A. shivering.
B. numbness.
C. drowsiness and slow breathing.
D. white, waxy skin.

120. Extreme hypothermia is characterized by
A. unconsciousness, absence of discernible vital signs.
B. shivering, numbness, drowsiness.
C. flaccid muscles.
D. rapid breathing.

121. The emergency care steps for a hypothermic patient who is alert and responding include all of the following except
A. keep the patient still.
B. keep the patient dry.
C. apply heat to the patient's body.
D. encourage the patient to walk.

122. After calming a snakebite victim and treating for shock, you locate the fang marks. Next, you should
A. immobilize the affected extremity.
B. conserve patient body heat.
C. cleanse the wound site.
D. apply a full tourniquet.

123. A patient who was working in a hot environment complains of severe muscle cramps in the legs and feels faint. You should move the patient to a cool place and begin care by
A. administering oxygen by nonrebreather.
B. transporting the patient immediately.
C. administering oxygen by nasal cannula.
D. giving the patient water.

124. The first step in caring for a rescued near-drowning victim is to
A. expel water from the victim's lungs.
B. provide positive pressure ventilation with oxygen.
C. establish an airway.
D. initiate chest compressions.

125. Your first step when called to care for any attempted suicide victim is to
A. gain access to the patient.
B. wait for police assistance.
C. survey for behavioral changes.
D. ensure your own safety.

126. You are unable to perform normal assessment and care procedures because the patient is aggressive and hostile. What action should you take?
A. Restrain the patient immediately.
B. Ask a family member to assist you.
C. Seek advice from medical direction.
D. Call the patient's physician.

127. When is the EMT-B allowed to use reasonable force?
A. only when the police are on the scene
B. to defend against attack by an emotionally disturbed patient
C. whenever a patient refuses treatment or transport
D. whenever alcohol abuse is suspected or observed

128. The developing unborn baby is called a
A. crowning.   C. placenta previa.
B. fetus.   D. stillborn.

129. The muscular organ in which the fetus develops is the
A. umbilical cord.   C. uterus.
B. placenta.   D. cervix.

130. The organ of pregnancy in which exchange of oxygen, nutrients, and wastes occurs between mother and fetus is the
A. placenta.   C. vagina.
B. cervix.   D. amniotic.

131. While developing, the fetus is protected by a thin, membranous "bag of waters" called the _____ sac.
A. uterine   C. amniotic
B. placental   D. peritoneal

132. When the presenting part of the baby first bulges from the vaginal opening, this is called
A. crowning.   C. labor.
B. dilating.   D. prolapsing.

133. The first stage of labor begins with
A. cervical dilation.
B. perineum.
C. uterine contractions.
D. afterbirth.

134. The second stage of labor ends with
A. cervical dilation.
B. infant delivery.

C. placental delivery.
D. uterine contractions.

135. The third stage of labor ends with
A. full cervical dilation.
B. perineum tearing.
C. delivery of the afterbirth.
D. delivery of infant.

136. If a woman is having her first baby, the first stage of labor will usually last _____ hours.
A. 4   C. 12
B. 8   D. 16

137. During the most active stage of labor, the uterus usually contracts every _____ minutes.
A. 1 to 2   C. 5 to 9
B. 2 to 3   D. 10 to 15

138. If the amniotic sac does not break during delivery, the EMT-B should
A. do nothing; it will break after birth.
B. quickly remove with sterile scissors.
C. puncture it with the finger.
D. transport the patient immediately.

139. To assist the mother in delivering the baby, gently
A. pull at the baby's shoulders.
B. support the baby's head.
C. rotate the baby to the left or right.
D. push your gloved hand into the vagina.

140. After the delivery, which of the following should be done first?
A. Clamp and cut the cord.
B. Suction the baby's mouth and nose.
C. Lay the baby on its back.
D. Lift the baby by the feet and slap its buttocks.

141. Following the delivery, if spontaneous respiration does not begin after suctioning the baby's mouth and nose, the EMT-B should first
A. begin mouth-to-mouth-and-nose resuscitation.
B. apply mechanical resuscitation with 100% oxygen.
C. vigorously rub the baby's back.
D. transport immediately, administering 100% oxygen.

142. The first clamp placed on the umbilical cord should be about _____ inches from the baby.
A. 2   C. 10
B. 5   D. 12

143. If bleeding continues from the umbilical cord after clamping and cutting, the EMT-B should
A. clamp the cord again.
B. unclamp the cord and tie.
C. apply a sterile dressing.
D. transport the baby immediately.

144. Which of the following is the maximum amount of time the EMT-B should wait for the placenta to be delivered before transporting the mother and infant?
A. 20 minutes   C. 1 hour
B. 45 minutes   D. 2 hours

145. Delivery of the placenta is usually accompanied by the loss of no more than _____ of blood.
A. 500 cc   C. 800 cc
B. 600 cc   D. 1000 cc

146. The first step to control vaginal bleeding after birth is to
A. apply a pressure dressing.
B. place a sanitary napkin over the vaginal opening.
C. massage the uterus.
D. pack the vagina with sterile gauze.

147. The presenting part of the baby in a breech birth is the
A. arms.   C. face.
B. buttocks or legs.   D. head.

148. If upon viewing the vaginal area, you see the umbilical cord presenting first, you should
A. gently push the cord back into the vagina.
B. gently push up on the baby's head or buttocks to keep pressure off the cord.
C. gently push on the cervix.
D. clamp and cut the cord.

149. If an arm presentation without a prolapsed cord is noted, the EMT-B should
A. reach up the vagina and turn the baby.
B. do nothing; the delivery will be normal.
C. transport immediately, providing oxygen.
D. insert the gloved hand and push back the vaginal wall.

150. A baby is considered premature if it weighs less than 5 pounds or is born before the _____ week of pregnancy.
A. 35th   C. 37th
B. 36th   D. 38th

Fill in the correct answer for each item. When scoring, note there are 150
questions valued at 0.666 points each.

1. [ ] A	[ ] B	[ ] C	[ ] D		37. [ ] A	[ ] B	[ ] C	[ ] D
2. [ ] A	[ ] B	[ ] C	[ ] D		38. [ ] A	[ ] B	[ ] C	[ ] D
3. [ ] A	[ ] B	[ ] C	[ ] D		39. [ ] A	[ ] B	[ ] C	[ ] D
4. [ ] A	[ ] B	[ ] C	[ ] D		40. [ ] A	[ ] B	[ ] C	[ ] D
5. [ ] A	[ ] B	[ ] C	[ ] D		41. [ ] A	[ ] B	[ ] C	[ ] D
6. [ ] A	[ ] B	[ ] C	[ ] D		42. [ ] A	[ ] B	[ ] C	[ ] D
7. [ ] A	[ ] B	[ ] C	[ ] D		43. [ ] A	[ ] B	[ ] C	[ ] D
8. [ ] A	[ ] B	[ ] C	[ ] D		44. [ ] A	[ ] B	[ ] C	[ ] D
9. [ ] A	[ ] B	[ ] C	[ ] D		45. [ ] A	[ ] B	[ ] C	[ ] D
10. [ ] A	[ ] B	[ ] C	[ ] D		46. [ ] A	[ ] B	[ ] C	[ ] D
11. [ ] A	[ ] B	[ ] C	[ ] D		47. [ ] A	[ ] B	[ ] C	[ ] D
12. [ ] A	[ ] B	[ ] C	[ ] D		48. [ ] A	[ ] B	[ ] C	[ ] D
13. [ ] A	[ ] B	[ ] C	[ ] D		49. [ ] A	[ ] B	[ ] C	[ ] D
14. [ ] A	[ ] B	[ ] C	[ ] D		50. [ ] A	[ ] B	[ ] C	[ ] D
15. [ ] A	[ ] B	[ ] C	[ ] D		51. [ ] A	[ ] B	[ ] C	[ ] D
16. [ ] A	[ ] B	[ ] C	[ ] D		52. [ ] A	[ ] B	[ ] C	[ ] D
17. [ ] A	[ ] B	[ ] C	[ ] D		53. [ ] A	[ ] B	[ ] C	[ ] D
18. [ ] A	[ ] B	[ ] C	[ ] D		54. [ ] A	[ ] B	[ ] C	[ ] D
19. [ ] A	[ ] B	[ ] C	[ ] D		55. [ ] A	[ ] B	[ ] C	[ ] D
20. [ ] A	[ ] B	[ ] C	[ ] D		56. [ ] A	[ ] B	[ ] C	[ ] D
21. [ ] A	[ ] B	[ ] C	[ ] D		57. [ ] A	[ ] B	[ ] C	[ ] D
22. [ ] A	[ ] B	[ ] C	[ ] D		58. [ ] A	[ ] B	[ ] C	[ ] D
23. [ ] A	[ ] B	[ ] C	[ ] D		59. [ ] A	[ ] B	[ ] C	[ ] D
24. [ ] A	[ ] B	[ ] C	[ ] D		60. [ ] A	[ ] B	[ ] C	[ ] D
25. [ ] A	[ ] B	[ ] C	[ ] D		61. [ ] A	[ ] B	[ ] C	[ ] D
26. [ ] A	[ ] B	[ ] C	[ ] D		62. [ ] A	[ ] B	[ ] C	[ ] D
27. [ ] A	[ ] B	[ ] C	[ ] D		63. [ ] A	[ ] B	[ ] C	[ ] D
28. [ ] A	[ ] B	[ ] C	[ ] D		64. [ ] A	[ ] B	[ ] C	[ ] D
29. [ ] A	[ ] B	[ ] C	[ ] D		65. [ ] A	[ ] B	[ ] C	[ ] D
30. [ ] A	[ ] B	[ ] C	[ ] D		66. [ ] A	[ ] B	[ ] C	[ ] D
31. [ ] A	[ ] B	[ ] C	[ ] D		67. [ ] A	[ ] B	[ ] C	[ ] D
32. [ ] A	[ ] B	[ ] C	[ ] D		68. [ ] A	[ ] B	[ ] C	[ ] D
33. [ ] A	[ ] B	[ ] C	[ ] D		69. [ ] A	[ ] B	[ ] C	[ ] D
34. [ ] A	[ ] B	[ ] C	[ ] D		70. [ ] A	[ ] B	[ ] C	[ ] D
35. [ ] A	[ ] B	[ ] C	[ ] D		71. [ ] A	[ ] B	[ ] C	[ ] D
36. [ ] A	[ ] B	[ ] C	[ ] D		72. [ ] A	[ ] B	[ ] C	[ ] D

73. [ ] A [ ] B [ ] C [ ] D	112. [ ] A [ ] B [ ] C [ ] D
74. [ ] A [ ] B [ ] C [ ] D	113. [ ] A [ ] B [ ] C [ ] D
75. [ ] A [ ] B [ ] C [ ] D	114. [ ] A [ ] B [ ] C [ ] D
76. [ ] A [ ] B [ ] C [ ] D	115. [ ] A [ ] B [ ] C [ ] D
77. [ ] A [ ] B [ ] C [ ] D	116. [ ] A [ ] B [ ] C [ ] D
78. [ ] A [ ] B [ ] C [ ] D	117. [ ] A [ ] B [ ] C [ ] D
79. [ ] A [ ] B [ ] C [ ] D	118. [ ] A [ ] B [ ] C [ ] D
80. [ ] A [ ] B [ ] C [ ] D	119. [ ] A [ ] B [ ] C [ ] D
81. [ ] A [ ] B [ ] C [ ] D	120. [ ] A [ ] B [ ] C [ ] D
82. [ ] A [ ] B [ ] C [ ] D	121. [ ] A [ ] B [ ] C [ ] D
83. [ ] A [ ] B [ ] C [ ] D	122. [ ] A [ ] B [ ] C [ ] D
84. [ ] A [ ] B [ ] C [ ] D	123. [ ] A [ ] B [ ] C [ ] D
85. [ ] A [ ] B [ ] C [ ] D	124. [ ] A [ ] B [ ] C [ ] D
86. [ ] A [ ] B [ ] C [ ] D	125. [ ] A [ ] B [ ] C [ ] D
87. [ ] A [ ] B [ ] C [ ] D	126. [ ] A [ ] B [ ] C [ ] D
88. [ ] A [ ] B [ ] C [ ] D	127. [ ] A [ ] B [ ] C [ ] D
89. [ ] A [ ] B [ ] C [ ] D	128. [ ] A [ ] B [ ] C [ ] D
90. [ ] A [ ] B [ ] C [ ] D	129. [ ] A [ ] B [ ] C [ ] D
91. [ ] A [ ] B [ ] C [ ] D	130. [ ] A [ ] B [ ] C [ ] D
92. [ ] A [ ] B [ ] C [ ] D	131. [ ] A [ ] B [ ] C [ ] D
93. [ ] A [ ] B [ ] C [ ] D	132. [ ] A [ ] B [ ] C [ ] D
94. [ ] A [ ] B [ ] C [ ] D	133. [ ] A [ ] B [ ] C [ ] D
95. [ ] A [ ] B [ ] C [ ] D	134. [ ] A [ ] B [ ] C [ ] D
96. [ ] A [ ] B [ ] C [ ] D	135. [ ] A [ ] B [ ] C [ ] D
97. [ ] A [ ] B [ ] C [ ] D	136. [ ] A [ ] B [ ] C [ ] D
98. [ ] A [ ] B [ ] C [ ] D	137. [ ] A [ ] B [ ] C [ ] D
99. [ ] A [ ] B [ ] C [ ] D	138. [ ] A [ ] B [ ] C [ ] D
100. [ ] A [ ] B [ ] C [ ] D	139. [ ] A [ ] B [ ] C [ ] D
101. [ ] A [ ] B [ ] C [ ] D	140. [ ] A [ ] B [ ] C [ ] D
102. [ ] A [ ] B [ ] C [ ] D	141. [ ] A [ ] B [ ] C [ ] D
103. [ ] A [ ] B [ ] C [ ] D	142. [ ] A [ ] B [ ] C [ ] D
104. [ ] A [ ] B [ ] C [ ] D	143. [ ] A [ ] B [ ] C [ ] D
105. [ ] A [ ] B [ ] C [ ] D	144. [ ] A [ ] B [ ] C [ ] D
106. [ ] A [ ] B [ ] C [ ] D	145. [ ] A [ ] B [ ] C [ ] D
107. [ ] A [ ] B [ ] C [ ] D	146. [ ] A [ ] B [ ] C [ ] D
108. [ ] A [ ] B [ ] C [ ] D	147. [ ] A [ ] B [ ] C [ ] D
109. [ ] A [ ] B [ ] C [ ] D	148. [ ] A [ ] B [ ] C [ ] D
110. [ ] A [ ] B [ ] C [ ] D	149. [ ] A [ ] B [ ] C [ ] D
111. [ ] A [ ] B [ ] C [ ] D	150. [ ] A [ ] B [ ] C [ ] D

Bleeding and Shock

MATCH TERMINOLOGY/DEFINITIONS

▶ **PART A**

A. Major artery of the upper arm

B. When the patient is developing shock, but the body is still able to maintain perfusion

C. Microscopic blood vessel in which oxygen/carbon dioxide and nutrient/waste exchange takes place

D. Shock resulting from uncontrolled bleeding

E. Condition that occurs when the body can no longer compensate for low blood volume or lack of perfusion; late signs, such as falling blood pressure, develop.

F. Major artery supplying the thigh

G. Severe bleeding; a major cause of shock

H. Lack of perfusion brought on by inadequate pumping action of the heart

I. Optimum time limit between time of injury and surgery at the hospital; survival rates are best if surgery takes place within this time period.

J. Blood vessel with thick, muscular walls that carries blood away from the heart

_____ **1.** Artery

_____ **2.** Brachial artery

_____ **3.** Capillary

_____ **4.** Cardiogenic shock

_____ **5.** Compensated shock

_____ **6.** Decompensated shock

_____ **7.** Femoral artery

_____ **8.** Golden hour

_____ **9.** Hemorrhage

_____ **10.** Hemorrhagic shock

A. Device that closes off all blood flow to and from an extremity

B. Blood vessel that has one-way valves and carries blood back to the heart

C. Adequate circulation of blood throughout the body, filling the capillaries and supplying the cells and tissues with oxygen and nutrients

D. Site where a large artery lies near the surface of the body and directly over a bone; pressure on such a location can control profuse bleeding in the extremities.

E. When the body has lost the battle to maintain perfusion to the organ systems; cell damage occurs, especially to the liver and kidneys.

F. Another name for hypoperfusion

G. Bulky dressing held in position with a tightly wrapped bandage to apply pressure to help control bleeding

H. Shock resulting from uncontrolled bleeding or plasma loss

I. Shock resulting from uncontrolled dilation of blood vessels due to nerve paralysis (sometimes caused by spinal cord injuries)

J. Inadequate circulation of the blood in which the body's cells and organs do not receive adequate supplies of oxygen and dangerous waste products build up

_____ 1. Hypoperfusion

_____ 2. Hypovolemic shock

_____ 3. Irreversible shock

_____ 4. Neurogenic shock

_____ 5. Perfusion

_____ 6. Pressure dressing

_____ 7. Pressure point

_____ 8. Shock

_____ 9. Tourniquet

_____ 10. Vein

MULTIPLE CHOICE REVIEW

_____ 1. Blood that has been depleted of oxygen and loaded with carbon dioxide empties into the _____ , which carry it back to the heart.
A. arteries
B. veins
C. capillaries
D. tissues

_____ 2. Cells and tissues of the brain, spinal cord, and _____ are the most sensitive to inadequate perfusion.
A. kidneys
B. lungs
C. stomach
D. heart

_____ 3. The use of _____ is essential whenever bleeding is discovered or anticipated.
A. full protective gear
B. BSI precautions
C. universal isolation precautions
D. Tyvek overalls

_____ 4. Bleeding is classified as all of the following except
A. arterial.
B. venous.
C. cellular.
D. capillary.

_____ 5. Which statement about arterial bleeding is correct?
A. Clot formation takes place rapidly.
B. It is often rapid and profuse.
C. It is the least difficult to control.
D. It causes the blood pressure to rise.

_____ 6. A steady flow of dark red or maroon blood is a result of _____ bleeding.
A. arterial
B. venous
C. capillary
D. pulmonary

_____ **7.** Bleeding described as oozing usually is a result of _____ bleeding.
   A. arterial
   B. venous
   C. capillary
   D. bronchiole

_____ **8.** When a large bleeding vein in the neck sucks in debris or an air bubble, this can cause
   A. an evisceration.
   B. heart stoppage.
   C. infection.
   D. severe bleeding.

_____ **9.** Sudden blood loss of _____ in an adult is considered serious.
   A. 250 cc
   B. 500 cc
   C. 600 cc
   D. 1000 cc

_____ **10.** Sudden blood loss of _____ in a child is considered serious.
   A. 200 cc
   B. 300 cc
   C. 400 cc
   D. 500 cc

_____ **11.** Sudden blood loss of _____ in a 1-year-old infant is considered serious.
   A. 25 cc
   B. 50 cc
   C. 100 cc
   D. 150 cc

_____ **12.** The body's natural responses to bleeding is constriction of the injured blood vessel and _____ .
   A. perfusion.
   B. hypoperfusion.
   C. compensation.
   D. clotting.

_____ **13.** The EMT-B's assessment of external bleeding includes all of the following items except
   A. estimating the amount of blood lost in order to predict potential shock.
   B. waiting for signs and symptoms of shock to appear before beginning treatment.
   C. triaging, or prioritizing, bleeding patients properly.
   D. identifying bleeding that must be treated during the initial assessment.

_____ **14.** The major methods used to control external bleeding include all of the following except
   A. direct pressure.
   B. elevation.
   C. pressure points.
   D. vessel clamps.

_____ **15.** Why is administration of supplemental oxygen an important treatment for any trauma patient?
   A. It enhances blood clotting.
   B. It improves oxygenation of the tissues.
   C. It constricts the blood vessels.
   D. All of the above.

_____ **16.** The most common and effective way to control external bleeding is by
   A. cold application.
   B. elevation.
   C. pressure points.
   D. direct pressure.

_____ **17.** The initial dressing should not be removed from a bleeding wound because it
   A. can become a biohazard.
   B. takes too long to remove.
   C. is a necessary part of clot formation.
   D. may increase the chance of infection.

_____ **18.** After controlling bleeding from an extremity using a pressure dressing, be sure to
   A. loosen the tourniquet.
   B. check the distal pulse.
   C. apply PASG (MAST).
   D. administer oxygen by nasal cannula.

_____ **19.** Elevation is used to assist in bleeding control for all of the following reasons except
   A. it slows bleeding.
   B. it raises the limb above the heart.
   C. it helps to reduce blood pressure in the limb.
   D. it speeds up the pulse rate.

_____ **20.** When is it inappropriate to use elevation to assist in bleeding control?
   A. as you apply direct pressure
   B. while trying to bandage an extremity
   C. if you suspect musculoskeletal injuries
   D. when a patient is found lying down

_____ **21.** A pressure point is a site where
   A. a main artery lies near the surface of the body directly over the bone.
   B. the blood pressure can be taken by auscultation.
   C. a large vein lies within the outer layer of the skin.
   D. excessive pressure causes the pulse rate to increase rapidly.

_____ **22.** Use of a pressure point may <u>not</u> be effective if the wound
   A. was caused by an impaled object.
   B. was accompanied by spinal injury.
   C. is at the distal end of a limb.
   D. is bleeding profusely.

_____ **23.** Which of the following is <u>true</u> about the use of an air splint?
   A. It is most effective for controlling venous and capillary bleeding.
   B. It should be used only if there is no suspected bone injury.
   C. It is most effective for controlling arterial bleeding.
   D. It should be used before other manual methods of bleeding control.

_____ **24.** Which of the following is <u>not</u> a helpful guideline when supplementing bleeding control with cold application?
   A. Wrap the ice pack in a cloth or towel.
   B. Do not apply directly onto the skin.
   C. Do not leave the cold pack in place for more than 20 minutes.
   D. Insert the ice directly into the wound.

_____ **25.** Many experts agree that the PASG (MAST) is useful for
   A. controlling bleeding from head trauma.
   B. controlling bleeding from the areas the garment covers.
   C. penetrating chest trauma.
   D. the patient in cardiogenic shock.

_____ **26.** Bleeding from a clean-edged amputation is usually initially cared for with
   A. a pressure dressing.   **C.** a tourniquet.
   B. cold application.   **D.** pneumatic anti-shock garment.

_____ **27.** Rough-edged amputations, usually produced by crushing or tearing injuries,
   A. are easily controlled by a pressure bandage.
   B. tend to stop bleeding on their own.
   C. often will bleed very heavily.
   D. will constrict quickly to control bleeding.

_____ **28.** Once a tourniquet is in place, it must
   A. not be removed or loosened unless ordered by medical direction.
   B. be covered immediately to prevent accidental removal.
   C. be loosened every 15 minutes to dislodge clots.
   D. be used under the pneumatic anti-shock garment.

_____ **29.** A blood pressure cuff
   A. can be used as a tourniquet if inflated to 70 mmHg.
   B. should never be used for bleeding control.
   C. can be used as a temporary tourniquet if inflated to 150 mmHg.
   D. should always be used to control arterial bleeding.

_____ **30.** If a patient has a head injury and you note bleeding or loss of cerebrospinal fluid from the patient's ears or nose, you should
   A. apply direct pressure to the skull.
   B. apply direct pressure to the ears and nose.
   C. apply cold packs to the ears and nose.
   D. allow the drainage to flow freely.

_____ **31.** The medical term for a nosebleed is
   A. hemorrhage.   **C.** epihemorrhage.
   B. epistaxis.   **D.** nostrium.

_____ **32.** To stop a nosebleed, try each of the following except
   A. place the patient in a sitting position, leaning forward.
   B. apply direct pressure by pinching the nostrils.
   C. keep the patient calm.
   D. apply cold packs to the bridge of the nose.

_____ **33.** The leading cause of internal injuries and bleeding is
   A. blunt trauma.   **C.** auto collisions.
   B. penetrating trauma.   **D.** large lacerations.

_____ **34.** Which is not an example of a penetrating trauma?
   A. blast injury   **C.** knife wound
   B. gunshot wound   **D.** ice pick wound

_____ **35.** Signs of internal bleeding include all of the following except
   A. vomiting a coffee ground-like substance.
   B. bradycardia and a flushed face.
   C. dark, tarry stools.
   D. tender, rigid, or distended abdomen.

_____ **36.** A patient who has internal bleeding may have all of the following except
   A. painful, swollen, or deformed extremities.
   B. signs and symptoms of shock.
   C. bright red blood in the stool.
   D. laceration to the forearm.

_____ **37.** Inadequate tissue perfusion is referred to as
   A. hyperperfusion.   **C.** hypoperfusion.
   B. hypoxia.   **D.** hypotension.

_____ **38.** Shock may develop as a result of all of the following except
   A. pump failure.   **C.** dilated blood vessels.
   B. lost blood volume.   **D.** injury to the head.

_____ **39.** The type of shock most commonly seen by EMT-Bs is _____ shock.
   A. cardiogenic   **C.** neurogenic
   B. irreversible   **D.** hypovolemic

_____ **40.** The most common mechanism of shock for a heart attack patient is
   A. vasoconstriction.   **C.** pump failure.
   B. fluid loss.   **D.** vasodilation.

_____ **41.** Shock caused by the failure of the nervous system to control the diameter of blood vessels is called _____ shock.
   A. hypovolemic   **C.** neurogenic
   B. cardiogenic   **D.** reversible

_____ **42.** When a patient is in shock but the body is still able to maintain perfusion to the vital organs, this is called
  A. compensated shock.   **C.** delayed shock.
  B. decompensated shock.   **D.** irreversible shock.

_____ **43.** Early signs of shock that are actually the body's compensating mechanisms include all of the following except
  A. increased heart rate.   **C.** pale, cool skin.
  B. increased respirations.   **D.** decreased capillary refill time.

_____ **44.** When the body has lost the battle to maintain perfusion to the organ systems, this is called
  A. shock.   **C.** decompensated shock.
  B. compensated shock.   **D.** irreversible shock.

_____ **45.** Why does a patient in shock feel nauseated?
  A. Blood is diverted from the digestive system.
  B. Blood rushes rapidly to the digestive system.
  C. Shock increases the production of digestive juices.
  D. The patient has swallowed a great amount of blood.

_____ **46.** The pulse of a patient in shock will
  A. decrease.   **C.** increase.
  B. be absent.   **D.** be irregular.

_____ **47.** A drop in blood pressure is
  A. an early sign of shock.   **C.** always present in shock.
  B. an early sign of shock in a child.   **D.** a late sign of shock.

_____ **48.** Additional signs of shock may include any of the following except
  A. thirst.
  B. dilated pupils.
  C. cyanosis around the lips and nailbeds.
  D. flushed, warm skin.

_____ **49.** The EMT-B should be especially careful when evaluating pediatric patients for shock because they
  A. cannot be administered oxygen at low flow rates.
  B. may display few signs/symptoms until a large percentage of blood volume is lost.
  C. will decompensate for blood loss in a short period of time.
  D. may exhibit erratic capillary refill times.

_____ **50.** Which of the following is the best description of the "platinum ten minutes?"
  A. maximum on-scene time when caring for a trauma or shock patient
  B. optimum time limit from the time of injury until surgery
  C. maximum time limit for controlling arterial bleeding before shock occurs
  D. optimum time limit for applying PASG to the shock patient

COMPLETE THE FOLLOWING

1. List the three major types of shock.

_____

_____

_____

2. List six of the signs and symptoms of shock.

_____

_____

_____

_____

_____

_____

EMT-BASIC SKILL PERFORMANCE CHECKLISTS

▶ BLEEDING CONTROL/SHOCK MANAGEMENT

❑ Take body substance isolation.

❑ Apply direct pressure to the wound.

❑ Elevate the extremity.

❑ Apply a dressing to the wound.

❑ Apply an additional dressing to the wound.

❑ Locate and apply pressure to appropriate arterial pressure point.

❑ Apply high concentration oxygen.

❑ Properly position the patient.

❑ Initiate steps to prevent heat loss from the patient.

❑ Indicate need for immediate transportation.

▶ APPLICATION OF PASG (MAST)

❑ Take body substance isolation.

❑ Assure patient meets local protocol criteria for PASG.

❑ Check for contraindications (e.g., pulmonary edema or penetrating chest injury).

❑ Remove clothing and check for sharp objects.

❑ Quickly assess areas that will be under the PASG.

❑ Position PASG with top of abdominal section at or below the last set of ribs.

❑ Secure PASG around patient.

❑ Attach hoses.

❑ Begin inflation sequence (do not actually inflate on a mock victim in classroom).

❑ Check blood pressure.

❑ Verbalize when to stop inflation sequence (106 mm Hg or pop off valves release).

❑ Operate PASG to maintain air pressure in device.

❑ Reassess patient's vital signs.

CASE STUDY

▶ **CONVENIENCE STORE SHOOTING**

You respond to a local convenience store where there has been an armed robbery. The call was dispatched as a shooting in which the police have secured the scene. A bystander who pulled up at the store just as the shooter was running out the front door states that she found the injured clerk sitting on the floor.

1. What is the importance of a secure scene?

2. As you enter the store, what other size-up procedures are important?

You find the 17-year-old male clerk holding the right upper quadrant of his abdomen with a piece of cloth soaked in blood. He is conscious and alert, knows his name, where he is, and the day of the week. His name is Tom. He complains of pain and says he is very thirsty. You reach down and feel for his radial pulse. You can barely feel it because it is so fast and weak.

3. What important information have you just found out about this patient?

4. What phase and what type of shock is your patient in based upon the information you know?

5. What is the relevance of his being thirsty?

When you check Tom's carotid pulse, it is about 120 per minute and thready. He has no radial pulse. His respirations are 24/shallow and regular. You quickly assess his chest and find no entry into the chest and equal breath sounds on both lungs. You immediately search for other injuries, ask him about other complaints, and find he has none. You do a very quick search from head to toe for additional external hemorrhage and an exit bullet wound. Your partner begins to control the bleeding and administer oxygen to the patient. Together, you and your partner carefully lay him down on a long spine board.

6. Since Tom was shot in the abdomen, what is the importance of listening to his lungs?

7. What device should be used and what liter flow rate should the regulator be set at for this patient?

8. Should an ALS unit be called for if one was not dispatched with you? If so, should you wait on the scene for ALS or arrange an intercept?

The patient is very pale and diaphoretic. He is beginning to get very anxious about dying. You and your partner rapidly move him to the ambulance.

9. On a call like this, what is the maximum time you should spend on the scene? What is this time frame commonly referred to as?

10. To give the surgeons a fighting chance to save Tom's life, what is the maximum time you should spend in assessment and transportation of the patient to the trauma center? What is this time frame commonly referred to as?

The patient is loaded in the ambulance, his level of consciousness is reassessed, and he is responding to painful stimuli only. ALS will intercept you en route.

11. Aside from reassessing the vitals, what airway care should be considered at this time?

12. Would the PASG (MAST) be indicated in this case?

13. Is this patient stable, unstable, or critical?

You meet up with the ALS unit; they jump aboard your ambulance with their portable equipment. The driver quickly continues to the hospital.

14. What procedures would you expect an ALS unit to do en route to the hospital?

15. Briefly write down the radio report that you would give to the hospital en route. The patient initially told you he has no allergies, takes no medications, and has been healthy; his last meal was lunch a few hours ago. The paramedics establish two large bore IVs and prepare to endotracheally intubate the patient. His pulse oximeter reading is 85 and his ECG is sinus tachycardia at a rate of 136.

Radio Report:

CHAPTER 26

Soft Tissue Injuries

MATCH TERMINOLOGY/DEFINITIONS

▶ **PART A**

A. Swelling caused by the collection of blood under the skin or in damaged tissues as a result of an injured or broken blood vessel

B. Outer layer of the skin

C. Any material used to hold a dressing in place

D. Cut that can be smooth or jagged

E. Intestine or other internal organ protruding through a wound in the abdomen

F. Internal injury in which there is no open pathway from the outside to the injured site

G. Burn in which all the layers of the skin are damaged; also called a third degree burn

H. Flap of skin or other tissue torn loose or pulled off completely

I. Any material used to cover a wound in an effort to control bleeding and help prevent additional contamination

J. Injury caused when force is transmitted from the body's exterior to its internal structures

K. Air bubble in the bloodstream

L. Layer of the skin found below the epidermis; it is rich in blood vessels, nerves, and specialized structures such as sweat glands, sebaceous (oil) glands, and hair follicles.

M. Bruise

N. Scrape or scratch in which the outer layer of the skin is damaged but all the layers are not penetrated

O. Surgical removal or traumatic severing of a body part, usually an extremity

_____ **1.** Abrasion

_____ **2.** Air embolus

_____ **3.** Amputation

_____ **4.** Avulsion

_____ **5.** Bandage

_____ **6.** Closed wound

_____ **7.** Contusion

_____ **8.** Crush injury

_____ **9.** Dermis

_____ **10.** Dressing

_____ **11.** Epidermis

_____ **12.** Evisceration

_____ **13.** Full thickness burn

_____ **14.** Hematoma

_____ **15.** Laceration

PART B

A. Large bulky dressing

B. Method for estimating the extent of a burn area in which areas on the body are assigned certain percentages of the body's total surface area.

C. Open chest wound in which air is "drawn" into the chest cavity

D. Burn in which the epidermis is burned through and the dermis is damaged; also called a second degree burn

E. Burn that involves only the epidermis, the outer layer of the skin; also called a first degree burn

F. Injury in which the skin is interrupted, or broken, exposing the tissue underneath

G. Layers of fat and soft tissues below the dermis

H. Any dressing that forms an airtight seal

I. Method for estimating the extent of a burn area; the palm of the patient's hand, which equals about 1% of the body's surface area, is compared with the patient's burn to estimate its size.

J. Open wound caused by a sharp, pointed object that tears through the skin and destroys underlying tissues

_____ 1. Occlusive dressing

_____ 2. Open wound

_____ 3. Partial thickness burn

_____ 4. Puncture wound

_____ 5. Rule of nines

_____ 6. Rule of palm

_____ 7. Subcutaneous layers

_____ 8. Sucking chest wound

_____ 9. Superficial burn

_____ 10. Universal dressing

MULTIPLE CHOICE REVIEW

_____ 1. The soft tissues of the body include all of the following except
   A. skin, fatty tissue, muscles.
   B. blood vessels and fibrous tissues.
   C. teeth, bones, cartilage.
   D. nerves, membranes, glands.

_____ 2. Which of the following is not a function of the skin?
   A. protection
   B. shock absorption
   C. temperature regulation
   D. blood insulation

_____ 3. The layers of the skin include all of the following except
   A. epidermis.
   B. dermis.
   C. subcutaneous.
   D. epithelial.

_____ 4. The layer of the skin called the _____ is composed of dead cells, which are rubbed off or sloughed off and are replaced continuously.
   A. epidermis
   B. dermis
   C. subcutaneous
   D. epithelial

_____ 5. Specialized nerve endings in the skin layer called the _____ are involved with the senses of touch, cold, heat, and pain.
   A. epidermis
   B. dermis
   C. subcutaneous layers
   D. epithelial cells

_____ 6. Shock absorption and insulation are major functions of which layer of the skin?
   A. epidermis
   B. dermis
   C. subcutaneous
   D. epithelial

_____ 7. Wounds that usually result from the impact of a blunt object are called
   A. stabbings.
   B. lacerations.
   C. closed.
   D. perforations.

_____ **8.** A closed wound that involves a large amount of tissue damage and a collection of blood at the injury site is called a

    A. crush injury.   **C.** contusion.

    B. hematoma.   **D.** penetration.

_____ **9.** A soft tissue injury caused by a force that can cause rupture or bleeding of internal organs is called a

    A. contusion.   **C.** crush injury.

    B. hematoma.   **D.** force injury.

_____ **10.** A(n) _____ is an injury in which the skin is interrupted, exposing the tissues underneath.

    A. hematoma   **C.** open wound

    B. closed wound   **D.** crush injury

_____ **11.** A minor ooze of blood from capillary beds is from an injury called a(n)

    A. amputation.   **C.** laceration.

    B. abrasion.   **D.** puncture.

_____ **12.** A wound caused by a sharp-edged object such as a razor blade or broken glass is called a(n)

    A. abrasion.   **C.** laceration.

    B. puncture.   **D.** avulsion.

_____ **13.** When a sharp, pointed object passes through the skin or other tissue, a(n) _____ wound has occurred.

    A. abrasion   **C.** amputation

    B. puncture   **D.** crush injury

_____ **14.** When the tip of the nose is cut or torn off, this is a(n)

    A. avulsion.   **C.** crush injury.

    B. penetration.   **D.** amputation.

_____ **15.** The priority when treating severe open wounds is to

    A. control bleeding.   **C.** prevent contamination.

    B. clean the wound.   **D.** bandage the wound.

_____ **16.** Care for a laceration includes

    A. applying a tourniquet

    B. applying a butterfly bandage; then releasing the patient.

    C. pulling apart the edges to inspect the wound.

    D. checking the pulse distal to the injury.

_____ **17.** Various types of guns fired at close range can cause all of the following except

    A. burns around the entry wound.   **C.** large contusion to the tissue.

    B. injection of air into the tissues.   **D.** damage to underlying tissue

_____ **18.** Care in the field for a patient with an impaled object in the leg involves all of the following except

    A. stabilize the object.   **C.** leave the object in place.

    B. use direct pressure.   **D.** carefully remove the object.

_____ **19.** Which of the following is not true about an injury caused by an impaled object?

    A. The object may be plugging bleeding from a major artery.

    B. Removal may cause further injury to the nerves, muscles, and soft tissue.

    C. Pressure should be applied to the object to stabilize it.

    D. All of the above.

_____ **20.** To control profuse bleeding resulting from an injury caused by an impaled object,
   A. position your gloved hands on either side of the object and exert downward pressure.
   B. use a pressure point distal to the injury to control the bleeding.
   C. let the blood flow freely from the wound left by removal of the object.
   D. stabilize the object with gloved hands and then immediately apply a tourniquet.

_____ **21.** Which of the following is <u>untrue</u> of an impaled object in the cheek?
   A. It should never be removed.
   B. It can create an airway obstruction.
   C. It can cause nausea and vomiting.
   D. It is pulled out in the direction it entered.

_____ **22.** If a patient has an impaled object in the eye, your care should include use of a
   A. pressure bandage placed over the eye.
   B. loose bandage placed over the eye.
   C. combination of 4 x 4s and a paper cup.
   D. combination of 3-inch gauze and a Styrofoam cup.

_____ **23.** When an avulsed flap of tissue has been torn loose but not off, the EMT-Basic should do all of the following <u>except</u>
   A. fold the skin back to its normal position.
   B. control bleeding and dress the wound.
   C. clean the wound surface.
   D. tear off the remainder of the flap and put it on ice.

_____ **24.** Avulsed parts torn from the body should be wrapped and placed in a
   A. cup of dry ice placed in an airtight container.
   B. plastic bag filled with ice.
   C. plastic bag on top of a sealed bag of ice.
   D. saline and ice solution.

_____ **25.** The most effective treatment for an amputation is to
   A. apply a tourniquet.
   B. place the amputated part in ice.
   C. place a snug pressure dressing over the stump.
   D. apply ice over the stump.

_____ **26.** When treating an amputation, whenever possible
   A. place the amputated body part in ice and transport before the patient.
   B. transport the patient and the amputated body part in the same ambulance.
   C. apply a tourniquet after completing a partial amputation.
   D. immerse the amputated part in saline and transport before the patient.

_____ **27.** An air bubble sucked into a large vein in the neck is called a(n)
   A. air embolus.   **C.** occlusion.
   B. blood clot.   **D.** case of the "bends."

_____ **28.** The treatment of neck vein injury is aimed at all of the following <u>except</u>
   A. tamponading the region of injury.   **C.** preventing cardiac arrest.
   B. preventing an embolus.   **D.** stopping bleeding.

_____ **29.** To treat a neck laceration, the EMT-B should use a(n)
   A. pressure bandage.   **C.** ACE bandage.
   B. thin dressing.   **D.** occlusive dressing.

_____ **30.** When applying pressure to a neck wound, be sure you do <u>not</u>
   A. apply pressure over the laceration.
   B. compress both carotids at the same time.
   C. administer oxygen to the patient.
   D. treat the patient for shock.

_____ **31.** The chest can be injured in a number of ways, including
    A. blunt trauma.
    B. penetrating objects.
    C. compression.
    D. All of the above.

_____ **32.** When the driver of a motor vehicle pitches forward after a head-on collision and strikes the chest on the steering column, this is called
    A. closed lung injury.
    B. penetrating trauma.
    C. compression injury.
    D. puncture trauma.

_____ **33.** All open wounds to the chest should be considered
    A. potentially infectious.
    B. life-threatening.
    C. a low priority.
    D. an indication for PASG (MAST).

_____ **34.** An injury which has both an entrance and an exit is called a _____ wound.
    A. puncture
    B. penetrating
    C. perforating puncture
    D. compression injury

_____ **35.** When the delicate pressure balance within the chest cavity is compromised, initially the
    A. diaphragm stops working.
    B. lung on the injured side will collapse.
    C. lung on the uninjured side will collapse.
    D. patient will stop breathing.

_____ **36.** When the chest cavity is open to the atmosphere, this is referred to as a
    A. flail chest.
    B. hemothorax.
    C. sucking chest wound.
    D. a rib fracture.

_____ **37.** The treatment for an open chest wound includes all of the following except
    A. maintaining an open airway.
    B. binding the chest tightly.
    C. administering high concentration oxygen.
    D. sealing the open wound.

_____ **38.** When air becomes trapped in the chest cavity, it can affect the body in all of the following ways except
    A. put pressure on the unaffected lung and heart.
    B. reduce cardiac output.
    C. affect oxygenation of the blood.
    D. increase the ventilatory volume of the chest.

_____ **39.** The signs of pneumothorax or tension pneumothorax include all of the following except
    A. tracheal deviation to the uninjured side.
    B. distended neck veins.
    C. uneven chest wall movement.
    D. increased depth of respiration.

_____ **40.** Which of the following is not a sign of traumatic asphyxia?
    A. distended neck veins
    B. coughed-up frothy blood
    C. head, neck, and shoulders that appear dark blue.
    D. bloodshot and bulging eyes

_____ **41.** When taping an occlusive dressing in place,
    A. have the patient inhale as you tape.
    B. have the patient forcefully exhale as you tape.
    C. tape between breaths.
    D. have the patient hold his breath.

_____ **42.** When an open wound to the abdomen is so large and deep that organs protrude through the opening, this is called an
    A. impaled object.
    B. evisceration.
    C. avulsion.
    D. amputed intestine.

_____ **43.** The signs of an abdominal injury include all of the following <u>except</u>
    A. lacerations and puncture wounds to the lower back.
    B. large bruised area on the abdomen.
    C. indications of developing shock.
    D. contusions over the upper ribs.

_____ **44.** Partially digested blood that is vomited looks like
    A. black and tarry material.   **C.** stained mucus.
    B. coffee grounds.   **D.** meconium staining.

_____ **45.** A rigid or tender abdomen is a sign of
    A. an evisceration.   **C.** gastric distension.
    B. patient guarding.   **D.** over inflation of the BVM.

_____ **46.** Which of the following is <u>not</u> a symptom of an abdominal injury?
    A. cramps.   **C.** headache.
    B. nausea.   **D.** thirst.

_____ **47.** Consider positioning the patient with an abdominal injury
    A. prone, with arms outstretched.   **C.** left lateral recumbent.
    B. supine, with legs flexed at knees.   **D.** supine, with legs straight.

_____ **48.** The treatment of an evisceration should <u>never</u> include
    A. using an occlusive dressing.
    B. cutting away the clothing.
    C. replacing or touching the exposed organ.
    D. applying a sterile, saline-soaked dressing.

_____ **49.** When covering an exposed abdominal organ, you should apply a(n)
    _____ directly over the wound site.
    A. plastic wrap   **C.** saline-moistened dressing
    B. occlusive dressing   **D.** aluminum foil wrap

_____ **50.** Burn injuries often involve structures below the skin, including muscles and
    A. nerves.   **C.** blood vessels.
    B. bones.   **D.** All of the above.

_____ **51.** In addition to the physical damage caused by burns, patients often suffer
    A. heart attacks.
    B. emotional and psychological problems.
    C. diabetic emergencies.
    D. delayed reactions such as cancer.

_____ **52.** When caring for a burn patient,
    A. think beyond the burn to possible medical causes and results.
    B. always begin transport before treatment.
    C. obtain the name of the product that caused the burn.
    D. determine the duration of the exposure.

_____ **53.** When caring for a burn patient,
    A. do not neglect assessment to begin burn care.
    B. transport immediately.
    C. take the patient to the closest hospital.
    D. run cold water on the patient for at least 20 minutes.

_____ **54.** Examples of agents causing burns include all of the following <u>except</u>
    A. AC current.   **C.** dry lime.
    B. hydrochloric acid.   **D.** distilled water.

_____ **55.** A burn that involves only the epidermis is called a _____ burn.
    A. superficial   **C.** full thickness
    B. partial thickness   **D.** epi-thickness

_____ **56.** Which of the following burns will result in deep intense pain, blisters, and mottled skin?
- **A.** superficial
- **B.** partial thickness
- **C.** full thickness
- **D.** medium layer

_____ **57.** To distinguish between a partial thickness burn and a full thickness burn, look for _____ , which indicate a full thickness burn.
- **A.** blisters
- **B.** mottled skin
- **C.** dry and white areas
- **D.** swelling

_____ **58.** Electrical burns are of special concern since they
- **A.** cause respiratory burns if superheated gas is inhaled.
- **B.** pose a great risk of severe internal injuries.
- **C.** may remain on the skin and continue to burn for hours.
- **D.** cause the patient to lose his/her hair over time.

_____ **59.** Chemical burns are of special concern since they
- **A.** cause respiratory burns if superheated gas is inhaled.
- **B.** pose a great risk of internal injury.
- **C.** may remain on the skin and continue to burn for hours.
- **D.** jump from one extremity to the other.

_____ **60.** Burns to the face are of special concern because they
- **A.** continue to burn for hours.
- **B.** can cause heart irregularities.
- **C.** increase the potential for shock.
- **D.** may involve airway injury.

_____ **61.** Burns that can interrupt circulation to distal tissues are called _____ burns.
- **A.** circulation
- **B.** radiation
- **C.** circumferential
- **D.** distal

_____ **62.** You are treating an adult patient who has partial thickness burns to the entire left arm, chest, face, and neck. Using the rule of nines, approximate the size of the burn area.
- **A.** 18 percent
- **B.** 22 percent
- **C.** 27 percent
- **D.** 32 percent

_____ **63.** You are treating an adult patient who has partial thickness burns totally covering the legs, chest, and abdomen. Using the rule of nines, approximate the size of the burn area.
- **A.** 18 percent
- **B.** 36 percent
- **C.** 45 percent
- **D.** 54 percent

_____ **64.** A burn the size of five palms would cover approximately _____ % of the body surface area.
- **A.** 5
- **B.** 10
- **C.** 15
- **D.** 20

_____ **65.** The age of the patient is an important factor in burns. Patients under _____ and over _____ years of age have the most severe body responses to burns.
- **A.** 3 : 50
- **B.** 5 : 55
- **C.** 10 : 65
- **D.** 15 : 70

_____ **66.** A partial thickness burn that involve less than 15% of the body surface is classified as a
- **A.** minor burn.
- **B.** moderate burn.
- **C.** critical burn.
- **D.** unnecessary to treat.

_____ **67.** A partial thickness burn that involves between 15% and 30% of the body surface area is classified as a _____ burn.
- **A.** minor
- **B.** moderate
- **C.** critical
- **D.** life-threatening

_____ **68.** A partial thickness burn that involves more than 30% of the body surface area is classified as a _____ burn.

    A. minor   **C.** critical

    B. moderate   **D.** fatal

_____ **69.** Critical burns include all of the following <u>except</u>

    A. circumferential burns.

    B. moderate burns in a infant or elderly patient.

    C. burns complicated by musculoskeletal injuries.

    D. partial thickness burns on the wrist.

_____ **70.** A partial thickness burn that involves between 10% and 20% of the body surface area of a child under 5 years of age is considered a _____ burn.

    A. minor   **C.** critical

    B. moderate   **D.** fatal

_____ **71.** Which of the following is <u>not</u> considered a critical burn?

    A. entire genitalia area

    B. full thickness burn to the entire chest and abdomen

    C. full thickness burn to the front of the right forearm

    D. partial thickness burn to both the lower extremities

_____ **72.** If a patient has a partial thickness burn to the entire back, the patient should be

    A. wrapped in a dry, sterile burn sheet.

    B. cooled down with ice for 15 minutes.

    C. wrapped in moist sterile dressings.

    D. dried and wrapped in an airtight dressing.

_____ **73.** The primary care for a patient with a chemical burn is to

    A. wrap the patient in a dry sterile burn sheet.

    B. wash away the chemical with flowing water.

    C. dry the patient and wrap in an airtight dressing.

    D. wrap the patient with moist sterile dressings.

_____ **74.** You are treating a patient who was burned. The patient is having visual difficulties, is restless and irritable, has an irregular pulse rate, and muscle tenderness. This patient probably has a _____ burn.

    A. chemical   **C.** electrical

    B. thermal   **D.** radiation

_____ **75.** An occlusive dressing is used to

    A. form an airtight seal.   **C.** control severe bleeding.

    B. stabilize an impaled object.   **D.** secure sprain injuries.

COMPLETE THE FOLLOWING

1. List eight signs of abdominal injury.

2. List the eleven locations of the 9% of the adult body used in the rule of nines.

3. List five signs and symptoms of an electrical injury.

LABEL THE DIAGRAM

Fill in the name of each type of burn and how the skin is damaged.

1.
2.
3.

4.
5.
6.

Epidermis
Dermis
Fat
Muscle

1. Superficial
2. Partial thickness
3. Full thickness
4. Skin reddened
5. Blisters
6. Charring

CHAPTER 27

Musculoskeletal Injuries

MATCH TERMINOLOGY/DEFINITIONS

A. Hard but flexible living structures that provide support for the body and protection for vital organs

B. Disruption or "coming apart" of a joint

C. Extremity injury in which the skin has been broken or torn through from the inside by an injured bone or from the outside by something that has caused a penetrating wound with associated injury to the bone

D. Special splint that applies constant pull along the length of the leg to help stabilize the fractured femur and reduce muscle spasms

E. Sound or feeling caused by broken bone ends rubbing together

F. Bands of connective tissue that bind muscles to bones

G. Any break in a bone

H. Portion of the skeleton that includes the clavicles, scapulae, arms, wrists, hands, pelvis, thighs, legs, ankles, and feet

I. Connective tissue that covers the outside of the bone ends and acts as a surface for articulation allowing for smooth movement at joints

J. Muscle injury caused by over-stretching or over-exertion of the muscle

K. Process of applying tension to straighten and realign a fractured limb before splinting

L. Places where bones articulate, or meet

M. Stretching and tearing of ligaments

N. Injury to an extremity in which the skin is not broken

O. Connective tissue that supports joints by attaching the bone ends and allowing for a stable range of motion

_____ **1.** Bones

_____ **2.** Cartilage

_____ **3.** Closed extremity injury

_____ **4.** Crepitus

_____ **5.** Dislocation

_____ **6.** Extremities

_____ **7.** Fracture

_____ **8.** Joints

_____ **9.** Ligaments

_____ **10.** Manual traction

_____ **11.** Open extremity injury

_____ **12.** Sprain

_____ **13.** Strain

_____ **14.** Tendons

_____ **15.** Traction splint

_____ **1.** As we age, our bones become
  A. deficient in magnesium.   **C.** high in iron.
  B. deficient in calcium.   **D.** high in potassium.

_____ **2.** The strong white fibrous material covering the bones is called the
  A. perineum.   **C.** periosteum.
  B. marrow.   **D.** shell.

_____ **3.** In children, the majority of the long bone growth occurs in the
  A. bone marrow.   **C.** periosteum.
  B. growth plate.   **D.** growth shaft.

_____ **4.** Musculoskeletal injuries are caused by direct, indirect, and _____ forces.
  A. positive   **C.** negative
  B. penetrating   **D.** twisting

_____ **5.** Fractures of the femur typically cause a _____ pint blood loss over the first two hours.
  A. 1   **C.** 3
  B. 2   **D.** 4

_____ **6.** The death rate from closed fracture of the femur dropped from 80% to 20% in the post WWI period due to the invention of the
  A. PASG (MAST).   **C.** traction splint.
  B. IV bag.   **D.** tourniquet.

_____ **7.** The coming apart of a joint is referred to as a
  A. dislocation.   **C.** sprain.
  B. fracture.   **D.** strain.

_____ **8.** The stretching or tearing of ligaments is called a
  A. dislocation.   **C.** sprain.
  B. fracture.   **D.** strain.

_____ **9.** A break in the continuity of the skin of a painful, swollen, deformed extremity is considered a(n) _____ bone or joint injury.
  A. simple   **C.** closed
  B. open   **D.** grating

_____ **10.** Proper splinting of a possible closed fracture is
  A. done with an airsplint and gentle traction.
  B. done with the pneumatic anti-shock garment.
  C. designed to prevent closed injuries from becoming open ones.
  D. completed in the hospital by a surgeon.

_____ **11.** The signs and symptoms of a bone or joint injury include all of the following except
  A. grating.   **C.** vomiting.
  B. swelling.   **D.** bruising.

_____ **12.** When a joint is locked into position, the EMT-B should
  A. splint the joint in the position found.
  B. pull traction and straighten the joint.
  C. use a long backboard as a full body splint.
  D. disregard splinting and transport immediately.

_____ **13.** Which procedure is done at least twice whenever a splint is applied?
  A. elevation of the injured extremity.
  B. manual stabilization of the injured extremity.
  C. assessment for pulses, sensation, and movement distal to the injury.
  D. application of gentle manual traction.

_____ **14.** The treatment of a painful, swollen, deformed extremity includes the steps below.
  1. Take BSI.
  2. Elevate the extremity.
  3. Splint the injury.
  4. Apply a cold pack.

What is the correct order of the steps?
  A. 2, 3, 4, 1   **C.** 3, 2, 4, 1
  B. 1, 3, 2, 4   **D.** 1, 4, 2, 3

_____ **15.** Multiple fractures, especially of the _____ , can cause life-threatening external and internal bleeding.
  A. radius   **C.** femur
  B. ulna   **D.** tibia

_____ **16.** Applying a cold pack to a possible fracture will
  A. help to reduce the swelling.
  B. stop bleeding from the bone.
  C. eliminate the need for a pressure bandage.
  D. stop all the pain and discomfort.

_____ **17.** If the initial assessment of a patient with a musculoskeletal injury reveals the patient is unstable, care should include all of the following except
  A. manage the ABCs.
  B. immobilize on a long spine board.
  C. transport immediately.
  D. splint each injury individually.

_____ **18.** A splint properly applied to a closed bone injury should help prevent all of the following except
  A. damage to muscles, nerves, or blood vessels.
  B. an open bone injury.
  C. motion of bone fragments.
  D. circulation to the extremity.

_____ **19.** Complications of bone injuries include all of the following except
  A. excessive bleeding.   **C.** paralysis of the extremity.
  B. increased pain from movement. **D.** increased distal circulation.

_____ **20.** The objective of realignment is to
  A. minimize blood loss and reduce pain.
  B. immobilize the bone ends and adjacent joints.
  C. assist in restoring circulation and to fit the extremity into a splint.
  D. prevent incorrect healing and avoid surgery.

_____ **21.** If there is a severe deformity of the distal extremity or it is cyanotic or pulseless, the EMT B should
  A. align with gentle traction before splinting.
  B. apply PASG (MAST) to align the extremity.
  C. delay splinting until en route to the hospital.
  D. contact medical direction immediately.

_____ **22.** The types of splints generally carried by EMT-Bs include
  A. rigid, formable, and traction.   **C.** padded, soft, and anatomical.
  B. PASG (MAST), board, and ladder.   **D.** air, cardboard, and vacuum.

_____ **23.** Which of the following is a false statement about rigid splints?
  A. They require the limb be moved into anatomical position.
  B. They tend to provide the greatest support.
  C. They are ideally used to splint long bones.
  D. They can immobilize joint injuries in the position found.

_____ **24.** Traction splints are used specifically for fractures of the _____ .
   A. pelvis   **C.** femur
   B. humerus   **D.** clavicle

_____ **25.** When splinting, the EMT-B should
   A. first move the patient to a stretcher.
   B. leave any open wounds exposed.
   C. replace protruding bones.
   D. immobilize the injury site and the joints above and below.

_____ **26.** To ensure proper immobilization and increase patient comfort
   when using a rigid splint,
   A. place the patient on a stretcher before splinting.
   B. place the patient on a long spine board before splinting.
   C. pad the spaces between the body part and the splint.
   D. ensure that the splint conforms to the body curves.

_____ **27.** The method of splinting is always dictated by
   A. the location of the injury and whether it is open or closed.
   B. the severity of the patient's condition and the priority decision.
   C. the number of available rescuers and the type of splints.
   D. All of the above.

_____ **28.** If the patient with a musculoskeletal injury is unstable, the EMT-B
   should do all of the following <u>except</u>
   A. care for life-threatening problems first.
   B. align the injuries in an anatomical position.
   C. immobilize the entire body to a long spine board.
   D. apply a fixation splint before immobilizing on long spine board.

_____ **29.** Hazards of improper splinting include
   A. aggravation of a bone or joint injury.
   B. reduced distal circulation.
   C. delay in transport of patient with life-threatening injury.
   D. All of the above.

_____ **30.** If the lower leg is cyanotic or lacks a pulse when a knee joint
   injury is assessed, the EMT-B should
   A. splint it in the position it was found.
   B. transport the patient to the hospital immediately.
   C. realign with gentle traction if no resistance is met.
   D. call for assistance from the paramedics.

_____ **31.** Examples of a bipolar traction splint include all of the following
   <u>except</u>
   A. Hare   **C.** Fernotrac
   B. Sagar   **D.** half-ring

_____ **32.** The amount of traction the EMT-Basic should pull when applying
   a Sager traction splint is
   A. enough until the patient verbalizes relief.
   B. about 10% of the patient's body weight up to 15 pounds.
   C. minimal since it doesn't require traction.
   D. about 15% of the patient's body weight up to 30 pounds.

_____ **33.** The indications for a traction splint are a painful, swollen,
   deformed mid-thigh with
   A. either knee or ankle involvement.
   B. no joint or lower leg injury.
   C. extensive blood loss.
   D. an open fracture.

_____ **34.** Whenever possible, _____ rescuers should be used to apply a traction splint.
    A. 2   **C.** 4
    B. 3   **D.** 5

_____ **35.** If the patient has multiple leg fractures and exhibits signs of shock (hypoperfusion), the EMT-B should
    A. apply two traction splints and pull tension to 30 pounds.
    B. align in a normal position and transport on a backboard.
    C. apply PASG (MAST) as a splint and treat for shock.
    D. apply a vacuum splint to each leg and transport quickly.

COMPLETE THE FOLLOWING

1. List eight signs and symptoms of musculoskeletal injury.

2. List eight signs and symptoms of a hip fracture.

LABEL THE DIAGRAM

Fill in the name of each bone on the line provided.

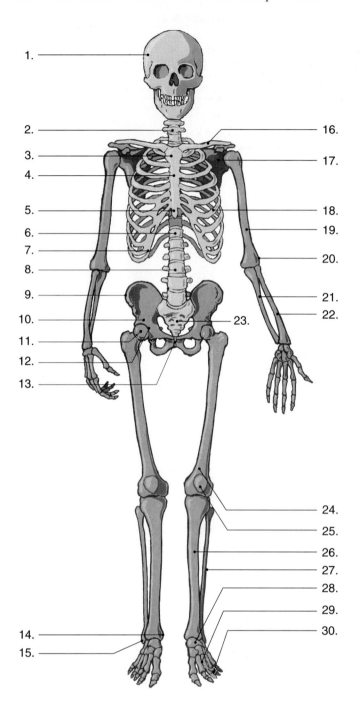

1. _Skull_
2. _Cervical Spine_
3. _Manubrium_
4. _Sternum_
5. _Xiphoid process_
6. _Thoracic Spine_
7. _Costal cartilage_
8. _Lumbar Spine_
9. _Iliac crest_
10. _Pelvis_
11. _Femur head_
12. _Acetabulum_
13. _Pubis_
14. _Medial malleolus_
15. _Lateral malleolus_
16. _Clavicle_
17. _Scapula_
18. _Ribs_
19. _Humerus_
20. _Elbow_
21. _Ulna_
22. _Radius_
23. _Sacral Spine_
24. _Femur_
25. _Patella_
26. _Tibia_
27. _Fibula_
28. _Tarsals_
29. _Metatarsals_
30. _Phalanges_

▶ **REALIGNING AN EXTREMITY**

❑ Take body substance isolation.

❑ Assess distal pulse, motor function, and sensation.

❑ One EMT-B grasps the distal extremity while a partner places one hand above and below the injury site.

❑ The partner supports the injury site while the first EMT-B pulls gentle manual traction in the direction of the long axis of the body. If resistance is felt or if it appears that bone ends will come through the skin, stop realignment and splint the extremity in the position found.

❑ If no resistance is felt, maintain gentle traction until the extremity is properly splinted.

❑ Reassess the distal pulse, motor function, and sensation.

▶ **IMMOBILIZATION: LONG BONE**

❑ Take body substance isolation.

❑ Direct application of manual stabilization.

❑ Assess distal pulse, motor function, and sensation.

❑ Measure splint.

❑ Apply splint.

❑ Immobilize joints above and below the injury site.

❑ Secure the entire injured extremity in a distal to proximal direction.

❑ Immobilize hand/foot in the position of function.

❑ Reassess distal pulse, motor function, and sensation.

▶ **IMMOBILIZATION: JOINT INJURY**

❑ Take body substance isolation.

❑ Direct application of manual stabilization of the injury.

❑ Assess distal pulse, motor function, and sensation.

❑ Select proper splinting material

❑ Immobilize the site of the injury and bones above and below.

❑ Reassess distal pulse, motor function, and sensation.

▶ IMMOBILIZATION: TRACTION SPLINTING

❑ Take body substance isolation.

❑ Direct manual stabilization of the injured leg.

❑ Assess distal pulse, motor function, and sensation.

❑ Direct application of manual traction.

❑ Adjust and position splint at the injured leg.

❑ Apply proximal securing device (e.g., ischial strap).

❑ Apply distal securing device (e.g., ankle hitch).

❑ Apply mechanical traction.

❑ Position and secure support straps.

❑ Re-evaluate the proximal/distal circulation.

❑ Reassess distal pulse, motor function, and sensation.

❑ Secure patient's torso and traction splint to long backboard for transport.

CHAPTER

Injuries to the Head and Spine

MATCH TERMINOLOGY/DEFINITIONS

A. Pairs of nerves that enter and exit the spinal cord between the vertebrae and the twelve pairs of cranial nerves that travel between the brain and organs without passing through the spinal cord, and all of the body's other motor and sensory nerves

B. Mild closed head injury without detectable damage to the brain

C. Body system that is divided into two sub-systems and that provides overall control of thought, sensation, and the voluntary and involuntary motor functions of the body

D. Cheek bone; also called the zygomatic bone

E. Bony bump on a vertebra that you can feel on a person's back

F. Bones of the spinal column

G. Movable joint formed between the mandible and the temporal bones; also called the TM joint

H. Bony structure making up the forehead, top, back, and upper sides of the skull

I. Fluid that surrounds the brain and spinal cord

J. Bruised brain caused when the force of a blow to the head is great enough to rupture blood vessels

K. Brain and the spinal cord

L. Bones that form part of the sides of the skull and floor of the cranial cavity

M. Bones that form the upper third, or bridge, of the nose

N. Bony structures, or sockets, around the eyes

O. Nervous system that consists of nerves that control involuntary functions such as the heartbeat and breathing

_____ **1.** Autonomic nervous system

_____ **2.** Central nervous system

_____ **3.** Cerebrospinal fluid (CSF)

_____ **4.** Concussion

_____ **5.** Contusion

_____ **6.** Cranium

_____ **7.** Malar

_____ **8.** Nasal bones

_____ **9.** Nervous system

_____ **10.** Orbits

_____ **11.** Peripheral nervous system

_____ **12.** Spinous process

_____ **13.** Temporal bones

_____ **14.** Temporomandibular joint

_____ **15.** Vertebrae

_____ **1.** The function of the spinal column is to
   A. produce cerebrospinal fluid.
   B. protect the spinal cord.
   C. allow for back movement in all directions.
   D. manufacture platelets.

_____ **2.** The spine is made up of _____ vertebrae.
   A. 35   **C.** 33
   B. 23   **D.** 38

_____ **3.** When a patient has a scalp injury,
   A. expect minimal bleeding.   **C.** expect profuse bleeding.
   B. determine the wound depth.   **D.** palpate the site with fingertips.

_____ **4.** A bruise behind the ear is called
   A. Cushing's syndrome.   **C.** Battle's sign.
   B. raccoon's eyes.   **D.** posturing syndrome.

_____ **5.** Discoloration of the soft tissues under both eyes is called
   A. Cushing syndrome.   **C.** Battle's sign.
   B. raccoon's eyes.   **D.** posturing syndrome.

_____ **6.** The signs and symptoms of a skull or brain injury include
   A. blood or fluid flowing from the ears and/or nose.
   B. yellow discoloration in the eyes.
   C. bruising around the base of the nose.
   D. pain at the base of the neck.

_____ **7.** Skull or brain injury may result in
   A. airway swelling and dizziness.
   B. altered mental status and unequal pupils.
   C. difficulty moving below the waist.
   D. headache and hypoperfusion.

_____ **8.** Which of the following is a late sign of brain or skull injury?
   A. temperature increase   **C.** irregular breathing patterns
   B. raccoon's eyes   **D.** Battle's sign

_____ **9.** Which of the following is generally <u>not</u> a sign of head injury except in infants?
   A. bleeding from the nose and ears   **C.** hypoperfusion
   B. unequal pupils   **D.** seizures

_____ **10.** What is the significance of an increase in carbon dioxide in the injured brain?
   A. It decreases the blood pressure.   **C.** It raises the heart rate.
   B. It causes brain tissue swelling.   **D.** It causes brain tissue shrinking.

_____ **11.** A patient with a GCS of less than _____ in most EMS systems is taken to a
   trauma center.
   A. 8   **C.** 12
   B. 10   **D.** 15

_____ **12.** If an object has penetrated a patient's skull, the EMT-B should
   A. shorten lengthy objects using any available tools.
   B. elevate the patient's legs immediately.
   C. remove it and quickly control the bleeding.
   D. stabilize the object with bulky dressings.

_____ **13.** The primary concern for emergency care of facial fractures or jaw injuries is
   A. the external bleeding.   **C.** the loss of teeth.
   B. the patient's airway.   **D.** a basilar skull fracture.

_____ 14. The vertebrae which are most frequently injured are the
A. lumbar and sacral.   C. coccygeal and thoracic.
B. thoracic and cervical.   D. cervical and lumbar.

_____ 15. When the spine is excessively pulled, which commonly occurs during a hanging, this is called a(n) _____ injury.
A. excessive rotation   C. distraction
B. lateral bending   D. compression

_____ 16. On your size-up of an automobile collision, you notice that both sides of the windshield have a spider-web crack. It is wise to call for a back up ambulance because
A. every collision should have a two ambulance response.
B. patients hitting their heads on the windshield will be critical.
C. both the driver and the passenger require spinal injury treatment.
D. It takes four EMS personnel to properly immobilize one patient.

_____ 17. Which of the following would <u>not</u> create a high index of suspicion of a spine injury?
A. motor vehicle or motorcycle accidents
B. falls that cause open fractures to the ankles
C. trauma patients who are found unconscious
D. a fall from two times the patient's height.

_____ 18. All of the following are examples of cervical spine injuries that can result from a diving accident <u>except</u>
A. excessive extension.   C. excessive flexion.
B. compression.   D. lateral bending.

_____ 19. The unconscious trauma patient should be
A. treated as if he has a potential spine injury.
B. rolled immediately to check for back injuries.
C. placed in the recovery position.
D. placed in a prone position for fluid to drain.

_____ 20. The most reliable sign of spinal cord injury in the conscious patient is
A. pain with movement   C. tenderness on the spine
B. impaired breathing   D. paralysis of the extremities

_____ 21. A lack of spinal pain does not rule out the possibility of spinal cord injury because
A. spinal injuries seldom cause pain.
B. other painful injuries may mask it.
C. spinal injuries are not painful until shock sets in.
D. a patient may feel the pain but cannot verbalize it.

_____ 22. When assessing a suspected spine-injured patient you note a reversal of the normal breathing pattern. This is likely a result of damage to the nerves that control the
A. rib cage.   C. abdomen.
B. diaphragm.   D. lungs.

_____ 23. If a patient is found on her back with arms extended above the head, this may indicate a _____ spine injury.
A. thoracic   C. sacral
B. lumbar   D. cervical

_____ 24. If a patient is up and walking around at the scene of a high-speed collision, the EMT-B should
A. assess for a potential spinal injury.
B. check with medical direction for orders.
C. check with bystanders about the patient's mental status.
D. assume that the patient is uninjured.

_____ **25.** If a responsive patient has the mechanism of injury for a spinal injury, the EMT-B should do all of the following <u>except</u>
    A. assess for spinal pain by asking the patient to move.
    B. keep the patient still while asking him questions.
    C. assess for equality of strength in the extremities.
    D. assess for tingling in the extremities.

_____ **26.** After performing the initial assessment and rapid trauma exam on a spine-injured patient, your next step is to
    A. determine the patient's priority.
    B. administer high-concentration oxygen.
    C. immobilize the patient on a long spine board.
    D. determine the mechanism of injury.

_____ **27.** If a suspected spine-injured patient complains of pain when you attempt to place the head in a neutral in-line position.
    A. pad the neck before immobilizing.
    B. steady the head in the position found.
    C. continue with the stabilization procedure.
    D. contact medical direction immediately.

_____ **28.** When treating a patient with a spine injury, one EMT-B should
    A. strap the patient's head, then the torso, to the long spine board.
    B. maintain constant manual in-line immobilization until the patient is secured to a backboard.
    C. assess for range of cervical spine motion.
    D. pad the neck before stabilizing.

_____ **29.** Which of the following statements about the rigid cervical collar is <u>false</u>?
    A. A wrong-sized collar can hyperextend the neck.
    B. Maintain manual stabilization when applying.
    C. It completely eliminates neck movement.
    D. The collar should never obstruct the airway.

_____ **30.** If a stable patient is found in a sitting position on the ground and is complaining about back pain, the EMT-B should
    A. apply a cervical collar and rapidly transport the patient.
    B. ask the patient to lie down, then immobilize.
    C. immobilize with a short spine board or extrication vest.
    D. perform a rapid take-down procedure with a long spine board.

_____ **31.** The rapid extrication procedure is used in all of the following situations <u>except</u>
    A. to rapidly move a patient from an unsafe scene.
    B. when a stable, low-priority patient must be immobilized.
    C. when more seriously injured patients must be accessed.
    D. to move a high priority patient.

_____ **32.** When immobilizing a 6-year-old-or-younger child on a long backboard,
    A. provide padding beneath the shoulder blades.
    B. it is unnecessary to apply a cervical collar.
    C. place a chin cup or chin strap on the patient.
    D. secure the head first, then secure the torso.

_____ **33.** All of the following are <u>appropriate</u> guidelines for helmet removal <u>except</u>
    A. Remove it if it interferes with breathing management.
    B. Remove it if it is a snug fit that allows no head movement.
    C. Remove it using a two-rescuer procedure.
    D. Remove it if it hinders immobilization.

_____ **34.** Which is the correct order of steps for applying a short spine immobilization device?
    1) Secure the device to patient's torso.
    2) Secure the patient's head to the device.
    3) Position device behind the patient.
    4) Evaluate torso fixation and pad behind neck as necessary.
    A. 3, 2, 1, 4   **C.** 4, 3, 1, 2
    B. 3, 1, 4, 2   **D.** 3, 4, 1, 2

_____ **35.** Prior to and after immobilization, the EMT-B should assess
    A. pulses in all extremities.   **C.** sensory function in all extremities.
    B. motor function in all extremities.   **D.** All of the above.

COMPLETE THE FOLLOWING

1. List six signs of a skull fracture and brain injury.

_____

_____

_____

_____

_____

_____

2. List three types of brain injuries.

_____

_____

_____

LABEL THE DIAGRAM

Fill in the name of each division of the spine on the line provided.

1. _____

2. _____

3. _____

4. _____

5. _____

▶ **SPINAL IMMOBILIZATION: SUPINE PATIENT**

❏ Take body substance isolation.

❏ Direct assistant to place/maintain head in neutral, in-line position and maintain manual immobilization of the head.

❏ Assess distal pulse, motor function, and sensation.

❏ Apply appropriate size extrication collar.

❏ Position the immobilization device appropriately.

❏ Move patient onto device without compromising the integrity of the spine. Apply padding to voids between torso and board as necessary.

❏ Immobilize patient's torso to the device.

❏ Evaluate and pad behind the patient's head as necessary.

❏ Pad and immobilize patient's head.

❏ Secure patient's legs to board.

❏ Secure patient's arms to board.

❏ Reassesses distal pulse, motor function, and sensation.

▶ **SPINAL IMMOBILIZATION: SEATED PATIENT**

❏ Take body substance isolation.

❏ Direct assistant to manually immobilize head in neutral, in-line position.

❏ Assess distal pulse, motor function, and sensation.

❏ Apply appropriate size extrication collar.

❏ Position immobilization device behind the patient.

❏ Secure device to the patient's torso.

❏ Evaluate and pad behind the patient's head as necessary.

❏ Secure patient's head to the device.

❏ Evaluate and adjust straps.

❏ Secure patient's wrists and legs and transfer to a long spine board.

❏ Reassess distal pulse, motor function, and sensation.

▶ RAPID TAKEDOWN TECHNIQUE: STANDING PATIENT

❑ Take body substance precautions.

❑ EMT-Basic A should be positioned behind the patient and hold manual in-line stabilization of the head and neck. Make sure the EMT-Basic in front of the patient explains the procedure to the patient so he/she does not move.

❑ EMT-Basic A behind the patient should not let go of the patient's head throughout the procedure.

❑ EMT-Basic B in front of the patient should quickly assess the sensory and motor function in all four extremities.

❑ EMT-Basic B applies a properly sized collar.

❑ EMT-Basic B positions long spine board behind the patient, being careful not to disturb the immobilization in any way.

❑ Two EMT-Basics, standing in front of the patient to each side, reach under the patient's armpit and grasp the spine board handholds at the level of the arm pit or higher. They both must hold the same level handhold.

❑ The same two EMT-Basics place their other hand on the patient's upper arm securing the patient to the spine board by holding their arm on the spine board.

❑ Slowly lower the patient back, communicating with the EMT-Basic behind the board so it is clear when the scapulae are beginning to rest on the spine board. Remember to lift with your legs, bending at the knees and not bending at the waist.

❑ EMT-Basic holding the head gently allows the head to come back to the spine board as the shoulders come back.

❑ Once the head is on the board, it never is lifted off the board again as the EMT-Basic kneels down at the patient's head.

❑ Reassess distal pulse, motor function, and sensation.

▶ RAPID EXTRICATION PROCEDURE

Assessment

❑ Take body substance isolation.

❑ EMT-Basic B: Manually stabilize the patient's head/neck.

❑ EMT-Basic A: Conduct initial assessment of patient and determine the need for rapid extrication based on patient status.

❑ EMT-Basic A: Assess distal pulse, motor function, and sensation in all four extremities.

Step One

❑ EMT-Basic B: Continue manual stabilization.

Step Two

❑ EMT-Basic A: Apply rigid collar.

Step Three

❑ EMT-Basic A: Hold patient's armpit and join hands with EMT-Basic C under the patient's thighs.

❑ EMT-Basic C: Hold patient by armpit and join hands with EMT-Basic A under patient's thighs.

Step Four

❑ EMT-Basic B: Call for a lift. Keep patient's head/neck stable in neutral position.

❑ EMT-Basic A: Lift patient approximately 2 inches off seat with EMT-Basic C.

❑ EMT-Basic C: Lift patient approximately 2 inches off seat with EMT-Basic A.

❑ Bystander (or 4th EMT-B) insert long spine board under patient on seat.

Step Five

❑ EMT Basic A: Reach across patient's chest and supports by both armpits.

❑ EMT-Basic B: While maintaining head/neck stabilization, call for a 1/4 turn so patient is moved perpendicular to the steering wheel ready to exit the car head first.

❑ EMT-Basic C: Free the patient's lower legs from any obstructions.

❑ EMT-Basic A: Begin to turn patient's back toward the door until EMT-Basic B says stop.

❑ EMT-Basic B: Turn patient. Call for stop turn just before being unable to hold patient's head anymore. This will be about a 1/4 turn.

❑ EMT-Basic C: Begin to turn patient's back toward door, freeing legs then sliding up to the thighs until EMT-Basic B says stop.

Step Six

❑ EMT-Basic A: Stop move and wait for EMT-Basic C. Then take over manual stabilization of the head/neck for EMT-Basic B.

❑ EMT-Basic B: Maintain head/neck stabilization until EMT-Basic A takes over allowing him/her to either exit car and work from outside or reach over the seat from inside if there is room or the roof has been removed.

❑ EMT-Basic C: Move hands from thighs to patient's armpits, then replace EMT-Basic A.

Step Seven

❑ Complete the patient turn another 1/4 turn.

Step Eight
❑ EMT-Basic A: Lower patient onto long backboard.

❑ EMT-Basic B: Call for move to lower patient's torso into a supine position on the spine board.

❑ EMT-Basic C: Lower patient onto long spine board.

❑ Bystander (or 4th EMT-B) stabilize the spine board.

Step Nine
❑ EMT-Basic A: Slide patient as a unit.

❑ EMT-Basic B: Call for move to slide patient toward head end of the spine board. Once in position tell partners to stop. Slide the chest as a unit.

❑ EMT Basic C: Slide pelvis as a unit until EMT-Basic B says to stop.

❑ Bystander (or 4th EMT-Basic) stabilize the head end of the long spine board.

Step Ten
❑ Crew carefully straps patient's torso and head, and then moves to the stretcher.

❑ Reassess distal pulse, motor function, and sensation.

▶ PEDIATRIC CHILD SAFETY SEAT IMMOBILIZATION

Assessment
❑ EMT-Basic A positions behind patient and holds manual in-line stabilization of the head/neck. This remains his/her job throughout the procedure.

❑ Based on the initial assessment and the patient's status, determine if the infant/toddler should be immobilized in the child safety seat or rapidly extricated from the seat.

❑ EMT-Basic B assesses distal pulses, motor function, and sensation in all four extremities before and after the immobilization.

▶ IMMOBILIZING IN A CHILD SAFETY SEAT

Step One
❑ EMT-Basic A: Stabilize child safety seat in an upright position. Continue manual head/neck stabilization.

❑ EMT-Basic B: Prepare equipment. Apply cervical collar or improvise with rolled hand towel for the newborn/infant.

Step Two
❑ EMT-Basic A: Maintain manual head/neck stabilization.

❑ EMT-Basic B: Place a small blanket or bath towel on the child's lap. Either strap or use wide tape to secure the pelvis and chest area to the seat.

Step Three
❑ EMT-Basic A: Maintain manual head/neck stabilization until the patient is completely taped and strapped securely in place. Carry child and seat to ambulance and strap onto the stretcher with the stretcher head raised.

❑ EMT-Basic B: Place a towel roll on both sides of the head to fill the voids. Tape the forehead in place. Then place tape across collar or maxilla. Avoid taping chin which would place pressure on the child's neck.

Assessment
❑ Have an EMT-Basic reassess distal pulse, motor function, and sensation.

▶ RAPID EXTRICATION FROM A CHILD SAFETY SEAT

Step One
❏ EMT-Basic A: Stabilize the child safety seat in upright position. Apply manual head/neck stabilization.

❏ EMT-Basic B: Prepare the equipment. Loosen or cut the seat straps and raise the front guard.

Step Two
❏ Apply the rigid collar or improvise with a rolled hand towel in the newborn/infant.

Step Three
❏ EMT-Basic A: Maintain manual head/neck stabilization.

❏ EMT-Basic B: Place the child safety seat on the center of the long spine board and slowly tilt it back into a supine position being careful not to allow the child to slide out of the chair. If the child has a large head, it is helpful to place a towel under the area where his/her shoulders will end up on the board.

Step Four
❏ EMT-Basic A: Maintain manual head/neck stabilization and call for a coordinated long axis move onto the board.

❏ EMT-Basic B: Grasp the chest and axilla with each hand and do a coordinated long axis move onto the board. Make sure the child is positioned at the end of the board and not in the middle.

Step Five
❏ EMT-Basic A: Maintain manual head/neck stabilization.

❏ EMT-Basic B: Place a rolled blanket on each side of the patient.

Step Six
❏ EMT-Basic B: Strap the pelvis and upper chest to the board. Do not strap abdomen down. Tape the lower legs to the board with wide tape.

Step Seven
❏ EMT-Basic A: Maintain manual head/neck stabilization until the patient is completely taped and strapped securely in place.

❏ EMT-Basic B: Place a towel roll on both sides of the head to fill the voids. Tape the forehead in place. Then place tape across the collar or the maxilla. Do not tape across the chin to avoid pressure on the child's neck.

Assessment
❏ Have an EMT-Basic do a reassessment of distal pulse, motor function, and sensation.

Infants and Children

MATCH TERMINOLOGY/DEFINITIONS

A. Child from 12 to 18 years of age

B. "Soft spot" at the front of an infant's skull where bones have not yet fused together

C. Flowing oxygen over the face of a small child so it will be inhaled

D. Child from 6 to 12 years of age

E. Child from 1 to 3 years of age

F. Feeding tube placed through the abdominal wall directly into the stomach

G. Child between birth and 1 year of age

H. Child from 3 to 6 years of age

I. Bacterial infection that produces swelling of the epiglottis and partial airway obstruction

J. Sudden unexplained death during sleep of an apparently healthy baby in its first year of life

K. Complication of a rapidly rising temperature

L. Group of viral illnesses that cause inflammation of the larynx, trachea, and bronchi

M. Tube placed through the neck into the trachea to create an open airway

N. Intravenous line that is placed close to the heart

O. Drainage device that runs from the brain to the abdomen to relieve excess cerebrospinal fluid

_____ **1.** Adolescent

_____ **2.** Blow-by oxygen

_____ **3.** Central line

_____ **4.** Croup

_____ **5.** Epiglottitis

_____ **6.** Febrile seizure

_____ **7.** Fontanelle

_____ **8.** Gastrostomy tube

_____ **9.** Newborn or infant

_____ **10.** Preschooler

_____ **11.** School-aged child

_____ **12.** Shunt

_____ **13.** SIDS

_____ **14.** Toddler

_____ **15.** Tracheostomy tube

MULTIPLE CHOICE REVIEW

_____ 1. When a child is considered a toddler, his/her age group is between
_____ years.
A. birth and 1
B. 1 and 3
C. 3 and 6
D. 6 and 12

_____ 2. When a child is considered school age, his/her age group is between
_____ years.
A. 1 and 3
B. 3 and 6
C. 6 and 12
D. 12 and 18

_____ 3. Which of the following is not appropriate when assessing the toddler?
A. Have the child sit on the parent's lap.
B. Avoid lying to the patient.
C. Explain what you are doing.
D. Perform the head exam first.

_____ 4. Until about age 4, a child's head is proportionately _____ than the adult's.
A. smaller and lighter
B. smaller and heavier
C. larger and heavier
D. larger and lighter

_____ 5. The soft spot on an infant's skull is called a _____ .
A. croup.
B. fontanelle.
C. depression.
D. shunt.

_____ 6. A sunken fontanelle may indicate
A. dehydration.
B. rising intracranial pressure.
C. external hemorrhage.
D. hypertension.

_____ 7. A bulging fontanelle may indicate
A. dehydration.
B. elevated intracranial pressure.
C. external hemorrhage.
D. hypertension.

_____ 8. Newborns usually breathe
A. over sixty times a minute.
B. less than eight times a minute.
C. through their mouths.
D. through their noses.

_____ 9. In an infant, hyperextension of the neck
A. is necessary to open the airway.
B. may result in airway obstruction.
C. is necessary if trauma is suspected.
D. is a procedure reserved for respiratory distress.

_____ 10. If the EMT-B suctions a child's airway for longer than a few seconds at a
time, this could lead to
A. gag reflex activation.
B. vagus nerve stimulation.
C. airway blockage.
D. cardiac arrest.

_____ 11. The tongues of infants and children are more likely than an adult's to fall
back into and block the airway because their tongues are
A. proportionately larger than the adult's.
B. larger than an adult's.
C. proportionately smaller than an adult's.
D. smaller than an adult's.

_____ 12. The insertion procedure for an oropharyngeal airway in an infant or child
is performed
A. much more quickly than in an adult.
B. with the tip pointing toward the tongue and throat.
C. the same way it is done for adults.
D. without inserting a tongue depressor.

_____ 13. When assessing the capillary refill of a child 5 years old or younger, peripheral perfusion is considered satisfactory if the color returns in less than _____ seconds.

A. 2   **C.** 4

B. 3   **D.** 5

_____ 14. Which of the following is not a sign of a partial airway obstruction in an infant or child?

A. pink skin   **C.** stridor and crowing

B. adequate peripheral perfusion   **D.** loss of consciousness

_____ 15. Signs of a severe partial airway obstruction or complete airway obstruction in an infant or child include all of the following except

A. cyanosis.   **C.** crying or coughing.

B. altered mental status.   **D.** inability to speak.

_____ 16. The effects of hypoxia on an infant and child are

A. slowed heart rate and improved mental status.

B. increased heart rate and decreased mental status.

C. slowed heart rate and altered mental status.

D. increased heart rate and coma.

_____ 17. All of the following are appropriate guidelines to follow when ventilating the infant or child except

A. avoid breathing too hard through the pocket face mask.

B. avoid using excessive bag pressure and volume.

C. use a properly sized mask to assure a good mask seal.

D. omit the use of infection control barriers.

_____ 18. The flow-restricted, oxygen-powered ventilation device is

A. used with caution in an infant.

B. contraindicated in infants and children.

C. preferred during the resuscitation of a child.

D. is only used with the pop-off valve engaged in children.

_____ 19. Common causes of shock in children include infection, trauma, blood loss, and

A. meningitis.   **C.** dehydration.

B. heart failure.   **D.** lack of insulin.

_____ 20. Less common causes of shock in a child include all of the following except

A. allergic reactions.   **C.** poisoning.

B. cardiac events.   **D.** croup.

_____ 21. The blood volume of infants and children is approximately _____ of the total body weight.

A. 6%   **C.** 10%

B. 8%   **D.** 12%

_____ 22. When children are in shock, they do all of the following except

A. compensate for a long time.

B. appear better than they actually are.

C. decompensate very rapidly.

D. decompensate very slowly.

_____ 23. When a child is bleeding internally, the EMT-Basic should avoid

A. administering too much oxygen.

B. transporting too quickly.

C. waiting for signs of decompensated shock before treating for shock.

D. placing the child in the Trendelenburg position if respiratory distress is not evident.

_____ **24.** Decreased urine output and absence of tears are signs of _____ in infants and children.
- **A.** epiglottitis
- **B.** shock
- **C.** hypothermia
- **D.** croup

_____ **25.** When treating a child in shock, unless there are injuries that would contraindicate it, the EMT-Basic should
- **A.** lower the patient's legs.
- **B.** elevate the patient' legs.
- **C.** have the patient sit up.
- **D.** have the patient lie supine.

_____ **26.** Because children have a large skin surface area in proportion to their body mass, they can easily become victims of
- **A.** hypothermia.
- **B.** high fever.
- **C.** airway obstruction.
- **D.** hypovolemia.

_____ **27.** If a child has an airway respiratory disease, it is very important that the EMT-Basic avoid
- **A.** opening the airway.
- **B.** inserting a tongue blade into the mouth.
- **C.** positioning the child in the parent's lap.
- **D.** administering blow-by oxygen.

_____ **28.** A child with signs of an airway disease should be transported as quickly as possible. The signs include all of the following except
- **A.** stridor on inspiration.
- **B.** breathing effort on exhalation.
- **C.** rapid breathing.
- **D.** wheezing.

_____ **29.** A viral illness that causes inflammation of the upper airway and bronchi which is often accompanied by a "seal bark" cough is called
- **A.** bronchitis.
- **B.** asthma.
- **C.** croup.
- **D.** epiglottitis.

_____ **30.** About _____ of all pediatric trauma deaths are related to airway mismanagement.
- **A.** one-fifth
- **B.** one-fourth
- **C.** one-third
- **D.** one-half

_____ **31.** Causes of fever in children include all of the following except
- **A.** upper respiratory infection.
- **B.** hypothermia.
- **C.** pneumonia.
- **D.** infection.

_____ **32.** In the prehospital setting, which of the following is not used to determine an infant's skin temperature?
- **A.** ungloved hand.
- **B.** rectal thermometer
- **C.** information from parents
- **D.** skin thermometer

_____ **33.** When treating an infant or child with a high fever,
- **A.** submerge the patient in cold water.
- **B.** use rubbing alcohol to cool the patient.
- **C.** monitor for shivering while cooling with tepid water.
- **D.** cover the patient with a towel soaked in ice water.

_____ **34.** Infants are more susceptible to _____ because, compared to adults, a greater percentage of their body is water.
- **A.** shock
- **B.** dehydration
- **C.** high fever
- **D.** All of the above.

_____ **35.** Which of the following is not true of seizures in the pediatric patient?
- **A.** Seizures require medical evaluation.
- **B.** Seizures should be considered life-threatening.
- **C.** Seizures are rarely caused by fever.
- **D.** Seizures may be a sign of an underlying condition.

_____ **36.** Severe aspirin poisoning in children can cause all of the following <u>except</u>
  A. seizures
  B. dehydration
  C. coma
  D. shock

_____ **37.** A common cause of lead poisoning in children is
  A. ingesting chips of lead-based paint.
  B. chewing on writing pencils.
  C. drinking water from a well.
  D. eating fish from fresh water lakes.

_____ **38.** You are treating a child who accidentally ingested a handful of her mother's vitamin tablets. Should you be concerned?
  A. No! The body eliminates excess vitamins.
  B. No! The child will just have diarrhea for a few days.
  C. Yes! Many vitamin pills contain iron which can be fatal to a child.
  D. Yes! Adult vitamins are too concentrated for children.

_____ **39.** The majority of meningitis cases occur between the ages of _____ and _____ .
  A. 1 month : 6 months
  B. 1 month : 1 year
  C. 1 month : 3 years
  D. 1 month : 5 years

_____ **40.** In cases of sudden infant death syndrome, the EMT-Basic should
  A. not deliver care and transport immediately.
  B. pronounce the infant's death.
  C. look for evidence of child neglect.
  D. provide resuscitation and transport.

_____ **41.** The number one cause of death in infants and children is
  A. respiratory arrest.
  B. trauma.
  C. cardiac arrest.
  D. child abuse.

_____ **42.** The child who has been struck by a vehicle may present with a triad of injuries that include head injury, lower extremity injury, and _____ injury.
  A. chest
  B. neck
  C. abdominal
  D. upper extremity

_____ **43.** Which of the following is <u>true</u> of a head-injury child?
  A. The most frequent sign is altered mental status.
  B. Respiratory arrest is a common secondary effect.
  C. Suspect internal injuries whenever the patient presents with shock.
  D. All of the above.

_____ **44.** Because the musculoskeletal structures of the chest are less developed in infants and children,
  A. they are able to maintain rapid respiratory rates for a long time.
  B. they are more likely than adults to fracture their ribs.
  C. the chest is less easily deformed.
  D. they are more likely to incur injury to structures beneath the ribs.

_____ **45.** Because the abdominal muscles of infants and small children are immature,
  A. they have less visible signs of breathing difficulty.
  B. they use their chest muscles for breathing.
  C. there is less protection for underlying organs.
  D. they rarely have distention of the abdomen.

_____ **46.** When using a PASG (MAST) on a pediatric patient, the EMT-B should remember
  A. to place the infant in the leg of an adult garment.
  B. the abdominal section is not generally used on children.
  C. it is contraindicated with pelvic instability.
  D. it is contraindicated in children younger than 12 years old.

_____ **47.** Guidelines for managing pediatric burn patients include all of the following except
  A. use the rule of nines to estimate the extent of burns.
  B. identify candidates for transportation to burn centers.
  C. cover the burn with sterile dressing.
  D. keep the patient cool to reduce pain.

_____ **48.** Indications that child abuse may be occurring, include all of the following except
  A. repeated responses to provide care for the same child or family.
  B. poorly healing wounds or improperly healed fractures.
  C. indications of past injuries.
  D. a parent who seems concerned about the child's injuries.

_____ **49.** When you respond to the home of a person that you think may be a child abuser, observe for all of the following except
  A. a family member who has trouble controlling anger.
  B. indications of alcohol and drug abuse.
  C. torn clothing on the child.
  D. any adult who appears in a state of depression.

_____ **50.** Which of the following is not a role of the EMT-B when child abuse is suspected?
  A. Control your emotions and hold back accusations.
  B. Gather information from parents/caregiver away from the child.
  C. Talk to the child separately and ask her if she has been abused.
  D. Report your suspicions of abuse to the emergency department.

COMPLETE THE FOLLOWING

1. List ten signs of respiratory distress in a child.

_____

_____

_____

_____

_____

_____

_____

_____

_____

_____

2. List five potential problems that can occur when caring for a special needs child with a tracheostomy tube.

_____

_____

_____

_____

_____

3. List four possible complications of central venous lines.

_____

_____

_____

_____

COMPLETE THE CHART

Fill in each numbered box to complete the chart.

Artificial Ventilation

	Child over 8 years	Child 1 to 8 years	Infant birth to 1 year
Ventilation duration	1.	2.	3.
Ventilation rate	4.	5.	6.

CASE STUDY ▬▬▬▬▬▬▬▬▬▬▬▬▬▬▬▬▬▬▬▬▬▬▬▬▬▬

Before completing this case study, review both Chapters 13 and 29.

▶ THE CASE OF THE POISONED JUICE

You are dispatched to a community day-care center that called 911 because a number of the children suddenly became ill after lunch. Upon arrival, you determine the scene is safe to enter and size-up the situation. There are at least six children of different ages, ranging from infant to six years old, who have become nauseated after drinking apple juice that was left over from a few days ago. They are vomiting and complaining of stomach cramps. You have decided to call for an ALS unit and another BLS unit for backup at this time.

1. What infection control precautions should you take?

2. How could you prepare for additional patients with the assistance of the day-care workers?

As your crew begins to evaluate each of the children, the day-care supervisor notifies you that all the parents of the sick children have been called and are on their way to the day-care center. It appears that all of the children are in various stages of vomiting and most also have diarrhea. Initial assessment doesn't reveal any patients who are high priority except one infant who normally requires special care.

3. What can be a complication of children vomiting and having diarrhea?

4. The infant who receives special care is normally healthy except she is closely watched because she has had a shunt installed since birth. What is a shunt and why are these frequently installed in infants?

The other ambulances arrive and the decision is made to immediately transport the infant with the shunt as a high priority and call for an additional ambulance to respond to the scene. Each of the EMT-Bs begins obtaining complete sets of vital signs on the remaining children. Most of the sixty children in the day-care center are being evaluated for complaints and a full set of vitals; a prehospital care report has been completed on each child. Most of the children are not sick; however, you are noticing a trend of "sympathy" pains from children who could not have possibly drank from the contaminated can of juice.

5. What would be the normal vital signs to expect from the infants?

6. What would be the normal vital signs to expect from the toddlers?

7. What would be the normal vital signs to expect from the preschoolers?

8. As you examine the infants, are there any assessment strategies which would be helpful?

9. As you examine the toddlers, are there any assessment strategies which would be helpful?

10. As you examine the preschoolers, are there any assessment strategies which would be helpful?

When the parents arrive, some of them decide to sign the appropriate documentation and to take their children to their pediatricians. Eight other parents have agreed to be transported with their children to the local hospital so the children can be examined further in the emergency department.

11. For the infants and toddlers who are being transported by ambulance, what is the safest way to transport them provided they are not unstable and their parents are nearby to assist?

12. For the infants being transported by ambulance, what is the best way to determine their level of consciousness with the assistance of their parents?

13. One of the paramedics suggest taking a sample of the juice that all the children drank. Why might this be helpful?

CHAPTER

Ambulance Operations

MATCH TERMINOLOGY/DEFINITIONS

A. EPA-registered, low-level disinfectant

B. Occlusive dressing used for sealing injuries to the chest

C. Legal term, which appears in most states' driving laws, referring to the responsibility of the emergency vehicle operator to drive safely and keep the safety of all others in mind at all times

D. Ambulance with a modular box on a pickup truck chassis conforming to the DOT specifications

E. Emergency Medical Dispatcher

F. Van ambulance with a raised roof conforming to the DOT specifications

G. Call in which the driver of the emergency vehicle responds with lights and siren because he/she is of the understanding that loss or life or limb is possible

H. Large, flat area without aerial obstruction in which a helicopter can land to pick up a patient

I. Ambulance with a van chassis and a modular box conforming to the DOT specifications

J. Special thermometer that is designed to go down to 82°F

K. Traction splint for the immobilization of a painful, swollen, deformed thigh

L. Automated external defibrillator

M. Head immobilizer (cervical immobilization device)

N. Automatic transport ventilator

O. Mechanical compressor for performing CPR that is especially helpful to services with transport time to the hospital over 15 minutes

_____ **1.** AED

_____ **2.** ATV

_____ **3.** CID

_____ **4.** Due regard

_____ **5.** EMD

_____ **6.** Hypothermia thermometer

_____ **7.** Landing zone (LZ)

_____ **8.** Lysol

_____ **9.** Sager

_____ **10.** Thumper

_____ **11.** True emergency

_____ **12.** Type I ambulance

_____ **13.** Type II ambulance

_____ **14.** Type III ambulance

_____ **15.** Vaseline gauze

_____ **1.** The federal agency that develops specifications for ambulance vehicle designs is the
  A. U.S. Department of Motor Vehicles.
  B. Food and Drug Administration.
  C. U.S. Department of Transportation.
  D. U.S. Department of Health, Education and Welfare.

_____ **2.** The purpose(s) for carrying an EPA-registered, intermediate-level disinfectant on the ambulance is to
  A. clean up blood spills.
  B. destroy mycobacterium tuberculosis.
  C. disinfect patient wounds.
  D. All of the above.

_____ **3.** Which of the following is not a piece of equipment that should be in the portable first-in kit to be taken directly to a patient's side?
  A. suction unit   **C.** blood pressure cuff
  B. rigid cervical collar   **D.** telemetry repeater

_____ **4.** Supplies used for the "C" step of the initial assessment of a trauma victim includes all of the following except
  A. blood pressure cuff.   **C.** the AED.
  B. occlusive dressings.   **D.** suction unit.

_____ **5.** Each of the following is a piece of equipment used to obtain vital signs except
  A. rubber bulb syringe.   **C.** sphygmomanometer kit.
  B. adult and pediatric stethoscope. **D.** penlight.

_____ **6.** A device used to carry patients over long distances is called a
  A. Stokes basket.   **C.** Reeves stretcher.
  B. scoop stretcher.   **D.** wheeled ambulance stretcher.

_____ **7.** Which of the following pieces of patient transfer equipment is incorrectly matched with its function?
  A. wheeled ambulance stretcher : transporting patients in sitting, supine, or Trendelenburg position
  B. folding stair chair : moving patients down stairs in a sitting position
  C. Reeves stretcher : carrying patients from a high-angle rescue
  D. scoop stretcher : picking up patients found in tight spaces

_____ **8.** Components of a typical fixed oxygen delivery system include
  A. 3,000-liter reservoir.
  B. a two-stage regulator.
  C. the necessary reducing valve and yokes.
  D. All of the above.

_____ **9.** Of the following devices carried on the ambulance for prehospital respiratory care, which is an optional item?
  A. six adult and four pediatric nasal cannula
  B. flow-restricted, oxygen-powered ventilation device
  C. automatic transport ventilator
  D. plastic cup for blow-by oxygen

_____ **10.** The fixed suction unit in the ambulance should
  A. provide an airflow of over 15 liters per minute.
  B. be usable by a person seated beside the patient.
  C. have a current hydrostat test date.
  D. reach a vacuum of at least 300 mmHg within 4 seconds.

_____ **11.** Which of the following pieces of equipment carried on ambulances for defibrillation or assisting with cardiopulmonary resuscitation is optional?
    A. short or long spine board   **C.** automated external defibrillator
    B. mechanical CPR compressor   **D.** kit with oral and nasal airways

_____ **12.** Equipment that is carried on an ambulance that is used for immobilization include all of the following except
    A. a Hare traction splint.   **C.** padded aluminum splints.
    B. triangular bandages.   **D.** a burn sheet.

_____ **13.** Chemical cold packs are carried on an ambulance primarily for use with _____ injuries.
    A. musculoskeletal   **C.** respiratory
    B. abdominal   **D.** cardiac

_____ **14.** Supplies used for wound care should include all of the following except
    A. sterile burn sheets.   **C.** self-adhering roller bandages.
    B. 5 × 9 inch combine dressings.   **D.** Hare traction device.

_____ **15.** What is the purpose of carrying sterilized aluminum foil on the ambulance?
    A. to wrap body parts in
    B. to maintain body heat
    C. to make a shield over an avulsed eye
    D. for warming minor abrasions

_____ **16.** The supplies for childbirth include all of the following except
    A. a rubber bulb syringe.   **C.** large safety pins.
    B. sanitary napkins.   **D.** sterile surgical gloves.

_____ **17.** Every shift, both you and your partner should
    A. wash and wax the ambulance.
    B. change the oil on the ambulance.
    C. complete the equipment checklist.
    D. do preventative maintenance on the ambulance.

_____ **18.** Of the following items checked on the ambulance, which is checked with the engine off?
    A. dash mounted gauges   **C.** windshield wiper operation
    B. battery   **D.** vehicle's warning lights

_____ **19.** The responsibilities of the Emergency Medical Dispatcher include all of the following except
    A. dispatching and coordinating EMS resources.
    B. interrogating the caller and prioritizing the call.
    C. coordinating with other public safety agencies.
    D. advising the caller that an ambulance is not needed.

_____ **20.** When an Emergency Medical Dispatcher questions a patient or caller, which of the following is not routinely asked?
    A. What is the exact location of the patient?
    B. What's the problem?
    C. Has the patient been in the hospital recently?
    D. How old is the patient?

_____ **21.** When speaking with a caller who is at the scene of a traffic collision, the Emergency Medical Dispatcher should ask all of the following except
    A. Is traffic moving?
    B. What brand vehicle was involved in the collision?
    C. How many lanes of traffic are open?
    D. Are any of the vehicles on fire?

_____ 22. To be a safe ambulance operator, the EMT-Basic should
    A. be tolerant of other drivers.
    B. always wear glasses or contact lenses if required.
    C. have a positive attitude about his/her ability as a driver.
    D. All of the above.

_____ 23. Every state has statutes that regulate the operation of emergency vehicles.
    Under certain circumstances, vehicle operators can do all of the following
    except
    A. park the vehicle anywhere so long as it does not damage personal
       property.
    B. proceed past red stop signals, flashing red stop signals, and stop signs.
    C. exceed the posted speed limit as long as life and property are not
       endangered.
    D. pass a school bus that has its red lights blinking.

_____ 24. At the scene of a collision, you examine a patient and find that he is stable.
    This situation is no longer a
    A. true emergency.   C. cold response.
    B. due regard.   D. priority one response.

_____ 25. Which guideline for the use of the ambulance siren is inappropriate?
    A. Use the siren sparingly.
    B. Never assume that all motorists will hear your signal.
    C. Be prepared for erratic movements of motorists.
    D. Keep it on until the call is completed.

_____ 26. Which of the following is true about the use of lights and sirens?
    A. Motorists are more inclined to give way to ambulances when sirens are
       continually sounded.
    B. The decision about their use should be based on the patient's medical
       condition.
    C. The use of the siren has little effect on the ambulance operator.
    D. Four-way flashers should be used in addition to emergency lights.

_____ 27. Use of escorts or multi-vehicle responses are a
    A. very quick and successful means of response.
    B. very dangerous means of response.
    C. means of decreasing the chance of collision.
    D. standard operating procedure in most communities.

_____ 28. Factors that can affect ambulance response include all of the following except
    A. time of the day.
    B. weather.
    C. road maintenance and construction.
    D. type of emergency.

_____ 29. You are the first vehicle on the scene of a auto collision in which one of
    the automobiles is on fire. You should park your vehicle
    A. 50 feet from the wreckage.   C. beyond the wreckage.
    B. in front of the wreckage.   D. downwind from the wreckage.

_____ 30. A sequence of operations to ready a patient for transfer is called
    A. stabilization.   C. transport.
    B. packaging.   D. removal.

_____ 31. An unconscious patient who has no potential spine injury should be
    positioned in the ambulance
    A. in the recovery position.   C. in the supine position.
    B. with legs raised 8 to 12 inches. D. sitting-up position.

_____ **32.** Which of the following is an action you would <u>not</u> perform en route to the hospital?
   A. Recheck the patient's bandages and splints.
   B. Form a general impression of the patient.
   C. Perform ongoing assessment and continue to monitor vital signs.
   D. Notify the receiving facility of your estimated time of arrival.

_____ **33.** If a patient develops cardiac arrest en route to the hospital, the EMT-B's <u>first</u> action should be to
   A. apply and operate the AED.
   B. begin cardiopulmonary resuscitation.
   C. notify the emergency department.
   D. tell the operator to stop the ambulance.

_____ **34.** When delivering the patient to the hospital, the EMT-Basic should <u>never</u>
   A. complete the prehospital care report at the hospital.
   B. simply move a patient onto the hospital stretcher and leave.
   C. transfer the patient's personal effects.
   D. obtain your release from the hospital.

_____ **35.** When approaching a helicopter, first wait for the pilot or medic to wave you in. Then approach from the
   A. rear of the craft.　　　　　　　**C.** front or side of the craft.
   B. uphill slope side of the craft.　**D.** downhill slope rear of the craft.

COMPLETE THE FOLLOWING

1. List the seven questions an EMD should ask a caller who is reporting a medical emergency.

_____

_____

_____

_____

_____

_____

_____

2. List seven factors that can affect an ambulance response.

_____

_____

_____

_____

_____

_____

_____

3. List the four major ways the EMT-Basic on the scene of a collision should describe the landing zone to the air rescue service.

- terrain
- major landmarks
- estimated distance to nearest town
- other pertinent information

LABEL THE PHOTOGRAPHS

Fill in the name of each level of disinfecting shown in the photo on the line provided.

1. low level

2. Inter-mediate

3. High - level

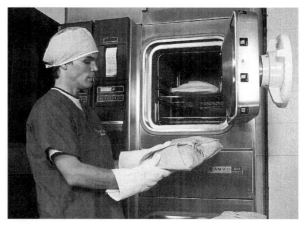

4. Sterilize

EMT-BASIC SKILLS PERFORMANCE CHECKLISTS

▶ **TRANSFERRING THE PATIENT**

❑ Take body substance isolation.

❑ Transfer the patient as soon as possible. In a routine admission or when an illness or injury is not life-threatening, first check to see what is to be done with the patient.

❑ An EMT-B should remain with the patient until transfer is complete.

❑ Assist the emergency department staff as required.

❑ Give a complete verbal report of the patient's condition and treatment administered.

❑ Complete your prehospital care report and turn a copy over to the hospital staff.

❑ Transfer the patient's personal effects.

❑ Obtain your release from the hospital, if required in you region.

▶ **ACTIONS TO BE TAKEN AT THE HOSPITAL**

❑ Take body substance isolation.

❑ Clean the ambulance interior as required by your service exposure control plan.

❑ Replace respiratory equipment as required.

❑ Replace expendable items according to local policies.

❑ Exchange equipment according to local policies.

❑ Make up the wheeled ambulance stretcher.

▶ **CHECKING THE AED***

❑ Check the defibrillator unit for cleanliness.

❑ Check the cables and connectors.

❑ Check the supplies carried with the AED.

❑ Check the power supply and its operation.

❑ Check the indicators on the ECG display.

❑ Check the ECG recorder operation.

❑ Check the charge display cycle with a simulator.

❑ Check the pacemaker feature if applicable.

❑ File a written report on the status of the AED.

*The specifics can be found on the FDA Automated Defibrillator: Operator's Shift Checklist.

CHAPTER 31

Gaining Access and Rescue Operations

MATCH TERMINOLOGY/DEFINITIONS

A. When moving towards the rear of the vehicle, the second post you see, which supports the roof

B. Glass used in an automobile's side and rear windows designed to break into small rounded pieces rather than sharp fragments

C. Named after a well-known consumer advocate, this case-hardened pin is held by the cams of an automobile's door locking system

D. Decreasing circles of voltage on the ground surrounding a point where a charged wire is down

E. When a patient is pinned and requires assistance, sometimes mechanical, to free him

F. To crib or block a vehicle or structure to prevent further unintended, uncontrolled movement

G. Gear designed to prevent the rescuer from being injured while working in the inner circle

H. Post in front of the driver's compartment which supports the roof and windshield

I. Safety glass used in the windshields of automobiles made of two sheets of plate glass bonded to a sheet of tough plastic

J. Blocks of hardwood usually 4 × 4 × 18-inch or 2 × 4 × 18-inch used to stabilize a vehicle

K. Area immediately around and including the wrecked vehicle

L. Using tools or special equipment to break an automobile window in order to reach the patient and perform an initial assessment of the patient

M. Three-part procedure used by rescue personnel to free a patient trapped in a vehicle

N. Process by which entrapped patients are rescued from vehicles, buildings, tunnels, or other places

O. Saw that is designed to cut laminated windshield glass

_____ **1.** A Post

_____ **2.** B Post

_____ **3.** Complex access

_____ **4.** Cribbing

_____ **5.** Disentanglement

_____ **6.** Entrapment

_____ **7.** Extrication

_____ **8.** Glas-Master

_____ **9.** Ground gradient

_____ **10.** Inner circle

_____ **11.** Laminated glass

_____ **12.** Nader Pin

_____ **13.** Protective gear

_____ **14.** Stabilization

_____ **15.** Tempered glass

MULTIPLE CHOICE REVIEW

_____ **1.** Trench, dive, ice, and high-angle rescue is frequently carried out by _____ .
    A. industrial rescue teams.   **C.** police rescue services.
    B. specialty rescue teams.   **D.** commercial rescue services.

_____ **2.** The phases of extrication include all of the following except
    A. gaining access to the patient.   **C.** disentangling the patient.
    B. defining patient care.   **D.** sizing up the situation.

_____ **3.** An important part of a rescue scene size-up is
    A. determining the extent of entrapment.
    B. starting IVs on the patient.
    C. removing shattered glass from around the patient.
    D. informing the patient about the extent of vehicle damage.

_____ **4.** During size-up of a collision, you must be able to read a collision and develop an action plan based on your knowledge of rescue operations and your
    A. previous experience at collision scenes.
    B. judgment of the extent of vehicle damage.
    C. estimate of the patient's condition and priority.
    D. evaluation of the resources available.

_____ **5.** When developing an action plan for patient extrication, always keep in mind the
    A. potential for observation by bystanders.
    B. "golden hour" concept of trauma management.
    C. cost of further damage to the vehicle.
    D. type of vehicle that is involved in the incident.

_____ **6.** If a vehicle has an air bag which deployed, the manufacturer recommends
    A. airing out the car for 15 minutes prior to treating the patient.
    B. placing masks on patients before treating.
    C. lifting the bag and examining the steering wheel and dash.
    D. using HEPA masks before gaining access.

_____ **7.** The unsafe act that contributes most to collision scene injuries is failure to
    A. eliminate or control hazards during operations.
    B. wear protective gear during rescue operations.
    C. recognize mechanisms of injury early on.
    D. select the proper tool for the task.

_____ **8.** Factors that may contribute to injuries of rescuers at a collision include all of the following except
    A. careless attitude toward personal safety.
    B. a lack of skill in tool and equipment use.
    C. physical problems that impede strenuous effort.
    D. limiting the inner circle to rescuers who are in protective gear.

_____ **9.** Good protective gear at the scene of a collision includes all of the following except
    A. firefighter or leather gloves.
    B. fire-resistant trousers or turnout pants.
    C. steel toe, high-top work shoes.
    D. plastic "bump caps."

_____ **10.** To ensure adequate eye protection at the collision scene, the EMT-B should wear
    A. safety goggles with a soft vinyl frame.
    B. a hinged plastic helmet shield.
    C. a thermal mask or shield.
    D. safety glasses with small lenses.

_____ 11. During an extrication, an aluminized rescue blanket may be used to
A. maintain the rescuer's body heat.
B. smother fire in the engine compartment.
C. protect the patient from poor weather and flying particles.
D. None of the above.

_____ 12. When using flares, the EMT-B should
A. watch for spilled fuel or other combustibles prior to igniting.
B. throw them out of the moving vehicle to save time.
C. use them as a traffic wand to divert traffic.
D. always walk with oncoming traffic while positioning them.

_____ 13. When there is an electrical hazard, the safe zone
A. should be established as soon as the power company arrives.
B. does not exist due to the numerous dangers of an electrical hazard.
C. should be far enough away to assure an arcing wire does not cause injury.
D. is located at least ten feet from the ground gradient.

_____ 14. A material or object that will carry electricity is
A. dangerous to stand near.   C. always energized.
B. not a hazard unless it is arcing. D. called a conductor.

_____ 15. If a vehicle collides with a broken utility pole with wires down, you should
A. ignore it since the vehicle will not conduct electricity.
B. tell the vehicle's occupants to stay in the vehicle.
C. immediately shut off the vehicle's ignition switch.
D. don full protective gear and remove downed wires.

_____ 16. In wet weather, a phenomenon known as _____ may provide your first clue that a wire is down.
A. an arc   C. lightning
B. ground gradient   D. flash point

_____ 17. As you approach a scene with an electrical hazard, you feel a tingling sensation in your legs and lower torso. Which action should you take?
A. Turn 180 degrees and shuffle with both feet together to safety.
B. Turn 90 degrees and walk as quickly as possible to safety.
C. Ask your partner for his hand and have him pull you to safety.
D. Turn 180 degrees and crawl to safety.

_____ 18. If there is a fire in the car's engine compartment and people are trapped in the vehicle, you should do all of the following except
A. quickly and carefully remove the patient.
B. assure that the fire department has been called.
C. don protective gear and use your fire extinguisher.
D. apply a short spine board to the driver right away.

_____ 19. When a vehicle's hood is closed and there is an engine fire, you should do all of the following except
A. use emergency moves to remove occupants.
B. let the fire department extinguish the fire.
C. fully open the hood to extinguish the fire.
D. let the fire burn under the closed hood.

_____ 20. When a vehicle rolls off the roadway into a field of dried grass, it is possible that a fire may be caused by the
A. catalytic converter.   C. ground gradient.
B. leaking radiator fluid. D. airbag deployment.

_____ 21. "Try Before You Pry" is the foundation for the _____ procedure.
A. disentanglement   C. simple access
B. stabilization   D. entanglement

22. Once a vehicle is stabilized and an entry point is gained, the EMT-B should immediately do all of the following <u>except</u>
   A. begin the initial assessment.
   B. crawl inside the vehicle.
   C. provide manual cervical stabilization.
   D. pull the patient out of the access hole.

23. If an unconscious patient is in a sitting position behind the wheel with legs pinned by the vehicle, which is the best approach to disentanglement?
   A. Displace the doors, cut the roof, then displace the dash.
   B. Pull the dash, cut the doors, then push the seat.
   C. Cut the roof, displace the doors, and then displace the dash.
   D. Cut the roof, displace the dash, then displace the doors.

24. Which of the following is <u>not</u> a reason for disposing of the roof to access a patient?
   A. It makes the entire interior of the vehicle accessible.
   B. It creates a large exitway through which to remove a patient.
   C. It provides fresh air and helps cool off the patient.
   D. It helps to quickly stabilize the vehicle.

25. An extrication involves displacing the dash or steering wheel but the air bag has not yet deployed. What should you do?
   A. Apply heat to the steering wheel.
   B. Drill a hole into the air bag module.
   C. Disconnect the battery cable.
   D. Displace the steering column.

COMPLETE THE FOLLOWING

1. List the ten phases of the rescue process.

_____

_____

_____

_____

_____

_____

_____

_____

_____

_____

2. List six factors that can increase the potential for an injury at a collision site.

_____

_____

_____

_____

_____

_____

LABEL THE PHOTOGRAPHS

Label each procedure on the lines provided.

1. _____

2. _____

3. _____

4. _____

5. _____

6. _____

CHAPTER 32

Special Operations

MATCH TERMINOLOGY/DEFINITIONS

A. Color-coded tag indicating the priority group to which a patient has been assigned

B. Area in which secondary triage takes place at a multiple-casualty incident

C. Process of quickly assessing patients in a multiple-casualty incident and assigning each a priority for receiving emergency care or transportation to definitive care

D. Person responsible for overseeing triage at a multiple-casualty incident

E. Area in which patient care is delivered at a multiple-casualty incident

F. Person responsible for overseeing treatment of patients who have been triaged at a multiple-casualty incident

G. Person responsible for communicating with sector officers and hospitals to manage transportation of patients to hospitals from the scene of a multiple-casualty incident

H. Area in which ambulances are parked and other resources are held until needed

I. Person responsible for overseeing and keeping track of ambulances and ambulance personnel at a multiple-casualty incident and who directs ambulances to treatment areas at the request of the transportation officer

J. Any medical or trauma event involving three or more patients that places a great demand on EMS equipment and personnel

K. System used for the management of a large-scale multiple-casualty incident, involving assumption of responsibility for command and designation and coordination of such elements as triage, treatment, transport, and staging

L. Senior EMS person on the scene who establishes an EMS command post and oversees the medical aspects of a multiple-casualty incident

M. Any substance or material in a form which poses an unreasonable risk to health, safety, and property when transported in commerce

N. Area immediately surrounding a dangerous goods incident that extends far enough to prevent adverse effects from released dangerous goods to personnel outside the zone

O. Area in which the command post and support functions that are necessary to control the incident are located

_____ **1.** Cold zone

_____ **2.** EMS Command

_____ **3.** Hazardous material

_____ **4.** Hot zone

_____ **5.** Incident Management System (IMS)

_____ **6.** Multiple-casualty incident (MCI)

_____ **7.** Staging officer

_____ **8.** Staging sector

_____ **9.** Transportation officer

_____ **10.** Treatment officer

_____ **11.** Treatment sector

_____ **12.** Triage

_____ **13.** Triage officer

_____ **14.** Triage sector

_____ **15.** Triage tag

_____ 1. Using the *North American Emergency Response Guidebook,* the EMT-B would find that ethyl acetate is a chemical that
  A. irritates the eyes and respiratory tract.
  B. destroys the bone marrow.
  C. damages internal organs.
  D. is extremely explosive.

_____ 2. Using the *North American Emergency Response Guidebook,* the EMT-B would find that Benzene (benzol) is a chemical that
  A. damages the eyes by eliminating moisture.
  B. has toxic vapors which can be absorbed through the skin.
  C. is used as an industrial blasting agent.
  D. is used in surgical techniques to control pain.

_____ 3. The regulations that require training in hazardous materials for responders to hazmat incidents are
  A. Ryan White CARE Act.   **C.** FEMA 1910.1030.
  B. NFPA 1200.   **D.** OSHA 1910.120

_____ 4. The level of training for those who initially respond to releases or potential releases of hazardous materials in order to protect people, property, and the environment is called
  A. First Responder Awareness.   **C.** Hazardous Materials Technician.
  B. First Responder Operations.   **D.** Hazardous Materials Specialist.

_____ 5. The level of training for those who are likely to witness or discover a hazardous substance release is called
  A. First Responder Awareness.   **C.** Hazardous Materials Technician.
  B. First Responder Operations.   **D.** Hazardous Materials Specialist.

_____ 6. The standard that deals with competencies for EMS personnel at a hazardous material incident is called
  A. OSHA 1910.1030.   **C.** NFPA 473.
  B. NFPA 472.   **D.** OSHA 1910.1200.

_____ 7. Which of the following is unlikely to be a potential hazardous material location?
  A. garden center   **C.** trucking terminal
  B. chemical plant   **D.** pet store

_____ 8. Unless EMS personnel are trained to the level of _____ , they must remain in the cold zone.
  A. First Responder Awareness.   **C.** Hazardous Materials Technician.
  B. First Responder Operations.   **D.** Hazardous Materials Specialist.

_____ 9. All victims leaving the _____ zone should be considered contaminated until proven otherwise.
  A. cold   **C.** hot
  B. warm   **D.** decontamination

_____ 10. What is the primary concern at the scene of a hazardous material incident?
  A. the safety of the EMT-B and crew, patients, and the public
  B. stabilizing the incident as fast as possible
  C. quickly removing all exposed patients from the scene
  D. determining the extent and cost of the damage

_____ 11. Upon arrival at a tanker truck crash where the vehicle has overturned and is rapidly leaking its contents onto the street, the EMT-B should
  A. quickly apply a short spine board to the truck driver in the tanker.
  B. isolate the area and call for the appropriate backup assistance.
  C. try to stop or seal the leak as quickly as possible.
  D. send the least senior EMT-B in to assess the patient.

_____ 12. The "safe zone" of a hazardous materials incident should be established in a _____ location.
   A. downwind/downhill
   B. upwind/same level
   C. downwind/same level
   D. upwind/downhill

_____ 13. The role of the incident commander at a hazardous material incident is to delegate responsibility for all of the following except
   A. directing bystanders to a safe area.
   B. establishing a perimeter.
   C. immediately initiating rescue attempts.
   D. evacuating people if necessary.

_____ 14. When a contaminated victim of a hazardous material incident comes in contact with other people who are not contaminated, this is referred to as _____ contamination.
   A. secondary
   B. chemical
   C. contact
   D. clone

_____ 15. The designations on the sides of tanker trucks are called hazardous material
   A. license plates.
   B. waybills.
   C. placards.
   D. shipping papers.

_____ 16. The commonly used placard system for fixed facilities is called the
   A. MSDS.
   B. NFPA 704.
   C. CHEM 369.
   D. UN Classification System.

_____ 17. All employers are required to post in an obvious spot the information about all the chemicals in the workplace on a form called a
   A. NFPA 704.
   B. MSDS.
   C. OSHA Chemical listing.
   D. Fair trade posting.

_____ 18. Resources that the EMT-B should use at a hazardous materials incident include all of the following except
   A. copies of NFPA rules.
   B. the local hazmat team.
   C. the _North American Emergency Response Guidebook._
   D. CHEM-TEL.

_____ 19. What is CHEMTREC?
   A. a 24-hour service for identifying hazardous materials
   B. a national hazmat training center
   C. a national hazmat response team
   D. a national aeronautical team

_____ 20. EMS personnel at the scene of a hazardous material incident are responsible for taking care of the injured and
   A. identifying and controlling the substance involved.
   B. monitoring and rehabilitating hazmat team members.
   C. decontaminating patients exiting the hot zone.
   D. moving patients from the hot zone to the warm zone.

_____ 21. Which of the following is not a characteristic of the rehab sector at a hazardous material incident?
   A. It should be located in the warm zone.
   B. It should be protected from the weather.
   C. It should be easily accessible to EMS.
   D. It should be free from exhaust fumes.

_____ 22. As soon as possible after a hazmat team member exits the hot zone, the EMT-B should
   A. have him drink a pint of water.
   B. remove his protective clothing.
   C. begin the decontamination process.
   D. reassess his vital signs.

_____ **23.** You are confronted with a patient at risk for causing secondary contamination in which treatment calls for irrigation with water. The hazmat team has not yet arrived. Which of the following actions is not recommended?
  A. Cut the patient's clothes off.
  B. Irrigate the patient with tepid water.
  C. Flush runoff water down the nearest drain.
  D. Use disposable equipment for treatment.

_____ **24.** Which of the following is not a feature of a good local disaster plan?
  A. All emergency responders should be familiar with the plan.
  B. The plan must be based on the actual availability of resources.
  C. The plan must be rehearsed to ensure it works correctly.
  D. The plan should be generic and meet national standards.

_____ **25.** Upon arrival of the first EMS unit at the scene of an MCI, the crew leader should do all of the following except
  A. assume EMS command.   **C.** call for backup.
  B. conduct a scene walk through.   **D.** begin patient treatment.

_____ **26.** Which of the following is not a principle of good communication at an MCI?
  A. The person responsible for incident management should have unique Command name.
  B. Responding units should be informed that a disaster plan is in effect.
  C. The majority of communications should be done via radio transmission.
  D. Communications between Command and sector officers should be face-to-face.

_____ **27.** If an MCI involves hazardous materials, which additional sector would be needed?
  A. hazmat sector   **C.** rehabilitation sector
  B. extrication sector   **D.** decontamination sector

_____ **28.** The individual at an MCI who is responsible for the sorting and prioritizing of the patients is the _____ officer.
  A. triage   **C.** transportation
  B. treatment   **D.** extrication

_____ **29.** Patients who are assessed to have decreased mental status at an MCI are considered Priority _____ .
  A. 1   **C.** 3
  B. 2   **D.** 4

_____ **30.** Patients who are assessed to have shock (hypoperfusion) at an MCI are considered Priority _____ .
  A. 1   **C.** 3
  B. 2   **D.** 4

_____ **31.** Patients who are assessed to have multiple-bone or joint injuries at an MCI are considered Priority _____ .
  A. 1   **C.** 3
  B. 2   **D.** 4

_____ **32.** Patients who are assessed to have died at the MCI scene are considered Priority _____ .
  A. 1   **C.** 3
  B. 2   **D.** 4

_____ **33.** The individual at an MCI who is responsible for maintaining a supply of vehicles and personnel at a location away from the incident site is the _____ officer.
  A. extrication   **C.** staging
  B. transportation   **D.** triage

_____ **34.** The individual at an MCI who is responsible for determining patient destinations and notifying the hospitals of the incoming patients is the _____ officer.

    A. triage   **C.** transportation

    B. treatment   **D.** extrication

_____ **35.** Patient transport decisions at an MCI are based upon all of the following except

    A. prioritization.   **C.** transportation resources.

    B. destination facilities.   **D.** patient's family preferences.

COMPLETE THE FOLLOWING

1. List the information you should be prepared to give when you call for assistance from CHEMTREC.

_____

_____

_____

_____

_____

_____

_____

_____

_____

_____

_____

_____

_____

_____

_____

_____

2. List four characteristics of the rehab sector at a hazardous material incident.

_____

_____

_____

_____

CHAPTER 32 Special Operations **255**

COMPLETE THE CHART

Fill in the blanks to complete the chart.

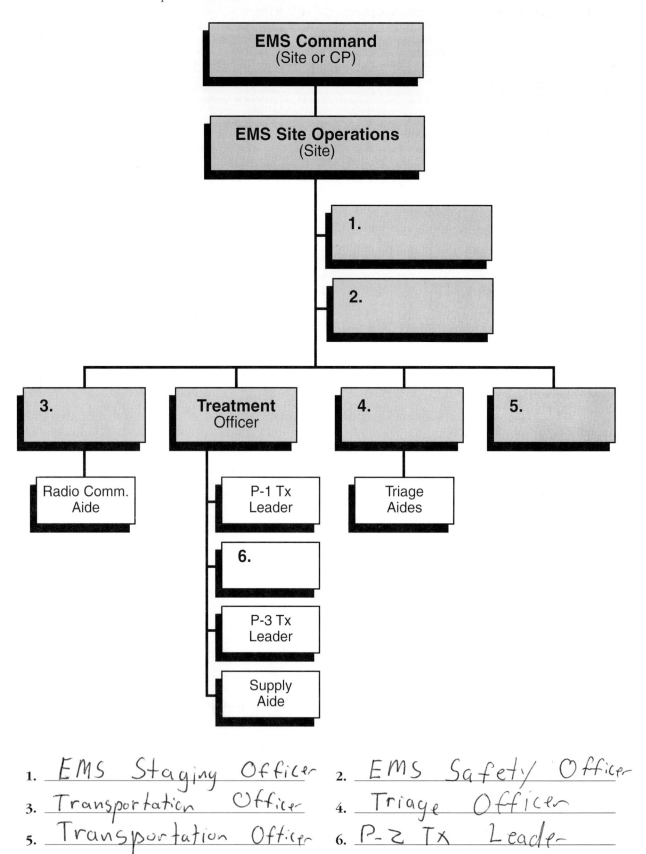

1. <u>EMS Staging Officer</u> 2. <u>EMS Safety Officer</u>
3. <u>Transportation Officer</u> 4. <u>Triage Officer</u>
5. <u>Transportation Officer</u> 6. <u>P-2 Tx Leader</u>

EMT-BASIC SKILLS PERFORMANCE CHECKLIST

▶ **ESTABLISHING COMMAND AT A MULTIPLE-CASUALTY INCIDENT**

❑ Perform an initial size-up of the situation.

❑ Locate the police and fire officers and establish a unified command post.

❑ Don the EMS command vest.

❑ Notify the EMS dispatcher you are declaring an MCI, inform dispatch of the extent of the incident, notify if it is ongoing or contained, approximate number of victims, and give the location of the command post.

❑ Request the number of BLS and ALS units needed.

❑ Designate a triage officer.

❑ Designate a staging officer and a location for staging and notify dispatcher to have all additional ambulances respond to staging.

❑ Request the dispatcher roll call the local hospitals for bed availability.

❑ Designate treatment officer and location for this sector (as needed).

❑ Designate transportation officer and location for this sector (as needed).

❑ Consider the need for extrication sector (if not already established).

❑ Consider the need for a safety officer (as needed).

❑ Consider the need for aeromedical evacuation and appropriate landing zone nearby the scene.

❑ Consider the usefulness of a school bus to transport the "walking wounded" low-priority patients. Make sure everyone on the bus is medically examined and that medical personnel also ride the bus.

❑ Consider the need for a follow-up CISD and rehab of personnel.

❑ Keep the dispatcher and other service chiefs in close contact throughout the incident.

❑ Along with the police and fire officers, consider the need for a public information officer to work with the arriving media representatives.

CASE STUDY

▶ THE SCHOOL BUS MCI

You are dispatched to a school-bus collision in a major intersection in town. En route the dispatcher notifies you that he has received numerous calls on the collision, and the police as well as the fire department are en route. Callers state that a large truck collided with the bus in an intersection at a high rate of speed, overturning the bus full of school children. As you near the center of town, the traffic is backed up in both directions for about five blocks. The police have arrived on the scene and are beginning to re-route the traffic after confirming that there are many injured children on and near the bus.

1. What would be your initial role as the crew leader of the first arriving ambulance at the scene?

2. **A)** Which vest from the MCI kit should you wear and, **B)** what are your responsibilities?

After declaring the MCI, confirming the incident with dispatch, and establishing contact with the police and fire officers, you begin to estimate the number of patients with the assistance of your two crew members.

3. What would be the most likely job to designate to one of your partners?

4. What are his/her specific functions?

Upon size-up of the situation, it is determined that there were forty children on the bus, half of which have numerous contusions and cuts and who are walking around the scene crying. You decide to designate a nearby store as the location for the P-3 patients. You have one of your partners make a PA announcement that the walking wounded should go to that location. In addition, you call for ten ambulances and another school bus to respond.

5. Where would be the best place to stage the ambulances?

6. What should be the role of the crew leader on the first ambulance arriving at the staging sector?

7. Should any ambulances report directly to the scene?

8. Are there any other sector officers needed at this time?

The fire department has cleared the bus for entry now that it is stabilized and no longer leaking any fuel. Inside there are fifteen patients who need to be removed from the bus. Many of the patients have head injuries, fractures, contusions, and glass cuts.

9. How should these patients be removed from the bus if it is possible?

10. Once removed from the bus, where should the patients be taken?

Prioritize the patients described below into the following categories: P-1 (critical and unstable), P-2 (potentially unstable), P-3 (stable walking wounded), P-4 (dead).

11. A 7-year-old female who complains of a swollen deformed right lower arm and a contusion to the head with no loss of consciousness. She is alert and has vital signs that are normal for her age.

12. A 9-year-old male who has a seizure disorder who has been unconscious since the collision and has already had two observed grand-mal seizures without a lucid interval.

13. A 10-year-old male who was thrown through the front window of the bus because he was standing up talking to the bus driver. He was ejected from the vehicle, was found approximately 50 feet from the bus, and has a large contusion, depressed skull fracture, and no vital signs.

14. A 8-year-old female who has a bruise on the left upper quadrant and the forehead. She denies any loss of consciousness but is pale, clammy, and tachycardia for her age.

The treatment officer has set up a treatment sector across the street from the collision in the gas station parking lot. He has set out a large yellow and a large red tarp. There is also a smaller black tarp inside the gas station for the P-4 patients. As the incident proceeds, you are able to obtain additional assistance from the firefighters at the scene for lifting the patients being removed from the bus and carried on backboards to the treatment sector. Also the area is becoming quite congested because a number of parents are arriving at the scene.

15. What is the best thing to do with the parents?

16. As a smooth flow of ambulances begins to arrive from the staging sector, who should coordinate the destinations of the patient transports and communicate with the hospitals?

17. What might this person want to know immediately from the local hospitals?

18. Other than the bus that was ordered for the P-3 patients, is there any other form of transportation that should be considered for this incident?

19. How should the decision be made as to who rides on the bus to a hospital?

20. As the incident is wrapped up, how could you, as the incident commander, deal with the media and the emotional and physical needs of your personnel?

INTERIM EXAM 3

Use the answer sheet on pages 273–274 to complete this exam. It is perforated so it can be easily removed from this book.

1. The circulation of blood throughout the body, filling the capillaries and supplying the cells and tissue with oxygen and nutrients is called
   A. physiology.
   B. perfusion.
   C. bleeding.
   D. metabolism.

2. With one exception, arteries carry _____ blood _____ the heart.
   A. deoxygenated : back to
   B. deoxygenated : away from
   C. oxygenated : back to
   D. oxygenated : away from

3. With one exception, veins carry _____ blood _____ the heart.
   A. deoxygenated : back to
   B. deoxygenated : away from
   C. oxygenated : back to
   D. oxygenated : away from

4. Once an adult loses approximately a _____ of blood, his/her condition is considered serious.
   A. quart
   B. gallon
   C. milliliter
   D. liter

5. Once a child loses approximately _____ of blood, his/her condition is considered serious.
   A. a milliliter
   B. 250 cc
   C. 500 ml
   D. 1 liter

6. Once an infant loses approximately _____ of blood volume, his/her condition is considered serious.
   A. 75 cc
   B. 150 cc
   C. 250 cc
   D. 500 cc

7. Since internal bleeding is not visible, the EMT-B must base severity of blood loss on
   A. signs and symptoms exhibited.
   B. what the patient tells you.
   C. the size of the contusion.
   D. advice from medical direction.

8. The factors on which severity of bleeding depends include all of the following except
   A. rate of bleeding and the amount of blood loss.
   B. patient's age and weight.
   C. ability of the patient's body to respond and defend against blood loss.
   D. the patient's history of diabetes.

9. Blood that oozes and is dark red is most likely from a
   A. vein.
   B. capillary.
   C. artery.
   D. lymphatic vessel.

10. You are treating a patient who has a slashed wrist which is spurting bright red blood. After trying direct pressure and elevation to control the bleeding, the next step would be to
    A. apply a tourniquet to the arm.
    B. apply an air splint to the arm.
    C. press on the brachial artery.
    D. press on the femoral artery.

11. When all other methods have failed to control bleeding, the EMT-B should
    A. apply the PASG (MAST).
    B. apply an air splint.
    C. press harder on the pressure point.
    D. apply a tourniquet.

12. Signs of internal bleeding include all of the following except
    A. painful, swollen, or deformed extremities.
    B. a tender rigid abdomen.
    C. vomiting bile.
    D. bruising.

13. Examples of penetrating trauma include all of the following except
    A. hand-gun bullet wound.
    B. carving-knife wound.
    C. fall from a height.
    D. screwdriver stab wound.

14. Examples of blunt trauma include all of the following except
    A. blast injuries.
    B. auto-pedestrian collisions.
    C. gunshot wounds.
    D. falls.

15. The signs and symptoms of internal bleeding are
    A. the same as those of hypovolemic shock.
    B. identical to those of external bleeding.
    C. usually not present in elderly patients.
    D. easy to stabilize in the field.

16. Which is not considered a type of shock?
    A. hypovolemic
    B. toxic
    C. cardiogenic
    D. neurogenic.

17. At a point when the body can no longer compensate for the low blood volume, _____ shock begins.
    A. compensated
    B. anaphylactic
    C. decompensated
    D. terminal

18. What are the major components of the central nervous system?
    A. cranial nerves
    B. peripheral nerves
    C. brain and spinal cord
    D. vessels and support tissue

19. Which of the following is not a division of the nervous system?
    A. central
    B. peripheral
    C. autonomic
    D. voluntary

20. The skull is made up of the cranium and the facial bones. The cranium consists of the _____ areas of the skull.
    A. temporal, mandible, maxilla, and superior
    B. frontal, parietal, occipital, and top
    C. anterior, forehead, and lateral
    D. forehead, top, back, and upper sides

21. All of the 14 irregularly shaped bones forming the face are fused with the exception of the _____ bone.
    A. temporal
    B. zygomatic
    C. mandible
    D. malar

22. The brain and spinal cord are bathed in
    A. cerebrospinal fluid.
    C. synovial fluid.
    B. lymphatic fluid.
    D. mucous secretion.

23. The spine is divided into sections called
    A. joints.
    B. vertebrae.
    C. coccygeal.
    D. compartments.

24. The lumbar area of the spine includes _____ vertebrae.
    A. 3
    B. 5
    C. 8
    D. 12

25. The cervical area of the spine includes _____ vertebrae.
    A. 3
    B. 5
    C. 7
    D. 9

26. When a patient strikes her head and states she feels groggy and has a headache, she most likely has a
    A. contusion.
    B. concussion.
    C. contrecoup.
    D. None of the above.

27. A 50-year-old male driver who was involved in an automobile collision states he did not loose consciousness. However, a bystander says he ran to the car after the collision and tried to talk to the driver, but said the driver "just sat there staring off into space for a few minutes." This patient may have any of the following except
    A. contusion.
    B. concussion.
    C. coup injury.
    D. attention deficit.

28. When a patient has some memory loss after a head injury, this is referred to as
    A. bruising.
    B. amnesia.
    C. verbally responsive.
    D. "seeing stars."

29. When a bruising of the brain occurs on the side of the injury, this is referred to as a _____ injury.
    A. contrecoup
    B. hematoma
    C. coup
    D. epidural

30. A collection of blood within the skull or the brain is called a _____ hematoma.
    A. subdural
    B. epidural
    C. intracerebral
    D. All of the above.

31. All of the following make a head injury worse except
    A. limited room for expansion inside the skull.
    B. increased pressure in the skull.
    C. increased carbon dioxide level in the brain.
    D. decreased respiration leading to increased cellular perfusion.

32. An assessment strategy used to check an extremity for injury or paralysis in a conscious patient is
    A. checking for a proximal pulse.
    B. assessing equality of strength.
    C. checking for foot wave.
    D. confirming sensitivity.

33. The type of immobilization device used for a patient depends on
    A. patient priority.
    B. availability.
    C. medical direction's advice.
    D. All of the above.

34. If a patient has a brain injury with skull fracture, the patient's pupils will tend to be
    A. equal.
    B. dilated.
    C. constricted.
    D. unequal.

35. Which of the following describes the blood pressure and pulse for a patient with a brain injury?
    A. decreased blood pressure, increased pulse
    B. decreased blood pressure, decreased pulse
    C. increased blood pressure, increased pulse
    D. increased blood pressure, decreased pulse

36. Consider the possibility of a cranial fracture whenever you note
    A. deep lacerations or severe bruises to the scalp or forehead.
    B. a LeForte fracture of the cranium.
    C. facial deformity.
    D. blood or other fluids in the airway.

37. The spinal column is made up of _____ shaped bones.
    A. 33 regularly
    B. 33 irregularly
    C. 24 regularly
    D. 12 irregularly

38. Any blunt trauma above the clavicles may damage the _____ vertebrae.
    A. lumbar
    B. cervical
    C. sacral
    D. thoracic

39. Priapism is
    A. a persistent erection of the penis.
    B. spasms to the hands and feet.
    C. apparent only in unconscious patients.
    D. uncontrolled muscle twitches of the thighs.

40. Often with a cervical spine injury, the patient in a supine position may have his arms
    A. straight out at his side.
    B. stretched out above his head.
    C. down at his side.
    D. across his chest.

41. The first step in the care of a scalp injury is to
    A. control bleeding.
    B. apply a sterile dressing.
    C. cut away hair around the site.
    D. apply a water-moistened dressing.

42. An unstable object impaled in the cheek wall should be
    A. stabilized from the outside.
    B. stabilized from the inside.
    C. pulled out if easily done.
    D. stabilized from the inside and the outside.

43. If possible, a patient with facial fractures should be transported on a long spine board in the _____ position.
    A. supine
    B. Trendelenburg
    C. head elevated
    D. prone

44. The pressure point for controlling bleeding from the leg is the
    A. carotid artery.
    B. brachial artery.
    C. subclavian vein.
    D. femoral artery.

45. Care for an open wound includes all of the following except
    A. pick embedded particles out of the cut.
    B. control bleeding.
    C. bandage the dressing in place.
    D. clean the wound surface.

46. The best method for control of nasal bleeding is
    A. packing the nose with cotton.
    B. pinching the nostrils together.
    C. packing the nose with gauze.
    D. applying pressure to the facial artery.

47. The first step in caring for possible internal bleeding after ensuring respiration and circulation and controlling life-threatening external bleeding is
    A. administering liquids by mouth to the patient.
    B. applying a bulky dressing.
    C. treating for shock.
    D. placing the patient in a sitting position.

48. A razor blade cut is an example of a(n)
    A. incision.
    B. abrasion.
    C. contusion.
    D. laceration.

49. The injury in which flaps of skin and tissues are torn loose or pulled off completely is called
    A. laceration.
    B. amputation.
    C. incision.
    D. avulsion.

50. If a patient has an object impaled in the forearm, after the control of profuse bleeding, you should
    A. remove the object.
    B. place a pressure dressing over the site.
    C. stabilize the object.
    D. apply firm pressure to a pressure point.

51. Which of the following is a sign of shock?
    A. high blood pressure
    B. constricted pupils
    C. slowed pulse rate
    D. pale, cool, clammy skin

52. An object impaled in the eye should be
    A. stabilized with gauze and protected with a disposable cup.
    B. removed carefully and a pressure dressing applied.
    C. shielded with a cup taped over the orbit.
    D. removed and a dressing applied with minimum pressure.

53. A lacerated eyelid or injury to the eyeball should be
   A. flushed with water.
   B. covered with a cold pack.
   C. covered with folded 4 × 4s.
   D. covered with dark patches.

54. All open wounds to the chest should be considered
   A. life-threatening.
   B. potentially infectious.
   C. a low priority.
   D. an indication for PASG (MAST).

55. Before moving a supine patient with possible spinal injuries onto a long spine board, you should always
   A. align the teeth and tape the jaw in place.
   B. apply a short spine board.
   C. apply a rigid collar.
   D. secure a KED to the patient.

56. The initial effort to control bleeding from a severed neck artery should be
   A. direct pressure or pinching.
   B. applying tape.
   C. pressure points.
   D. occlusive dressing.

57. The most reliable sign of spinal cord injury in conscious patients is
   A. pain without movement.
   B. paralysis of extremities.
   C. pain with movement.
   D. tenderness along the spine.

58. When caring for an open abdominal wound with evisceration,
   A. replace the organ but cover with occlusive material.
   B. replace the organ but cover with a bulky dressing.
   C. do not replace the organ but cover with occlusive material.
   D. do not replace the organ but cover with a moistened dressing.

59. A patient in acute abdominal distress without vomiting should be transported
   A. in the Trendelenburg position with legs straight.
   B. in the coma position.
   C. face up with the knees bent.
   D. in the recumbent position with one knee bent.

60. When a joint is locked into position, the EMT-Basic should
   A. pull traction on the extremity.
   B. straighten it.
   C. splint it in the position found.
   D. skip splinting and transport immediately.

61. A splint properly applied to an extremity should prevent all of the following except
   A. circulation to the extremity.
   B. an open bone injury.
   C. motion of bone fragments.
   D. damage to muscles and blood vessels.

62. A fractured clavicle is best cared for with a
   A. padded splint.
   B. sling and swathe.
   C. wrist sling.
   D. bulky pressure dressing.

63. A fracture to the humerus shaft is best cared for by immobilizing with a(n)
   A. wrist sling.
   B. rigid splint or sling and swathe.
   C. air-inflated splint.
   D. sling and swathe.

64. A fracture to the proximal end of the humerus is best cared for by immobilizing with a(n)
   A. wrist sling and swathe.
   B. padded board, sling, and swathe.
   C. air-inflated splint.
   D. sling and swathe.

65. The best way to immobilize a fractured elbow when the arm is found in the bent position and there is a distal pulse is to
   A. straighten the arm and apply an air-inflated splint.
   B. keep the arm in its found position and apply a short padded board splint.
   C. keep the arm in its found position and apply an air-inflated splint.
   D. straighten the arm and apply a wire-ladder splint.

66. When splinting, if a severe deformity exists or distal circulation is compromised, you should
   A. push protruding bones back into place.
   B. align to anatomical position under gentle traction.
   C. immediately move the patient to a stretcher.
   D. immobilize in the position found.

67. The first step in immobilizing a fractured wrist with distal pulse is to
   A. correct angulation of the wrist.
   B. secure a padded board splint to the wrist.
   C. place the broken hand in its position of function.
   D. tape the wrist.

68. A patient with a fractured pelvis should be immobilized on an orthopedic stretcher or long spine board with
   A. legs bound together with wide cravats.
   B. long padded boards secured down each side of the body.
   C. stabilizing sandbags placed between the legs.
   D. straps securing the torso and pelvis.

69. A fractured femur is best immobilized with a(n) _____ splint.
   A. long padded   C. rigid vacuum
   B. air-inflated   D. traction

70. Before immobilizing a fractured knee,
   A. assess distal PMS function.
   B. straighten the angulation.
   C. apply firm traction.
   D. flex the leg at the knee.

71. The best method for immobilizing a suspected ankle fracture is a(n) _____ splint.
   A. traction   C. padded board
   B. pillow splint   D. air-inflated

72. A sprain is an injury in which
   A. tendons are torn.
   B. ligaments are torn.
   C. cartilage is crushed.
   D. muscles spasm.

73. Which of the following is <u>not</u> true of open extremity injuries?
   A. The skin has been broken or torn.
   B. There is increased likelihood of infection.
   C. Definitive care is provided in the prehospital setting.
   D. Such injuries require surgery at the hospital.

74. Muscle is attached to bone by
   A. cartilage.   C. smooth muscles.
   B. ligaments.   D. tendons.

75. A second degree burn involves the
   A. epidermis.
   B. epidermis and dermis.
   C. epidermis, dermis, and subcutaneous layers.
   D. epidermis, dermis, subcutaneous layers, and muscles.

76. The entire back of an adult patient's right arm and her entire chest have been burned. What percentage of surface burn would you report?
   A. 13.5%   C. 27%
   B. 18%   D. 36%

77. A moderate burn involves
   A. second or third degree burns of the face and hands.
   B. third degree burns over less than 2% of the body surface.
   C. first degree burns covering more than 50% of the body surface .
   D. first degree burns covering less than 20% of the body surface.

78. Second degree burns cause
   A. swelling and blistering.
   B. nerve damage.
   C. slight swelling.
   D. scarring.

79. A patient is suffering from chemical burns to the skin caused by dry lime. Your first step should be to
   A. wash the area with running water.
   B. remove the lime with phenol.
   C. remove the lime with alcohol.
   D. brush away the lime.

80. Acid burns to the eyes should be washed for at least _____ minute(s).
   A. 1   C. 10
   B. 5   D. 20

81. A method for estimating the extent of a burn is the
   A. rule of nines.
   B. rule of percentages.
   C. rule of degree.
   D. burn assessment rule.

82. The number one priority for all EMS personnel at a collision scene is
   A. wearing the appropriate protective clothing.
   B. keeping the bystanders clear of the scene.
   C. assuring the patient's safety first.
   D. contacting medical control for instructions.

83. When arriving at the scene of a collision, the <u>first</u> thing an EMT-B should do is
   A. evaluate hazards and calculate the need for additional support.
   B. determine whether patients are low or high priority.
   C. check to see if the vehicles involved have deployed air bags.
   D. determine the extent of patient entrapment and the means of extrication.

84. The EMT-B is responsible for protecting the patient from all of the following except
   A. broken glass from the wrecked car.
   B. sharp metal in the wrecked car.
   C. the environment.
   D. injuries sustained by not wearing a seatbelt.

85. At the scene of an auto collision, the EMT-B should try to do all of the following except
   A. keep the patient's safety in mind.
   B. inform the patient of the unique aspects of the extrication.
   C. keep his/her personal safety in mind.
   D. describe the extrication procedures to bystanders.

86. A vehicle involved in a collision that is determined to be a simple access will
   A. not require towing.
   B. not require stopping traffic.
   C. not require equipment to get to the patient.
   D. require only basic air-powered tools.

87. Which of the following is untrue of applying a short spine board?
   A. Secure the torso first, and then the head.
   B. Pad between the patient's head and the spine board.
   C. Apply a single chin strap prior to moving the patient.
   D. Reassess the patient after the device is placed.

88. To assist with patient access, the EMT-B should initially do each of the following except
   A. try opening each car door.
   B. roll down windows.
   C. ask the patient to unlock the doors.
   D. pull the patient out the side windows.

89. What dictates the specific technique used for spinal immobilization of a patient at a collision extrication?
   A. requirements for speed of removal
   B. how many rescuers are available for removal
   C. whether an air bag has deployed
   D. None of the above.

90. Which step in the phases of the rescue process is out of order 1) sizing up the situation, 2) gaining the access, 3) disentangling the patient, 4) stabilizing the vehicle?
   A. 1   C. 3
   B. 2   D. 4

91. Considerations for size-up of a collision include all of the following except
   A. potential hazards.
   B. need for additional EMS units.
   C. the number of patients involved.
   D. the number of ambulances in the region.

92. To minimize injuries at a collision, the EMT-B should
   A. use a limited number of tools and make them work for the task.
   B. deactivate the safety guards on tools.
   C. wear highly visible clothing.
   D. wait until the police arrive on the scene.

93. The vehicle's catalytic converter can be a source of ignition at a collision because it
   A. often emits sparks.
   B. is often over 1200°F.
   C. may leak gasoline.
   D. pumps high pressure fumes.

94. The three-step process of disentanglement described in the text includes all of the following except
   A. open the trunk and cut the battery cable.
   B. create exitways by displacing doors and roof posts.
   C. disentangle occupants by displacing front end.
   D. gain access by disposing of the roof.

95. Which of the following is true about dealing with a collision vehicle's electrical system?
   A. It should be disabled by cutting a battery cable.
   B. If it must be disrupted, disconnect the ground cable form the battery.
   C. Cutting the battery cable can assist in rescue operations.
   D. Disconnecting the ground cable will produce a spark that can ignite battery gases.

96. When positioning flares, use a formula that includes the stopping distance for the posted speed plus the
   A. angle of the road.
   B. radius of the danger zone.
   C. reaction distance.
   D. margin of safety.

97. Once the vehicle has been stabilized, the second part of an extrication procedure for patient rescue is to
   A. dispose of the vehicle's roof.
   B. displace the front end of the vehicle.
   C. displace doors and roof posts.
   D. None of the above.

98. The Emergency Medical Dispatcher has told you the exact location of a collision, how many and what kinds of vehicles are involved, and any known hazards. What other information would you like the EMD to provide concerning this collision?
A. how many persons are injured
B. the direction designator
C. how to contact the person who reported the collision
D. the nature of the emergency

99. Which of the following is an <u>unnecessary</u> question for the Emergency Medical Dispatcher to ask when receiving a call for help?
A. How old is the patient?
B. What's the patient's sex?
C. What's the patient's name?
D. Is the patient conscious?

100. When operating a siren, be aware that
A. the continuous sound of a siren could worsen a patient's condition.
B. all motorists will hear and honor your signal.
C. the siren must be used continuously when carrying injured patients.
D. it's necessary to pull up close to vehicles and sound the siren.

101. All of the following are factors that affect an ambulance's response to a scene <u>except</u>
A. day of the week.   C. detours.
B. time of the day.   D. danger zones.

102. If a patient develops cardiac arrest during transport, have the operator of the ambulance
A. adjust the ambulance's speed.
B. stop the ambulance.
C. contact the hospital emergency department.
D. assist you with CPR.

103. When transferring a non-emergency patient to the emergency department personnel, you should
A. wait for emergency staff to call for the patient.
B. off-load, wheel to the designated area, and stay with the patient.
C. check to see what is to be done with the patient.
D. off-load, wheel to the designated area, and leave the patient.

104. The last step when transferring a patient is to
A. wait to help the emergency department staff.
B. transfer the patient's valuables.
C. obtain your release.
D. transfer patient information.

105. At the hospital, as soon as you are free from patient care activities, you should
A. notify dispatch you are back in service.
B. quickly clean the vehicle's patient compartment.
C. prepare the prehospital care report.
D. check on patient status with the emergency department.

106. Which of the following is <u>not</u> a biohazard?
A. suction catheters.
B. contaminated dressings.
C. blood-soaked linen.
D. unopened gauze bandages.

107. Which of the following is <u>not</u> a benefit of an EMS/hospital equipment exchange program?
A. Patients are not subjected to injury-aggravating movement.
B. Delay of the crew at the hospital is prevented.
C. Ambulances can return to quarters fully equipped.
D. Completeness and operability of equipment is ensured.

108. Vigorous cleaning of the ambulance while parked at the hospital is prevented or restricted by all of the following limitations <u>except</u>
A. time.   C. space.
B. equipment.   D. law.

109. While en route to your quarters,
A. radio dispatch that you are returning.
B. disinfect and decontaminate the ambulance.
C. clean and sanitize the patient compartment.
D. clean any equipment that touched the patient.

110. When you return to quarters, do all of the following <u>except</u>
A. replenish oxygen cylinders.
B. prepare for service.
C. clean the interior of the ambulance.
D. air the ambulance if necessary.

111. A poison-control kit should include all of the following except
   A. paper cups.
   B. activated charcoal.
   C. drinking water.
   D. antivenin solution.

112. Which of the following is not a piece of equipment in the first-in kit?
   A. stethoscope
   B. penlight
   C. fixed suction system
   D. rigid cervical collar

113. The first thing to inspect on the ambulance when the engine is off is the
   A. body of the vehicle.
   B. battery.
   C. siren.
   D. fuel level.

114. Rescue tools should always be examined for
   A. electrolyte levels.   C. water pressure.
   B. rust and dirt.   D. dead batteries.

115. Along with physical and mental fitness, ambulance operators should be able to
   A. move other vehicles off the roadway.
   B. perform under stress.
   C. always be up for a run.
   D. justify feelings of superiority.

116. When driving an ambulance, you should realize that there are no state laws that grant the
   A. use of controlled additional speed.
   B. passage through traffic signals.
   C. privilege of special parking at the scene.
   D. absolute right of way.

117. The headlights of an ambulance should be turned on
   A. only at night.
   B. whenever the vehicle is on the road.
   C. during the day, but only when raining.
   D. and off in a blinking fashion.

118. When a car collides with a utility pole, the EMT-B should assume all of the following except
   A. obviously dead wires could be energized at any moment.
   B. that severed conductors may be energizing every wire.
   C. wires may be charged at the highest voltage present.
   D. there is no electrical hazard.

119. The easiest way to break tempered window glass is with a
   A. blunt object.
   B. spring-loaded center punch.
   C. Glas Master window saw.
   D. sledge hammer.

120. Which of the following signs is not an indication that a child has an airway disease?
   A. wheezing
   B. breathing effort on exhalation
   C. rapid breathing
   D. lack of airway passage swelling

121. The soft spot on top of an infant's head is called a
   A. contusion.   C. fontanelle.
   B. depression site.   D. suture.

122. Small children are referred to as _____ breathers.
   A. neck   C. head
   B. abdominal   D. chest

123. A child's compensating mechanisms for shock fails at approximately _____ blood loss.
   A. 10%   C. 30%
   B. 20%   D. 40%

124. In cases of sudden death syndrome, the EMT-Basic should
   A. hunt for evidence of child abuse.
   B. hold off on care and simply transport the body.
   C. declare the patient dead.
   D. provide resuscitation and transport to the hospital.

125. Which injuries might lead you to consider child abuse?
   A. multiple skinned knees.
   B. a burn from chewing an electric cord.
   C. injuries to the center of the back and upper arms.
   D. both ankles are sprained.

126. A child who is hypoxic will
   A. have a slowed heart rate.
   B. have an increased heart rate.
   C. forget to breathe.
   D. complain of neck pain.

127. Artificial ventilations for an infant or child under 8 years of age should be provided at a rate of _____ per minute.
   A. 8   C. 16
   B. 12   D. 20

128. If you suspect respiratory distress in a conscious toddler, you should <u>not</u>
   A. administer high-concentration oxygen.
   B. insert anything into the patient's mouth.
   C. open the airway.
   D. allow the child to sit up.

129. How do children usually get lead poisoning?
   A. eating pencils
   B. eating fish
   C. eating paint chips
   D. breathing asbestos

130. Common causes of shock in children include infections, trauma, blood loss, and
   A. meningitis.   C. dehydration.
   B. heart failure   D. lack of insulin.

131. A sunken fontanelle may indicate
   A. elevated intracranial pressure.
   B. hypertension.
   C. dehydration.
   D. fever.

132. Flowing oxygen over the face of a small child so it will be inhaled is referred to as the _____ technique.
   A. blow-by   C. supplemental
   B. rebreather   D. flow-by

133. A complication of a rapidly rising temperature in a child is often
   A. hyperactivity.
   B. a seizure.
   C. vomiting.
   D. ringing in the ears.

134. A group of viral illnesses that results in inflammation of the larynx, trachea, and bronchi is called
   A. meningitis.   C. asthma.
   B. anaphylaxis.   D. croup.

135. A child ages three to six is referred to as
   A. trouble.   C. preschooler.
   B. preadolescent. D. toddler.

136. The strong, white, fibrous material covering the bones is called the
   A. shell.   C. marrow.
   B. perineum.   D. periosteum.

137. The coming apart of a joint is referred to as a
   A. fracture.   C. dislocation.
   B. sprain.   D. strain.

138. Over-stretching or over-exertion of a muscle is called a
   A. strain.   C. dislocation.
   B. sprain.   D. fracture.

139. Proper splinting of a closed fracture is
   A. done with the PASG (MAST).
   B. designed to prevent closed injuries from becoming open ones.
   C. completed in the hospital by a surgeon.
   D. done with an air splint.

140. Any force strong enough to fracture the pelvis also can cause injury to the
   A. clavicle.   C. rib cage.
   B. spine.   D. tibia.

141. Examples of a bipolar traction splint include all of the following <u>except</u>
   A. Hare.   C. half-ring.
   B. Fernotrac.   D. Sager.

142. The indications for a traction splint are painful, swollen, deformed mid-thigh with
   A. an open fracture of the lower leg.
   B. extensive blood loss and shock.
   C. no joint or lower leg injury.
   D. either ankle or knee involvement.

143. The level of training established by OSHA for those who actually plug, patch, or stop the release of a hazardous material is called
   A. First Responder Awareness.
   B. First Responder Operations.
   C. Hazardous Materials Technician.
   D. Hazardous Materials Specialist.

144. At a hazardous materials accident site, the "safe zone" should be located _____ .
   A. downwind/downhill
   B. downwind/same level
   C. upwind/same level
   D. upwind/downhill

145. A resource that must be maintained at the work site by the employer and that must be available to all employees working with hazardous materials is called
   A. NFPA 704.
   B. *Material Safety Data Sheet*
   C. *North American Emergency Response Guidebook.*
   D. shipping manifest.

146. The responsibilities of EMS personal at a hazmat incident include caring for the injured and
   A. staging personnel and equipment in the warm zone.
   B. monitoring and rehabilitating the hazmat team members.
   C. decontaminating those exiting the hot zone.
   D. notifying medical direction about the incident.

147. When a patient is categorized as Priority 1 at a MCI, this means the patient
  A. is serious, but does not have life-threatening injuries or illness.
  B. has minor musculoskeletal or soft-tissue injuries.
  C. is dead or fatally injured.
  D. has treatable life-threatening illness or injuries.

148. The MCI officer responsible for communicating with each treatment sector to determine the number and priority of the patients in that sector is called the _____ officer.
  A. staging
  B. triage
  C. treatment
  D. transportation

149. When identifying a patients treatment priority at an MCI, a Priority 2 patient would be color-coded as _____ .
  A. black
  B. green
  C. yellow
  D. red

150. At an MCI, patients who are assessed to have minor injuries should be categorized as Priority _____ .
  A. 1
  B. 2
  C. 3
  D. 4

INTERIM EXAM 3: ANSWER SHEET

Fill in the correct answer for each item. When scoring, note there are 150 questions valued at 0.666 points each.

	A	B	C	D			A	B	C	D
1.	[ ]	[ ]	[ ]	[ ]	37.	[ ]	[ ]	[ ]	[ ]
2.	[ ]	[ ]	[ ]	[ ]	38.	[ ]	[ ]	[ ]	[ ]
3.	[ ]	[ ]	[ ]	[ ]	39.	[ ]	[ ]	[ ]	[ ]
4.	[ ]	[ ]	[ ]	[ ]	40.	[ ]	[ ]	[ ]	[ ]
5.	[ ]	[ ]	[ ]	[ ]	41.	[ ]	[ ]	[ ]	[ ]
6.	[ ]	[ ]	[ ]	[ ]	42.	[ ]	[ ]	[ ]	[ ]
7.	[ ]	[ ]	[ ]	[ ]	43.	[ ]	[ ]	[ ]	[ ]
8.	[ ]	[ ]	[ ]	[ ]	44.	[ ]	[ ]	[ ]	[ ]
9.	[ ]	[ ]	[ ]	[ ]	45.	[ ]	[ ]	[ ]	[ ]
10.	[ ]	[ ]	[ ]	[ ]	46.	[ ]	[ ]	[ ]	[ ]
11.	[ ]	[ ]	[ ]	[ ]	47.	[ ]	[ ]	[ ]	[ ]
12.	[ ]	[ ]	[ ]	[ ]	48.	[ ]	[ ]	[ ]	[ ]
13.	[ ]	[ ]	[ ]	[ ]	49.	[ ]	[ ]	[ ]	[ ]
14.	[ ]	[ ]	[ ]	[ ]	50.	[ ]	[ ]	[ ]	[ ]
15.	[ ]	[ ]	[ ]	[ ]	51.	[ ]	[ ]	[ ]	[ ]
16.	[ ]	[ ]	[ ]	[ ]	52.	[ ]	[ ]	[ ]	[ ]
17.	[ ]	[ ]	[ ]	[ ]	53.	[ ]	[ ]	[ ]	[ ]
18.	[ ]	[ ]	[ ]	[ ]	54.	[ ]	[ ]	[ ]	[ ]
19.	[ ]	[ ]	[ ]	[ ]	55.	[ ]	[ ]	[ ]	[ ]
20.	[ ]	[ ]	[ ]	[ ]	56.	[ ]	[ ]	[ ]	[ ]
21.	[ ]	[ ]	[ ]	[ ]	57.	[ ]	[ ]	[ ]	[ ]
22.	[ ]	[ ]	[ ]	[ ]	58.	[ ]	[ ]	[ ]	[ ]
23.	[ ]	[ ]	[ ]	[ ]	59.	[ ]	[ ]	[ ]	[ ]
24.	[ ]	[ ]	[ ]	[ ]	60.	[ ]	[ ]	[ ]	[ ]
25.	[ ]	[ ]	[ ]	[ ]	61.	[ ]	[ ]	[ ]	[ ]
26.	[ ]	[ ]	[ ]	[ ]	62.	[ ]	[ ]	[ ]	[ ]
27.	[ ]	[ ]	[ ]	[ ]	63.	[ ]	[ ]	[ ]	[ ]
28.	[ ]	[ ]	[ ]	[ ]	64.	[ ]	[ ]	[ ]	[ ]
29.	[ ]	[ ]	[ ]	[ ]	65.	[ ]	[ ]	[ ]	[ ]
30.	[ ]	[ ]	[ ]	[ ]	66.	[ ]	[ ]	[ ]	[ ]
31.	[ ]	[ ]	[ ]	[ ]	67.	[ ]	[ ]	[ ]	[ ]
32.	[ ]	[ ]	[ ]	[ ]	68.	[ ]	[ ]	[ ]	[ ]
33.	[ ]	[ ]	[ ]	[ ]	69.	[ ]	[ ]	[ ]	[ ]
34.	[ ]	[ ]	[ ]	[ ]	70.	[ ]	[ ]	[ ]	[ ]
35.	[ ]	[ ]	[ ]	[ ]	71.	[ ]	[ ]	[ ]	[ ]
36.	[ ]	[ ]	[ ]	[ ]	72.	[ ]	[ ]	[ ]	[ ]

73. [ ] A	[ ] B	[ ] C	[ ] D	112. [ ] A	[ ] B	[ ] C	[ ] D
74. [ ] A	[ ] B	[ ] C	[ ] D	113. [ ] A	[ ] B	[ ] C	[ ] D
75. [ ] A	[ ] B	[ ] C	[ ] D	114. [ ] A	[ ] B	[ ] C	[ ] D
76. [ ] A	[ ] B	[ ] C	[ ] D	115. [ ] A	[ ] B	[ ] C	[ ] D
77. [ ] A	[ ] B	[ ] C	[ ] D	116. [ ] A	[ ] B	[ ] C	[ ] D
78. [ ] A	[ ] B	[ ] C	[ ] D	117. [ ] A	[ ] B	[ ] C	[ ] D
79. [ ] A	[ ] B	[ ] C	[ ] D	118. [ ] A	[ ] B	[ ] C	[ ] D
80. [ ] A	[ ] B	[ ] C	[ ] D	119. [ ] A	[ ] B	[ ] C	[ ] D
81. [ ] A	[ ] B	[ ] C	[ ] D	120. [ ] A	[ ] B	[ ] C	[ ] D
82. [ ] A	[ ] B	[ ] C	[ ] D	121. [ ] A	[ ] B	[ ] C	[ ] D
83. [ ] A	[ ] B	[ ] C	[ ] D	122. [ ] A	[ ] B	[ ] C	[ ] D
84. [ ] A	[ ] B	[ ] C	[ ] D	123. [ ] A	[ ] B	[ ] C	[ ] D
85. [ ] A	[ ] B	[ ] C	[ ] D	124. [ ] A	[ ] B	[ ] C	[ ] D
86. [ ] A	[ ] B	[ ] C	[ ] D	125. [ ] A	[ ] B	[ ] C	[ ] D
87. [ ] A	[ ] B	[ ] C	[ ] D	126. [ ] A	[ ] B	[ ] C	[ ] D
88. [ ] A	[ ] B	[ ] C	[ ] D	127. [ ] A	[ ] B	[ ] C	[ ] D
89. [ ] A	[ ] B	[ ] C	[ ] D	128. [ ] A	[ ] B	[ ] C	[ ] D
90. [ ] A	[ ] B	[ ] C	[ ] D	129. [ ] A	[ ] B	[ ] C	[ ] D
91. [ ] A	[ ] B	[ ] C	[ ] D	130. [ ] A	[ ] B	[ ] C	[ ] D
92. [ ] A	[ ] B	[ ] C	[ ] D	131. [ ] A	[ ] B	[ ] C	[ ] D
93. [ ] A	[ ] B	[ ] C	[ ] D	132. [ ] A	[ ] B	[ ] C	[ ] D
94. [ ] A	[ ] B	[ ] C	[ ] D	133. [ ] A	[ ] B	[ ] C	[ ] D
95. [ ] A	[ ] B	[ ] C	[ ] D	134. [ ] A	[ ] B	[ ] C	[ ] D
96. [ ] A	[ ] B	[ ] C	[ ] D	135. [ ] A	[ ] B	[ ] C	[ ] D
97. [ ] A	[ ] B	[ ] C	[ ] D	136. [ ] A	[ ] B	[ ] C	[ ] D
98. [ ] A	[ ] B	[ ] C	[ ] D	137. [ ] A	[ ] B	[ ] C	[ ] D
99. [ ] A	[ ] B	[ ] C	[ ] D	138. [ ] A	[ ] B	[ ] C	[ ] D
100. [ ] A	[ ] B	[ ] C	[ ] D	139. [ ] A	[ ] B	[ ] C	[ ] D
101. [ ] A	[ ] B	[ ] C	[ ] D	140. [ ] A	[ ] B	[ ] C	[ ] D
102. [ ] A	[ ] B	[ ] C	[ ] D	141. [ ] A	[ ] B	[ ] C	[ ] D
103. [ ] A	[ ] B	[ ] C	[ ] D	142. [ ] A	[ ] B	[ ] C	[ ] D
104. [ ] A	[ ] B	[ ] C	[ ] D	143. [ ] A	[ ] B	[ ] C	[ ] D
105. [ ] A	[ ] B	[ ] C	[ ] D	144. [ ] A	[ ] B	[ ] C	[ ] D
106. [ ] A	[ ] B	[ ] C	[ ] D	145. [ ] A	[ ] B	[ ] C	[ ] D
107. [ ] A	[ ] B	[ ] C	[ ] D	146. [ ] A	[ ] B	[ ] C	[ ] D
108. [ ] A	[ ] B	[ ] C	[ ] D	147. [ ] A	[ ] B	[ ] C	[ ] D
109. [ ] A	[ ] B	[ ] C	[ ] D	148. [ ] A	[ ] B	[ ] C	[ ] D
110. [ ] A	[ ] B	[ ] C	[ ] D	149. [ ] A	[ ] B	[ ] C	[ ] D
111. [ ] A	[ ] B	[ ] C	[ ] D	150. [ ] A	[ ] B	[ ] C	[ ] D

CHAPTER 33

Advanced Airway Management

MATCH TERMINOLOGY/DEFINITIONS

▶ PART A

A. Fork at the lower end of the trachea where the two mainstem bronchi branch

B. Insertion of a tube

C. Tube designed to be inserted into the trachea; oxygen, medication, or a suction catheter can be directed into the trachea through an endotracheal tube.

D. Area directly above the openings of both the trachea and the esophagus

E. Inadequate oxygenation, or oxygen starvation

F. Opening to the trachea

G. Tube that leads from the pharynx to the stomach

H. To provide ventilations at a higher rate to compensate for oxygen not delivered during intubation or suctioning

I. Leaf-shaped structure that acts as covering to the opening of the trachea and that prevents food and foreign matter from entering it

J. Ring-shaped structure that circles the trachea at the lower portion of the larynx

K. Two large sets of branches that come off the trachea and enter the lungs

L. Voice box

M. Microscopic sacs of the lungs where exchange of oxygen and carbon dioxide takes place

N. Illuminating instrument that is inserted into the pharynx to permit visualization of the pharynx and larynx

O. Esophageal intubation detector device that may be used to detect incorrect placement (or to verify correct placement) of the endotracheal tube

_____ **1.** Alveoli

_____ **2.** Bronchi

_____ **3.** Carina

_____ **4.** Cricoid cartilage

_____ **5.** EIDD

_____ **6.** Endotracheal tube

_____ **7.** Epiglottis

_____ **8.** Esophagus

_____ **9.** Glottic opening

_____ **10.** Hyperventilate

_____ **11.** Hypopharynx

_____ **12.** Hypoxia

_____ **13.** Intubation

_____ **14.** Laryngoscope

_____ **15.** Larynx

PART B

A. Placement of an endotracheal tube through the mouth and into the trachea

B. "Windpipe"; structure that connects the pharynx to the lungs

C. Two thin folds of tissue within the larynx that vibrate as air passes between them, producing sounds

D. Long, thin, flexible metal probe

E. Either of the two (right or left) large sets of branches that come off the trachea and enter the lungs

F. Groove-like structure anterior to the epiglottis

G. Tube designed to be passed through the nose, nasopharynx, and esophagus. It is used to relieve distention of the stomach in an infant or child patient.

H. Area directly posterior to the nose

I. Area directly posterior to the mouth

J. Pressure applied to the cricoid cartilage to suppress vomiting and bring the vocal cords into view; also called cricoid pressure

_____ **1.** Mainstem bronchi

_____ **2.** Nasogastric tube (NG tube)

_____ **3.** Nasopharynx

_____ **4.** Oropharynx

_____ **5.** Orotracheal intubation

_____ **6.** Sellick's maneuver

_____ **7.** Stylet

_____ **8.** Trachea

_____ **9.** Vallecula

_____ **10.** Vocal cords

MULTIPLE CHOICE REVIEW

_____ **1.** The area directly above the openings of both the trachea and the esophagus is called the
    A. vallecula.   **C.** hypopharynx.
    B. larynx.   **D.** oropharynx.

_____ **2.** The groove-like structure anterior to the epiglottis is called the
    A. carina.   **C.** epiglottis.
    B. vallecula.   **D.** vocal cord.

_____ **3.** Why is food more apt to be aspirated into the right mainstem bronchus rather than the left mainstem bronchus?
    A. It splits off the carina at more of an angle than the left.
    B. It splits off the carina at less of an angle than the left.
    C. It is much larger in diameter than the left.
    D. It is much smaller in diameter than the left.

_____ **4.** The brain's center for respiratory control is located in the
    A. brainstem.   **C.** pons.
    B. cerebellum.   **D.** cerebrum.

_____ **5.** The endotracheal tube is primarily intended to
    A. be placed into the esophagus.
    B. provide a medication route.
    C. be inserted into the trachea.
    D. be used as a means of suctioning the hypopharynx.

_____ **6.** Orotracheal intubation allows direct ventilation of the lungs, bypassing the
    A. entire upper airway.   **C.** vocal cords.
    B. entire lower airway.   **D.** oropharynx.

_____ **7.** When placing the endotracheal tube, EMT-Bs use
    A. a rapid-sequence technique.   **C.** direct visualization.
    B. a blind technique.   **D.** a surgical technique.

_____ 8. The advantage of orotracheal intubation is that it offers complete control of the airway and it
A. minimizes the risk of aspiration.
B. allows for better oxygen delivery.
C. allows for deeper suctioning of the airway.
D. All of the above.

_____ 9. All of the following are complications of orotracheal intubation <u>except</u>
A. hypoxia from prolonged intubation attempts.
B. soft tissue trauma to the lips, gums, or airway structures.
C. increased heart rate from vagal stimulation.
D. gagging and vomiting from airway stimulation.

_____ 10. When the endotracheal tube is advanced too deeply, this commonly results in
A. vallecula injury.
B. right-mainstem intubation.
C. esophageal intubation.
D. left-mainstem intubation.

_____ 11. The <u>most</u> serious complication of endotracheal intubation is
A. left-mainstem intubation.
B. bradycardia from airway stimulation.
C. esophageal intubation.
D. airway trauma.

_____ 12. The EMT-B should reassess endotracheal tube placement each time the patient is moved to prevent disastrous complications from
A. accidental extubation.
B. vomiting.
C. right mainstem intubation.
D. occlusion of the ET tube.

_____ 13. Most adult patients can be intubated using a size _____ straight blade or size _____ curved blade.
A. 0 or 1 : 1
B. 1 or 2 : 2
C. 2 or 3 : 3
D. 3 or 4 : 4

_____ 14. The straight blade is designed so that the tip of the blade is placed
A. into the vallecula.
B. into the carina.
C. under the epiglottis.
D. behind the epiglottis.

_____ 15. The curved blade is designed so the tip of the blade is inserted
A. into the carina.
B. under the epiglottis.
C. into the glottis.
D. into the vallecula.

_____ 16. The cuff at the distal end of the endotracheal tube
A. usually seals with 8 to 10 cc of air.
B. is called the pilot balloon.
C. has a standard 15 millimeter adapter.
D. holds 5 cc of air in an infant tube.

_____ 17. When using an endotracheal tube on an infant or child less than eight years of age, do not expect to see
A. the child's vocal cords.
B. a Murphy eye.
C. a cuff on the tube.
D. a variety of tube sizes.

_____ 18. No matter what the internal diameter of the endotracheal tube, it
A. will always fit into a large adult.
B. has a standard 15-millimeter adapter.
C. will have an inflation valve.
D. will have a pilot balloon.

_____ 19. It is generally accepted that the adult male should receive either a(n) _____ mm tube.
A. 6.0 or 6.5
B. 7.0 or 7.5
C. 8.0 or 8.5
D. 9.0 or 9.5

_____ 20. In an adult, the properly placed tube will have the _____ cm mark at the teeth.
   A. 18
   B. 20
   C. 22
   D. 24

_____ 21. Once the lubricated stylet is inserted, the endotracheal tube should be shaped like a
   A. hairpin.
   B. horseshoe.
   C. "C".
   D. hockey stick.

_____ 22. Prior to securing an endotracheal tube, do all of the following except
   A. insert an oral airway as a bite block.
   B. listen to both lungs.
   C. listen over the epigastrium.
   D. suction down the tube.

_____ 23. Items that should be checked prior to an intubation attempt include all of the following except the
   A. laryngoscope light bulb.
   B. cuff on the tube.
   C. length of the tube.
   D. shape of the tube and stylet.

_____ 24. The laryngoscope is designed to be
   A. used as a fulcrum pivoting on the teeth.
   B. placed in the left corner of the patient's mouth.
   C. held in the left hand.
   D. held in the right hand.

_____ 25. The Sellick's maneuver is designed to help
   A. reduce the risk of vomiting.
   B. move the vallecula into view.
   C. move the carina into view.
   D. compress the trachea.

_____ 26. The correct order for verifying tube placement by auscultation is
   A. right, then left, then epigastrium.
   B. epigastrium, then left, then right.
   C. epigastrium, then right, then left.
   D. left, then right, then epigastrium.

_____ 27. If the breath sounds are diminished or absent on the left but present on the right, it is likely the tube has advanced into the
   A. esophagus.
   B. left lung.
   C. right mainstem bronchus.
   D. carina.

_____ 28. It is recommended that the EMT-B make no more than _____ attempt(s) at orotracheal intubation.
   A. one
   B. two
   C. three
   D. four

_____ 29. The narrowest point of the infant's or small child's airway is the
   A. glottic opening.
   B. carina.
   C. epiglottis.
   D. cricoid ring.

_____ 30. The preferred laryngoscope blade size in infants and small children is
   A. #2 straight.
   B. #1 straight.
   C. #5 curved.
   D. #2 curved.

_____ 31. A nasogastric tube is commonly used in an infant or child patient to
   A. suction out the esophagus.
   B. perform deep and extensive suctioning.
   C. decompress the stomach and proximal bowel.
   D. provide a means of ventilating the patient.

_____ 32. When you are unable to adequately ventilate the pediatric patient due to distention of the stomach, you should consider the use of a
   A. nasotracheal tube.
   B. nasogastric tube.
   C. shunt.
   D. tracheal tube.

_____ **33.** The major contraindication for a nasogastric tube placement in the infant or child is
  A. pulmonary edema.   **C.** trauma to the chest.
  B. an inflated stomach.   **D.** head or major facial trauma.

_____ **34.** The nasogastric tube should be measured from the
  A. tip of the nose around the ear to below the xiphoid process.
  B. bottom of the earlobe to the stomach.
  C. tip of the nose and directly to the xiphoid process.
  D. nose to the angle of the jaw and then to the umbilicus.

_____ **35.** Once the nasogastric tube is passed gently downward along the nasal floor, the EMT-B should do all of the following except
  A. confirm tube placement by aspirating stomach contents.
  B. secure the tube in place with tape.
  C. confirm placement by auscultating the epigastrium while injecting 10–20 cc of air.
  D. hook the tube up to the suction unit.

COMPLETE THE FOLLOWING

1. List four indications for when to perform orotracheal intubation.

_____

_____

_____

_____

2. List six complications of deep suctioning that can be avoided by hyperventilation.

_____

_____

_____

_____

_____

_____

LABEL THE DIAGRAM

Fill in the name of each part of the endotracheal tube on the numbered line provided.

1. Inflation valve
2. 10 cc Syringe
3. pilot balloon
4. 15 mm adapter
5. open - end (top)
6. open - end (bottom)
7. Cuff
8. Murphy eye

EMT-BASIC SKILL PERFORMANCE CHECKLISTS

▶ VENTILATORY MANAGEMENT AND ENDOTRACHEAL INTUBATION

❑ Take body substance isolation.

❑ Open airway manually.

❑ Elevate tongue and insert simple airway adjunct (oropharyngeal or nasopharyngeal airway).

❑ Ventilate the patient immediately using a BVM device unattached to oxygen.

❑ Hyperventilate the patient with room air.

❑ Attach the oxygen reservoir to the BVM.

❑ Attach BVM to high flow oxygen.

❑ Ventilate the patient at the proper volume and rate (800–1200 ml per breath/10 to 20 breaths per minute).

❑ Direct assistant to hyperventilate the patient.

❑ Identify and select proper equipment for intubation.

❑ Check equipment (cuff for leaks, laryngoscope operation, and bulb tightness).

❑ Position the head properly.

❑ Insert the laryngoscope blade while displacing the tongue.

❑ Elevate the mandible with the laryngoscope.

❑ Introduce the ET tube and advance it to the proper depth.

❑ Inflate the cuff to the proper pressure and disconnect the syringe.

❑ Direct ventilation of the patient.

❑ Confirm proper placement by auscultation over the epigastrium and bilaterally over the lungs.

❑ Secure the ET tube.

▶ INSERTION OF THE NASOGASTRIC TUBE

❑ Take body substance isolation.

❑ Prepare and assemble the equipment.

❑ Oxygenate the patient.

❑ Measure tube from the tip of the nose, around the ear, to below the xiphoid process.

❑ Lubricate the end of the tube and pass the tube gently downward along the nasal floor into the stomach.

❑ To confirm correct placement, auscultate over the epigastrium. Listen for rush of air while injecting 10 to 20 cc of air into the tube.

❑ Use suction to aspirate stomach contents.

❑ Secure the tube in place with tape.

APPENDIX

ALS-Assist Skills

MATCH TERMINOLOGY/DEFINITIONS

A. Drip chamber used when minimal flow of fluid is needed (with children, for example)

B. Stop cock located below the drip chamber that can be pushed up or down to start, stop, or control the flow rate

C. Chamber from which the drops of IV fluid flow

D. Drip chamber used when a higher flow of fluid is needed (for a multi-trauma victim in shock, for example)

E. Measurement of the electrical activity of the heart on a graph

F. Photoelectric device that monitors the amount of oxygen circulating in the blood

G. Gently pressing the thumb and index finger just to either side of the medial throat and over the cricoid cartilage to bring the patient's vocal cords into view

H. Intravenous line inserted into a vein so that blood, fluids, or medications can be administered directly into a patient's circulation

I. Opening below the flow regulator on an IV set into which medication is injected

J. When an IV needle has either punctured a vein and exited the other side or has pulled out of the vein and the fluid is flowing into the surrounding tissues instead of into the vein

_____ **1.** Cricoid pressure

_____ **2.** Drip chamber

_____ **3.** ECG

_____ **4.** Flow regulator

_____ **5.** Infiltration

_____ **6.** IV

_____ **7.** Macro drip

_____ **8.** Mini drip

_____ **9.** Needle port

_____ **10.** Pulse oximeter

MULTIPLE CHOICE REVIEW

_____ **1.** The "gold standard" of airway care is the
    A. jaw-thrust maneuver.
    B. ATV.
    C. endotracheal tube.
    D. nasal airway.

_____ **2.** Typical patients who need an endotracheal tube inserted include all of the following except
    A. pulmonary or cardiopulmonary arrest patients.
    B. trauma patients in need of airway control.
    C. patients with respiratory failure due to overdose.
    D. patients with third degree burns to the extremities.

_____ **3.** Prior to an intubation attempt, you may be asked to
    A. hyperventilate the patient.
    B. insert a gastric tube.
    C. flex the neck.
    D. press on the neck.

_____ **4.** During the intubation attempt, you may be asked to do any of the following <u>except</u>
   A. shock the patient.
   B. stand by and be prepared to begin ventilations.
   C. gently press on the sides of the cricoid cartilage.
   D. maintain neck stabilization.

_____ **5.** Once the endotracheal tube is inserted in the trachea and the cuff is inflated, the paramedic should
   A. extend the patient's neck.
   B. use an esophageal intubation detector.
   C. tape the endotracheal tube in place.
   D. insert an oral airway as a bite block.

_____ **6.** After inserting the tube, the intubator should listen with a stethoscope in all of the following locations <u>except</u> the
   A. left lung.   **C.** epigastrium.
   B. right lung.   **D.** lower abdomen.

_____ **7.** If during the movement of the patient the ET tube is moved, you should
   A. notify the paramedic, who will immediately recheck placement.
   B. apply the pulse oximeter to the patient.
   C. increase the oxygen concentration.
   D. quickly pull out the tube and replace it.

_____ **8.** If you are ventilating a breathing patient with a BVM, you should
   A. increase the liter flow to at least 25 lpm.
   B. time your ventilations with the patient's respiratory efforts.
   C. decrease the oxygen concentration.
   D. ventilate at a faster rate than you normally would.

_____ **9.** If when ventilating you feel a sudden change in the resistance, this could be caused by
   A. shock.
   B. anaphylaxis.
   C. air escaping through a hole in the lungs.
   D. a sucking chest injury.

_____ **10.** When ventilating a patient in cardiac arrest with a BVM, with each defibrillation attempt you should
   A. drop the bag and move back.   **C.** lower the ventilation rate.
   B. remove the bag from the tube.   **D.** continue ventilations.

_____ **11.** Why is it important to note the mental status changes of patients who are intubated?
   A. They may not be getting enough oxygen.
   B. They may wake up and bite on the tube.
   C. They may need to be hypoventilated.
   D. They may need a larger tube.

_____ **12.** After the paramedic injects some medication down the tube, if you are assigned to ventilations, you may be asked to
   A. hyperventilate the patient.
   B. turn up the oxygen concentration.
   C. reassess the tube placement.
   D. hyperventilate the neck.

_____ **13.** If the patient has a suspected cervical spine injury, your role will be to
   A. hold the patient's chin forward during the intubation attempt.
   B. hand the paramedic the equipment for intubation.
   C. maintain in-line spinal stabilization throughout the procedure.
   D. place your fingers on the patient's throat throughout the procedure.

_____ **14.** A standard procedure used to alert EMS personnel to life-threatening heart rhythm disturbances is the
    A. myelogram.   **C.** ECG.
    B. EEG.   **D.** AED.

_____ **15.** The EMT-B should know how to turn on the ECG monitor and do all of the following except
    A. change the battery.   **C.** record an ECG strip.
    B. change the roll of paper.   **D.** interpret the ECG.

_____ **16.** When assisting with an ECG, you should try to get in the habit of applying the
    A. electrode to the patient right away.
    B. leads to the electrode and then to the patient.
    C. electrode to the patient and then the leads to the electrodes.
    D. defibrillator to the patient to monitor the ECG.

_____ **17.** Which of the following is not part of preparing the patient's skin for ECG electrodes?
    A. drying the area   **C.** shaving excessive hair
    B. removing oil   **D.** applying alcohol

_____ **18.** In the most common electrode configuration, the red electrode is placed
    A. under the center of the left lower chest.
    B. under the center of the left clavicle.
    C. on the right lower chest.
    D. on the left lower chest.

_____ **19.** In the most common electrode configuration, the green or black electrode is placed
    A. under the center of left lower chest.
    B. under the center of the left clavicle.
    C. on the right clavicle.
    D. on the left lower chest.

_____ **20.** The pulse oximeter should be used with
    A. patients who have carbon monoxide poisoning.
    B. patients complaining of respiratory problems.
    C. any patient who is hypothermic.
    D. any patient suffering from severe shock.

_____ **21.** The pulse oximeter is helpful because it
    A. encourages you to be more aggressive about providing oxygen therapy.
    B. helps you decide when you should not give oxygen.
    C. indicates when a patient is about to become hypothermic.
    D. gives an indication that the patient is a heavy smoker.

_____ **22.** The oximeter will produce falsely high readings in patients with
    A. hypoxia.   **C.** carbon monoxide poisoning.
    B. barbiturate poisoning.   **D.** croup.

_____ **23.** Chronic smokers may have a pulse oximeter reading that is
    A. lower than normal.   **C.** 20 to 25% off.
    B. higher than normal.   **D.** difficult to read.

_____ **24.** A mini drip IV administration set produces _____ drops for every cc.
    A. 15   **C.** 45
    B. 30   **D.** 60

_____ **25.** A macro drip IV administration set produces _____ drops for every cc.
    A. 10 to 15   **C.** 30 to 40
    B. 20 to 30   **D.** 40 to 50

26. When inspecting an IV fluid bag, always check for
    A. expiration date.   **C.** leaks in the bag.
    B. clarity of the fluid.   **D.** All of the above.

27. When removing the protective covering from the port of the fluid bag and the protective covering from the spiked end of the tubing,
    A. be very careful to maintain sterility.
    B. only touch the ends with gloves.
    C. hold the bag lower than the tubing.
    D. it is not necessary to protect the end of this tubing.

28. Why is the IV line flushed prior to using it on a patient?
    A. It prevents the patient from developing a blood clot.
    B. It prevents introducing an air embolism.
    C. It helps to maintain sterility of the entire system.
    D. The fluid will run much faster without air in the line.

29. Interruptions in the flow of an IV can be caused by each of the following except
    A. a closed flow regulator.
    B. a constricting band left on the patient's arm.
    C. a rise in the patient's blood pressure.
    D. kinked tubing.

30. When an IV needle has punctured both walls of the vein and fluid is leaking out around the vein, this is called
    A. evisceration.   **C.** infiltration.
    B. necrosis.   **D.** overinflation.

COMPLETE THE FOLLOWING

1. List four steps that you may be asked to perform in the process of applying electrodes.

_____

_____

_____

_____

2. List four types of patients for which the pulse oximeter reading may prove inaccurate.

_____

_____

_____

_____

EMT-BASIC SKILL PERFORMANCE CHECKLISTS

▶ USING THE PULSE OXIMETER

❑ Take body substance isolation.

❑ Review the instruction manual for the specific unit you are using.

❑ Properly assemble finger clip sensor and extension to the pulse oximeter.

❑ Properly affix finger clip sensor to the index finger. (It may be necessary to quickly remove fingernail polish.)

❑ Turn on the pulse oximeter and record the heart and oxygen saturation readings. Spot check mode and extended mode (30 minutes).

❑ Demonstrate how to shut off the unit; disassemble and store the wiring and accessories in the pouch provided.

❑ Explain the operation of all the display indicators, pulse amplitude, low battery, pulse search, oxygen saturation, and pulse rate.

❑ Explain all controls (i.e., measure button, battery check button, printer on/off, printer paper advance).

❑ Change the battery and paper print out if necessary.

▶ SETTING UP AND RUNNING AN IV LINE

❑ Take body substance isolation.

❑ Inspect the fluid bag for clarity, expiration date, and leaks. Remove the outer wrapper and gently squeeze the bag.

❑ Select the proper administration set, uncoil the tubing, and do not let the ends touch the ground.

❑ Connect an extension set if using a mini drip (macro drips should not have an extension set).

❑ Make sure the flow regulator is closed by rolling the stopcock away from the direction of the fluid bag.

❑ Remove the protective coverings from the port of the fluid bag and the spiked end of the tubing. Insert the spiked end of the tubing into the fluid bag with a quick twist.

❑ Hold the fluid bag higher than the drip chamber. Squeeze the drip chamber one or two times to start the flow. Fill the chamber to the marker line (one-third full).

❑ Open the flow regulator and allow the fluid to flush all the air from the tubing. You may need to loosen the cap at the lower end to get the fluid to flow. Be very careful to maintain sterility and to replace the cap.

APPENDIX

Stress in EMS

MATCH TERMINOLOGY/DEFINITIONS

A. State of physical and/or psychological arousal to a stimulus

B. Hormone that influences your metabolism and your immune response

C. Any situation that triggers a strong emotional response

D. Post traumatic stress disorder which may occur at any time, days to years, following a critical incident; also called PTSD

E. Reaction that is a result of prolonged recurring stressors in our work or private lives

F. First stage of the body's response to stress in which the sympathetic nervous system increases its activity in what is known as the "fight or flight" syndrome

G. Shorter and less structured form of debriefing usually led by a peer support member

H. Formal, highly structured process employed to assist individuals who are experiencing acute stress reactions; it includes six phases: fact, thought, reaction, symptom, teaching, and re-entry.

I. During this phase of grief, the dying person comes to peace with impending death.

J. Emotional reaction to a loss that includes the process of recovery and adjustment to the loss

_____ **1.** Acceptance

_____ **2.** Alarm reaction

_____ **3.** Cortisol

_____ **4.** Critical incident

_____ **5.** Cumulative stress reaction

_____ **6.** Debriefing

_____ **7.** Defusing

_____ **8.** Delayed stress reaction

_____ **9.** Grief

_____ **10.** Stress

MULTIPLE CHOICE REVIEW

_____ **1.** Stressors that you are exposed to as an EMT-B may be the result of any of the following <u>except</u>
   A. environmental factors.
   B. predictable factors that can be avoided.
   C. your dealings with other people.
   D. your self-image or performance expectations.

_____ **2.** The three stages of the general adaptation syndrome as described by Dr. Hans Selye include alarm reaction, resistance, and
   A. exhaustion.   **C.** denial
   B. acceptance.   **D.** bargaining.

_____ 3. Cortisol, which influences your metabolism and immune response under stress, is produced by which body system?
   A. respiratory
   B. digestive
   C. endocrine
   D. nervous

_____ 4. The stress triad, which occurs late in the exhaustion phase, involves all of the following except
   A. enlargement of the adrenal glands.
   B. wasting of the lymph nodes.
   C. development of cancer.
   D. bleeding gastric ulcers.

_____ 5. What is another name for burnout?
   A. PTSD
   B. cumulative stress reaction
   C. delayed stress reaction
   D. acute stress reaction

_____ 6. Which of the following signs and symptoms of acute stress reaction is unlikely to require intervention?
   A. acute chest pain
   B. long periods of uncontrollable crying
   C. continuous abnormal heart rhythms
   D. overeating for a 24-hour period

_____ 7. The late signs of cumulative stress reaction include all of the following except
   A. headaches and stomach ailments.
   B. sleep disturbances.
   C. loss of emotional control.
   D. boredom or apathy.

_____ 8. The ultimate key to preventing or managing cumulative stress lies in
   A. ongoing psychological help.
   B. seeking balance in one's life.
   C. replacing EMS with another career.
   D. drugs and alcohol use.

_____ 9. Which of the following statements does not support the viewpoint that critical incidents can be developmental rather than pathogenic?
   A. People come out of incidents just as they were going into them.
   B. A sound, routine incident command structure can prevent many critical incidents.
   C. Informal critiques should be conducted following every incident.
   D. Organizational and functional factors have minimal effect on job-related stress.

_____ 10. The phases of grief generally follow which order?
   1. anger, 2. bargaining, 3. depression, 4. denial and isolation, 5. acceptance
   A. 1, 2, 3, 4, 5
   B. 5, 4, 1, 2, 3
   C. 4, 1, 2, 3, 5
   D. 3, 2, 1, 4, 5

COMPLETE THE FOLLOWING

1. List five of the signs and symptoms associated with an acute stress reaction that may require intervention.

_____

_____

_____

_____

_____

2. List the six phases of a CISD.

_____

_____

_____

_____

_____

_____

Basic Cardiac Life Support Review

Before beginning your EMT-Basic course, you are required to have completed a course in cardiopulmonary resuscitation. The elements of CPR are tested here as "extra value" for your review.

MATCH TERMINOLOGY/DEFINITIONS

A. Providing artificial ventilations to a person who has stopped breathing or whose breathing is inadequate

B. Manual thrusts to the abdomen used to dislodge an airway obstruction

C. When breathing and heartbeat stop

D. Pulse felt between the groove of the Adam's apple and the muscles located along the side of the neck

E. Requirement that the amount of time you spend compressing the patient's chest should be the same as the time spent for release

F. Bulging of the stomach that may be caused by forcing air into the patient's stomach during rescue breathing

G. When brain cells die

H. Short triangular piece of cartilage (tough, elastic gristle) that extends from the bottom of the sternum

I. General term for the area of the lower border of the sternum

J. Maneuver that provides for maximum opening of the airway

K. Pulse measured by feeling the major artery of the arm; the absence of this pulse is used as a sign, in infants, that heartbeat has stopped and CPR should begin.

L. Actions you take to revive a person—or at least temporarily prevent biological death—by keeping the person's heart and lungs working

M. Maneuver used to open the airway of a patient with a suspected spine injury

N. Red or purple skin discoloration that occurs when gravity causes the blood to sink to the lowest parts of the body and collect there

O. Lying the patient on his side to allow for drainage from the mouth and to prevent the tongue from falling backward

_____ **1.** Biological death

_____ **2.** Brachial pulse

_____ **3.** Cardiopulmonary resuscitation

_____ **4.** Carotid pulse

_____ **5.** Clinical death

_____ **6.** 50 : 50 rule

_____ **7.** Gastric distention

_____ **8.** Head-tilt, chin lift maneuver

_____ **9.** Heimlich maneuver

_____ **10.** Jaw-thrust maneuver

_____ **11.** Line of lividity

_____ **12.** Recovery position

_____ **13.** Rescue breathing

_____ **14.** Substernal notch

_____ **15.** Xiphoid process

_____ **1.** When a patient's breathing and heartbeat stop, the _____ cells will begin to die after 4 to 6 minutes.
    A. heart   **C.** liver
    B. brain   **D.** kidney

_____ **2.** Once clinical death occurs, how long does it usually take for biological death to occur?
    A. 4 minutes   **C.** 8 minutes
    B. 6 minutes   **D.** 10 minutes

_____ **3.** In the ABC method of cardiopulmonary resuscitation, the A stands for
    A. air flow.   **C.** airway.
    B. arterial pulse.   **D.** aorta.

_____ **4.** In the ABC method of cardiopulmonary resuscitation, the C stands for
    A. cardiac.   **C.** circulation.
    B. compression.   **D.** carotid.

_____ **5.** To determine if an adult or child is pulseless, the EMT-B should check for a pulse at the _____ artery.
    A. femoral   **C.** radial
    B. brachial   **D.** carotid

_____ **6.** To determine pulselessness in an infant, the EMT-B should use the _____ artery.
    A. brachial   **C.** femoral
    B. carotid   **D.** apical

_____ **7.** If you are alone, after determining unresponsiveness in the adult, the next thing you should do before starting CPR is
    A. reposition the patient.   **C.** establish an open airway.
    B. activate EMS.   **D.** check for breathing.

_____ **8.** When an unconscious patient's head flexes forward, the _____ could cause an airway obstruction.
    A. hypopharynx   **C.** tongue
    B. uvula   **D.** larynx

_____ **9.** One of the best methods to relieve an airway obstruction due to the positioning of the patient's tongue is the
    A. jaw-thrust maneuver.   **C.** head-tilt, chin-lift maneuver.
    B. abdominal-thrust maneuver.   **D.** jaw-lift maneuver.

_____ **10.** The head-tilt, chin-lift maneuver should <u>not</u> be used on a
    A. stroke victim.
    B. diabetic patient.
    C. diving accident victim.
    D. patient who had a seizure in bed.

_____ **11.** The recommended maneuver for opening the airway of a patient with possible cervical spine injury is the _____ maneuver.
    A. jaw-thrust   **C.** head-tilt, chin-lift
    B. mouth-to-nose   **D.** jaw-lift

_____ **12.** After opening the airway in a patient who requires rescue breathing, the EMT-B should inflate the patient's lung with
    A. one quick, full breath.   **C.** one half breath.
    B. two slow breaths.   **D.** four slow breaths.

13. Initial ventilations did not result in chest rise. Your next step is to
   A. continue standard mouth-to-mask ventilations.
   B. administer oxygen.
   C. perform airway clearance techniques.
   D. deliver four quick breaths.

14. A common problem in the resuscitation of infants and children caused by improper head position or too quick ventilations is
   A. spinal injury.
   B. gastric distension.
   C. pulmonary trauma.
   D. airway injury.

15. Adult rescue breathing should be provided at a rate of _____ breaths per minute.
   A. 5–7
   B. 10–12
   C. 15–20
   D. 21–25

16. Infants should be ventilated at the rate of one breath every _____ seconds.
   A. 3
   B. 5
   C. 8
   D. 10

17. When a patient has a distended abdomen due to air being forced into the stomach, the EMT-B should
   A. manually press on the abdomen to relieve the distention.
   B. decrease the oxygen concentration being administered to the patient.
   C. be prepared to suction should the patient vomit.
   D. increase the force of the ventilation.

18. Why is the recovery position used?
   A. It protects the airway and allows for drainage from the mouth.
   B. It forces the mouth to remain open at all times.
   C. It protects the patient's head during a seizure.
   D. It makes oxygen administration possible in the unconscious patient.

19. When delivering chest compressions during CPR, which of the following should be avoided?
   A. Keep your elbows straight.
   B. Keep your hands on the sternum.
   C. Deliver compressions with a stabbing motion.
   D. Move from your hips.

20. The CPR compression point is located on the lower half of the _____ , centered from side to side.
   A. clavicle
   B. substernal notch
   C. ribs
   D. sternum

21. Before beginning artificial ventilation, assess the patient's breathing for _____ seconds.
   A. 3–5
   B. 5–10
   C. 15–20
   D. 25–30

22. For an adult, the one-rescuer compressions-to-ventilations ratio is
   A. 5 : 1.
   B. 5 : 2.
   C. 10 : 2.
   D. 15 : 2.

23. The adult CPR compression rate in one-rescuer CPR is _____ times a minute.
   A. 30–60
   B. 60–80
   C. 80–100
   D. 100–130

24. The adult CPR compressions rate in two-rescuer CPR is _____ times a minute.
   A. 60–80
   B. 80–100
   C. 50–70
   D. 100–130

_____ **25.** In two-rescuer CPR, the ratio of compressions to ventilations is
  A. 5 : 1.   **C.** 10 : 1.
  B. 5 : 2.   **D.** 10 : 2.

_____ **26.** When performing CPR on an adult, the sternum is depressed
  A. $1/2$ to $3/4$ inch.   **C.** $1 1/2$ to 2 inches.
  B. $3/4$ to 1 inch.   **D.** $2 1/2$ to 3 inches.

_____ **27.** When performing CPR on an infant, the sternum is depressed
  A. $1/4$ to $1/2$ inch.   **C.** $3/4$ to $1 1/2$ inches.
  B. $1/2$ to 1 inch.   **D.** 1 to $1 1/2$ inches.

_____ **28.** When performing CPR on a child, the sternum is compressed
  A. $1/4$ to $1/2$ inch.   **C.** $3/4$ to $1 1/2$ inches.
  B. $1/2$ to $3/4$ inch.   **D.** 1 to $1 1/2$ inches.

_____ **29.** The compression rate when performing CPR on an infant is at least
  _____ times a minute.
  A. 70   **C.** 90
  B. 80   **D.** 100

_____ **30.** When opening the airway of an infant, use a
  A. full head-tilt method.   **C.** slight head-tilt.
  B. jaw-thrust method.   **D.** neck hyperextension method.

_____ **31.** With effective CPR, the patient's pupils may
  A. dilate.
  B. constrict.
  C. assume a ground-glass appearance.
  D. begin to move.

_____ **32.** CPR compressions are delivered to children
  A. in the same manner as to adults.
  B. with the fingertips of index and middle fingers.
  C. with the palm of one hand.
  D. with the heel of one hand.

_____ **33.** With the exceptions of endotracheal tube placement or moving the patient, CPR should not be interrupted for more than
  A. a few seconds.   **C.** 15 seconds.
  B. 10 seconds.   **D.** 20 seconds.

_____ **34.** If you are treating a patient with a partial airway obstruction, poor air exchange, and gray skin, you should
  A. wait for the patient to stop breathing, then ventilate.
  B. treat the patient for a complete airway obstruction.
  C. increase the delivered oxygen concentration.
  D. None of the above.

_____ **35.** Complete airway obstruction in a conscious patient is indicated by
  A. crowing sounds.   **C.** gurgling sounds.
  B. an inability to speak.   **D.** snoring sounds.

_____ **36.** When you recognize complete airway obstruction in a conscious adult patient, you should immediately
  A. place the patient in the supine position.
  B. deliver four back blows in rapid succession.
  C. deliver a series of five rapid manual abdominal thrusts.
  D. attempt to ventilate the patient.

_____ **37.** To deliver abdominal thrusts to an unconscious patient, place the patient in the _____ position.
   A. upright
   B. prone
   C. coma
   D. supine

_____ **38.** You are treating an unresponsive adult patient with a complete airway obstruction. You have been unsuccessful in your initial attempts to ventilate the patient. Which is the correct sequence to continue your effort?
   A. finger sweeps, back blows, manual thrusts.
   B. manual thrusts, finger sweeps, back blows.
   C. ventilations, finger sweeps, manual thrusts.
   D. manual thrusts, finger sweeps, ventilations.

_____ **39.** When treating an 8-month pregnant female who has a complete airway obstruction, the EMT-B should
   A. use the Heimlich maneuver.
   B. only use the back blows.
   C. use chest thrusts.
   D. start CPR immediately.

_____ **40.** If a patient has a partial airway obstruction and is able to speak and cough forcefully, you should
   A. perform the Heimlich maneuver.
   B. carefully watch the patient.
   C. perform the chest thrust.
   D. position the patient on the floor.

_____ **41.** A major difference between the adult and child obstructed airway procedure is
   A. chest thrusts are used with children.
   B. back blows are administered to adults.
   C. blind finger sweeps are not used with children.
   D. the number of abdominal thrusts is greater in the adult.

_____ **42.** While you are trying to clear an adult's obstructed airway, the patient loses consciousness. You open the airway, perform finger sweeps, and attempt to ventilate. If this fails,
   A. deliver five chest thrusts.
   B. retilt the head and again attempt to ventilate.
   C. deliver four back blows.
   D. attempt another finger sweep.

_____ **43.** You have been unsuccessful in initially ventilating an unconscious infant. You reposition the infant's head and attempt to ventilate again but are unsuccessful. Your next step is to perform
   A. a series of chest thrusts.
   B. back blows and chest thrusts.
   C. the Heimlich maneuver.
   D. a tongue-jaw lift.

_____ **44.** Which of the following is <u>not</u> a sign of choking in an infant?
   A. ineffective cough
   B. agitation
   C. wheezing
   D. strong cry

_____ **45.** To correct a complete airway obstruction in an infant, position the patient in the _____ position.
   A. upright
   B. supine
   C. head-down
   D. prone

COMPLETE THE FOLLOWING

1. List the special circumstances in which the EMT-Basic should not initiate CPR even though the patient is pulseless.

_____

_____

_____

_____

_____

2. List situations in which the EMT-Basic may stop CPR.

_____

_____

_____

_____

_____

EMT-BASIC CHECKLISTS

▶ MOVING WHILE DOING CPR*

❏ Take body substance isolation.

❏ Begin CPR immediately per American Heart Association's one- or two-person skill performance sheet (see next pages).

❏ Place a spine board under the patient, interrupting CPR for a maximum of 7 seconds.

❏ Resume CPR and prepare to lift on EMT-B's signal.

❏ On signal, quickly transfer patient and spine board to litter.

❏ Move litter slowly so effective CPR can continue.

❏ Before moving down stairs, pause briefly at landings to continue CPR.

❏ On signal, move quickly to next landing and resume CPR for a maximum of 30 seconds.

❏ Rescuer guides EMT-B to back down stairs.

❏ Begin CPR again.

*NOTE: Be extremely careful and prevent dislodging the IV or endotracheal tube when moving the patient who has received ALS care.

▶ Using the Thumper

❑ Take body substance isolation.

❑ Assure CPR is in progress and effective.

❑ Attach the Thumper base plate to long backboard.

❑ Stop CPR momentarily to slide the long backboard under the patient.

❑ Restart CPR and attach shoulder straps to patient.

❑ Slide the Thumper piston plate into position on the base plate (away from the chest).

❑ Stop CPR and quickly pivot the piston arm into place measuring the anterior/posterior and middle sternum placement.

❑ Slowly adjust the depth of compression to the appropriate diagram.

❑ Adjust the ventilations.

❑ Demonstrate the procedure for pulse check, a defibrillation, and how to power down the unit. (Always remember to store the unit with the compression depth turned down to the minimum setting).

▶ American Heart Association CPR Guidelines

The next ten pages include the American Heart Association's CPR guidelines and are reproduced with permission from the American Heart Association. They include the steps for Basic Life Support for varying circumstances:
1) 1- or 2-rescuer CPR; 2) CPR victim as adult, child, or infant; and
3) conscious or unconscious victim with obstructed airway.

Skill Performance Sheet
Adult One-Rescuer CPR

American Heart
Association

Student Name _____ Date _____

Performance Guidelines	Performed
1. Establish unresponsiveness. Activate the EMS system.	
2. Open airway (head tilt—chin lift or jaw thrust). Check breathing (look, listen, feel).*	
3. Give 2 slow breaths (1 1/2 to 2 seconds per breath), watch chest rise, allow for exhalation between breaths.	
4. Check carotid pulse. If breathing is absent but pulse is present, provide rescue breathing (1 breath every 5 seconds, about 12 breaths per minute).	
5. If no pulse, give cycles of 15 chest compressions (rate, 80 to 100 compressions per minute) followed by 2 slow breaths.	
6. After 4 cycles of 15:2 (about 1 minute), check pulse.* If no pulse, continue 15:2 cycle beginning with chest compressions.	

*If victim is breathing or resumes effective breathing, place in recovery position.

Comments _____

_____

_____

Instructor _____

Circle one: **Complete**   **Needs more practice**

Skill Performance Sheet
Adult Two-Rescuer CPR

American Heart
Association

Student Name _____   Date _____

Performance Guidelines	Performed
1. Establish unresponsiveness. EMS system has been activated.	
RESCUER 1	
2. Open airway (head tilt—chin lift or jaw thrust). Check breathing (look, listen, feel).*	
3. Give 2 slow breaths (1 1/2 to 2 seconds per breath), watch chest rise, allow for exhalation between breaths.	
4. Check carotid pulse.	
RESCUER 2	
5. If no pulse, give cycles of 5 chest compressions (rate, 80 to 100 compressions per minute) followed by 1 slow breath by Rescuer 1.	
6. After 1 minute of rescue support, check pulse.* If no pulse, continue 5:1 cycles.	

*If victim is breathing or resumes effective breathing, place in recovery position.

Comments _____

_____

_____

Instructor _____

Circle one: **Complete**   **Needs more practice**

Skill Performance Sheet
Adult Foreign-Body Airway
Obstruction—Conscious

American Heart
Association

Student Name _____   Date _____

Performance Guidelines	Performed
1. Ask "Are you choking?"	
2. Give abdominal thrusts (chest thrusts for pregnant or obese victim).	
3. Repeat thrusts until effective or victim becomes unconscious.	
Adult Foreign-Body Airway Obstruction— Victim Becomes Unconscious	
4. Activate the EMS system.	
5. Perform a tongue-jaw lift followed by a finger sweep to remove the object.	
6. Open airway and try to ventilate; if still obstructed, reposition head and try to ventilate again.	
7. Give up to 5 abdominal thrusts.	
8. Repeat steps 5 through 7 until effective.*	

*If victim is breathing or resumes effective breathing, place in recovery position.

Comments _____

_____

_____

Instructor _____

Circle one: **Complete**   **Needs more practice**

© Reproduced with permission. *Basic Life Support Heartsaver Guide*, 1993.
Copyright American Heart Association.

Skill Performance Sheet
Adult Foreign-Body Airway
Obstruction—Unconscious

American Heart
Association

Student Name _____ Date _____

Performance Guidelines	Performed
1. Establish unresponsiveness. Activate the EMS system.	
2. Open airway and try to ventilate; if still obstructed, reposition head and try to ventilate again.	
3. Give up to 5 abdominal thrusts.	
4. Perform a tongue-jaw lift followed by a finger sweep to remove the object.	
5. Repeat steps 2 through 4 until effective.*	

*If victim is breathing or resumes effective breathing, place in recovery position.

Comments _____

_____

_____

Instructor _____

Circle one: **Complete**   **Needs more practice**

Skill Performance Sheet
Child One-Rescuer CPR

American Heart
Association

Student Name _____ Date _____

Performance Guidelines	Performed
1. Establish unresponsiveness. If second rescuer is available, have him or her activate the EMS system.	
2. Open airway (head tilt—chin lift or jaw thrust). Check breathing (look, listen, feel).*	
3. Give 2 slow breaths (1 to 1 1/2 seconds per breath), watch chest rise, allow for exhalation between breaths.	
4. Check carotid pulse. If breathing is absent but pulse is present, provide rescue breathing (1 breath every 3 seconds, about 20 breaths per minute).	
5. If no pulse, give 5 chest compressions (100 compressions per minute), open airway, and provide 1 slow breath. Repeat this cycle.	
6. After about 1 minute of rescue support, check pulse.* If rescuer is alone, activate the EMS system. If no pulse, continue 5:1 cycles.	

*If victim is breathing or resumes effective breathing, place in recovery position.

Comments _____

_____

_____

Instructor _____

Circle one: **Complete**   **Needs more practice**

Skill Performance Sheet
Child Foreign-Body Airway
Obstruction—Conscious

American Heart
Association

Student Name _____   Date _____

Performance Guidelines	Performed
1. Ask "Are you choking?"	
2. Give abdominal thrusts.	
3. Repeat thrusts until effective or victim becomes unconscious.	
Child Foreign-Body Airway Obstruction— Victim Becomes Unconscious	
4. If second rescuer is available, have him or her activate the EMS system.	
5. Perform a tongue-jaw lift, and if you see the object, perform a finger sweep to remove it.	
6. Open airway and try to ventilate; if still obstructed, reposition head and try to ventilate again.	
7. Give up to 5 abdominal thrusts.	
8. Repeat steps 5 through 7 until effective.*	
9. If airway obstruction is not relieved after about 1 minute, activate the EMS system	

*If victim is breathing or resumes effective breathing, place in recovery position.

Comments _____

_____

_____

Instructor _____

Circle one: Complete   Needs more practice

© Reproduced with permission. *Basic Life Support Heartsaver Guide,* 1993.
  Copyright American Heart Association.

Skill Performance Sheet
Child Foreign-Body Airway
Obstruction—Unconscious

American Heart
Association

Student Name _____ Date _____

Performance Guidelines	Performed
1. Establish unresponsiveness. If second rescuer is available, have him or her activate the EMS system.	
2. Open airway and try to ventilate; if still obstructed, reposition head and try to ventilate again.	
3. Give up to 5 abdominal thrusts.	
4. Perform a tongue-jaw lift, and if you see the object, perform a finger sweep to remove it.	
5. Repeat steps 2 through 4 until effective.*	
6. If airway obstruction is not relieved after about 1 minute, activate the EMS system.	

*If victim is breathing or resumes effective breathing, place in recovery position.

Comments _____

_____

_____

Instructor _____

Circle one: **Complete**   **Needs more practice**

Skill Performance Sheet
Infant One-Rescuer CPR

American Heart
Association

Student Name _____   Date _____

Performance Guidelines	Performed
1. Establish unresponsiveness. If second rescuer is available, have him or her activate the EMS system.	
2. Open airway (head tilt—chin lift or jaw thrust). Check breathing (look, listen, feel).*	
3. Give 2 slow breaths (1 to 1 1/2 seconds per breath), watch chest rise, allow for exhalation between breaths.	
4. Check brachial pulse. If breathing is absent but pulse is present, provide rescue breathing (1 breath every 3 seconds, about 20 breaths per minute).	
5. If no pulse, give cycles of 5 chest compressions (rate, at least 100 compressions per minute) followed by 1 slow breath.	
6. After about 1 minute of rescue support, check pulse.* If rescuer is alone, activate the EMS system. If no pulse, continue 5:1 cycles.	

*If victim is breathing or resumes effective breathing, place in recovery position.

Comments _____

_____

_____

Instructor _____

Circle one: **Complete**   **Needs more practice**

Skill Performance Sheet
Infant Foreign-Body Airway
Obstruction—Conscious

American Heart
Association

Student Name _____ Date _____

Performance Guidelines	Performed
1. Confirm complete airway obstruction. Check for serious breathing difficulty, ineffective cough, *no* strong cry.	
2. Give up to 5 back blows and 5 chest thrusts.	
3. Repeat step 2 until effective or victim becomes unconscious.	
Infant Foreign-Body Airway Obstruction— Victim Becomes Unconscious	
4. If second rescuer is available, have him or her activate the EMS system.	
5. Perform a tongue-jaw lift, and if you see the object, perform a finger sweep to remove it.	
6. Open airway and try to ventilate; if still obstructed, reposition head and try to ventilate again.	
7. Give up to 5 back blows and 5 chest thrusts.	
8. Repeat steps 5 through 7 until effective.*	
9. If airway obstruction is not relieved after about 1 minute, activate the EMS system.	

*If victim is breathing or resumes effective breathing, place in recovery position.

Comments _____

_____

_____

Instructor _____

Circle one: **Complete**   **Needs more practice**

Skill Performance Sheet
Infant Foreign-Body Airway
Obstruction—Unconscious

American Heart
Association

Student Name _____   Date _____

Performance Guidelines	Performed
1. Establish unresponsiveness. If second rescuer is available, have him or her activate the EMS system.	
2. Open airway and try to ventilate; if still obstructed, reposition head and try to ventilate again.	
3. Give up to 5 back blows and 5 chest thrusts.	
4. Perform a tongue-jaw lift, and if you see the object, perform a finger sweep to remove it.	
5. Repeat steps 2 through 4 until effective.*	
6. If airway obstruction is not relieved after about 1 minute, activate the EMS system.	

*If victim is breathing or resumes effective breathing, place in recovery position.

Comments _____

_____

_____

Instructor _____

Circle one: **Complete**   **Needs more practice**

National Registry Skill Sheets

The National Registry of Emergency Medical Technicians is an organization founded in 1970, one of whose goals is to establish nationwide professional standards for EMTs. Many state EMS systems use examinations developed by the National Registry to establish certification of EMTs.

The National Registry has prepared a certification examination correlated to the 1994 Department of Transportation Emergency Medical Technician-Basic: National Standard Curriculum. The examination includes both a written portion and a practical portion that consists of a series of performance-based skill stations.

To assist students in preparing for the skill stations that are part of the EMT-Basic examination, as well as to establish guidelines and parameters for those who will evaluate students' performance at the skill stations, the National Registry has developed a series of skill sheets. Each skill sheet contains a set of directions, the skill criteria, and the critical criteria that if not met by the student result in immediate failure of the station.

In studying for the National Registry examination, you should use these skills sheets in conjunction with the material presented in the textbook and not as the sole means of learning the individual skills. The skill sheets will aid you in organizing the steps necessary to perform each skill and in identifying the criteria that will be used to evaluate your performance. You can use these sheets to evaluate your own performance when practicing these skills and preparing for your practical skills evaluation.

Note: Three skill sheets regarding advanced airway management are included. The use of these skills will vary based on your medical director, training program, and local protocol.

ORGANIZATION OF THE NATIONAL REGISTRY EXAMINATION

The practical examination consists of six stations, five mandatory stations and one random basic skill station, consisting of both skill-based and scenario-based testing. The random skill station is conducted so the candidate is totally unaware of the skill to be tested until he or she arrives at the test site.

The candidate will be tested individually in each station and will be expected to direct the actions of any assistant EMTs who may be present in the station. The candidate should pass or fail the examination based solely on his or her actions and decisions.

On the next page is a list of the stations and their established time limits. The maximum time is determined by the number and difficulty of tasks to be completed.

INSTRUCTIONS TO THE CANDIDATE

▶ PATIENT ASSESSMENT/MANAGEMENT— TRAUMA

This station is designed to test your ability to perform a patient assessment of a victim of multi-system trauma and voice-treat all conditions and injuries discovered. You must conduct your assessment as you would in the field, including communicating with your patient. You may remove the patient's clothing down to shorts or swimsuit if you feel it is necessary. As you conduct your assessment, you should state everything you are assessing. Clinical information not obtainable by visual or physical inspection, for example, blood pressure, will be given to you after you demonstrate how you would normally gain that information. You may assume that you have two EMTs working with you and that they are correctly carrying out the verbal treatments you indicate. You have (10) ten minutes to complete this skill station. Do you have any questions?

▶ PATIENT ASSESSMENT/MANAGEMENT— MEDICAL

This station is designed to test your ability to perform a patient assessment of a victim with a chief complaint of a medical nature and voice-treat all conditions and injuries discovered. You must conduct your assessment as you would in the field, including communicating with your patient. As you conduct your assessment, you should state everything you are assessing. Clinical information not obtainable by visual or physical inspection, for

Station 1:	Patient Assessment/Management—Trauma	10 min
Station 2:	Patient Assessment/Management—Medical	10 min
Station 3:	Cardiac Arrest Management/AED	15 min
Station 4:	Bag-Valve-Mask Apneic Patient	10 min
Station 5:	Spinal Immobilization Station	
	Spinal Immobilization—Supine Patient	10 min
	Spinal Immobilization—Seated Patient	10 min
Station 6:	Random Basic Skill Verification	
	Long Bone Injury	5 min
	Joint Injury	5 min
	Traction Splint	10 min
	Bleeding Control/Shock Management	10 min
	Upper Airway Adjuncts and Suction	5 min
	Mouth-to-Mask with Supplemental Oxygen	5 min
	Supplemental Oxygen Administration	5 min

example, blood pressure, will be given to you after you demonstrate how you would normally gain that information. You may assume that you have two EMTs working with you and that they are correctly carrying out the verbal treatments you indicate. You have (10) ten minutes to complete this skill station. Do you have any questions?

▶ **CARDIAC ARREST MANAGEMENT/AED**

This station is designed to test your ability to manage a pre-hospital cardiac arrest by integrating CPR skills, defibrillation, airway adjuncts, and patient/scene management skills. There will be an EMT assistant in this station. The EMT assistant will only do as you instruct him. As you arrive on the scene you will encounter a patient in cardiac arrest. A first responder will be present performing single rescuer CPR. You must immediately establish control of the scene and begin resuscitation of the patient with an automated external defibrillator. At the appropriate time, you must control the airway and ventilate the victim using adjunctive equipment. You may not delegate this action to the EMT assistant. You may use any of the supplies available in this room. You have (15) fifteen minutes to complete this skill station. Do you have any questions?

▶ **AIRWAY, OXYGEN, VENTILATION SKILLS BAG-VALVE-MASK APNEIC PATIENT WITH PULSE**

This station is designed to test your ability to ventilate a patient using a bag-valve mask. As you enter the station you will find an apneic patient with a palpable central pulse. There are no bystanders and artificial ventilation has not been initiated. The only patient intervention required is airway management and ventilatory support using a bag-valve mask. You must initially ventilate the patient for a minimum of 30 seconds. You will be evaluated on the appropri-

ateness of ventilator volumes. I will inform you that a second rescuer has arrived and will instruct you that you must control the airway and the mask seal while the second rescuer provides ventilation. You may use only the equipment available in this room. You have (10) ten minutes to complete this procedure. Do you have any questions?

▶ **SPINAL IMMOBILATION—SUPINE PATIENT**

This station is designed to test your ability to provide spinal immobilization on a patient using a long spine immobilization device. You arrive on the scene with an EMT assistant. The assistant EMT has completed the scene size-up as well as the initial and focused assessments. As you begin the station there are no airway, breathing, or circulatory problems. You are required to treat the specific, isolated problem of an unstable spine using a long spine immobilization device. When moving the patient to the device, you should use the help of the assistant EMT and the evaluator. The assistant EMT should control the head and cervical spine of the patient while you and the evaluator move the patient to the immobilization device. You are responsible for the direction and subsequent action of the EMT assistant. You may use any equipment available in this room. You have (10) ten minutes to complete this procedure. Do you have any questions?

▶ **SPINAL IMMOBILIZATION—SEATED PATIENT**

This station is designed to test your ability to provide spinal immobilization on a patient using a half spine immobilization device. You arrive on the scene with an EMT assistant. The assistant EMT has completed the scene size-up, initial and focused assessments. As you begin the station, there are no airway, breathing, or circulatory problems. You are required to treat the specific, isolated problem of an unstable spine using a half spine immobilization device. Continued assessment of airway, breathing, and central circulation is not necessary. You are responsible for the direction and subsequent actions of the EMT assistant.

Transferring the patient to the long spine board should be accomplished verbally. You may use any equipment available in this room. You have (10) ten minutes to complete this procedure. Do you have any questions?

▶ IMMOBILIZATION—LONG BONE INJURY

This station is designed to test your ability to properly immobilize a closed, non-angulated long bone injury. You are required to treat only the specific, isolated injury. The scene size-up and initial assessment have been completed and during the focused assessment a closed, non-angulated injury of the _____ (radius, ulna, tibia, fibula) was detected. Ongoing assessment of the patient's airway, breathing, and central circulation is not necessary. You may use any equipment available in this room. You have (5) five minutes to complete this procedure. Do you have any questions?

▶ IMMOBILIZATION—JOINT INJURY

This station is designed to test your ability to properly immobilize a non-complicated shoulder injury. You are required to treat only the specific, isolated injury. The scene size-up and initial assessment have been accomplished on the victim and during the focused assessment a shoulder injury was detected. Ongoing assessment of the patient's airway, breathing, and central circulation is not necessary. You may use any equipment available in this room. You have (5) five minutes to complete this procedure. Do you have any questions?

▶ IMMOBILIZATION—TRACTION SPLINTING

This station is designed to test your ability to properly immobilize a mid-shaft femur injury with a traction splint. You will have an EMT assistant to help you in the application of the device by applying manual traction when directed to do so. You are required to treat only the specific, isolated injury. The scene size-up and initial assessment have been accomplished on the victim, and during the focused assessment a mid-shaft femur deformity was detected. Ongoing assessment of the patient's airway, breathing, and central circulation is not necessary. You may use any equipment available in this room. You have (10) ten minutes to complete this procedure. Do you have any questions?

▶ BLEEDING CONTROL/SHOCK MANAGEMENT

This station is designed to test your ability to control hemorrhage. This is a scenario-based testing station. As you progress through the scenario, you will be offered various signs and symptoms appropriate for the patient's condition. You will be required to manage the patient based on these signs and symptoms. A scenario will be read aloud to you, and you will be given an opportunity to ask clarifying questions about the scenario; however, you will not receive answers to any questions about the actual steps of the procedures to be performed. You may use any of the supplies and equipment available in this room. You have (10) ten minutes to complete this skill station. Do you have any questions?

▶ AIRWAY, OXYGEN, VENTILATION SKILLS UPPER AIRWAY ADJUNCTS AND SUCTION

This station is designed to test your ability to properly measure, insert, and remove an oropharyngeal and a nasopharyngeal airway as well as suction a patient's upper airway. This is an isolated skills test comprised of three separate skills. You may use any equipment available in this room. You have (5) five minutes to complete this skill station. Do you have any questions?

▶ AIRWAY, OXYGEN, VENTILATION SKILLS MOUTH-TO-MASK WITH SUPPLEMENTAL OXYGEN

This station is designed to test your ability to ventilate a patient with supplemental oxygen using a mouth-to-mask technique. This is an isolated skills test. You may assume that mouth-to-mouth ventilation is in progress and that the patient has a central pulse. The only patient management required is ventilatory support using a mouth-to-mask technique with supplemental oxygen. You must ventilate the patient for at least 30 seconds. You will be evaluated on the appropriateness of ventilatory volumes. You may use any equipment available in this room. You have (5) five minutes to complete this skill station. Do you have any questions?

▶ AIRWAY, OXYGEN, VENTILATION SKILLS SUPPLEMENTAL OXYGEN ADMINISTRATION

This station is designed to test your ability to correctly assemble the equipment needed to administer supplemental oxygen in the pre-hospital setting. This is an isolated skills test. You will be required to assemble an oxygen tank and regulator and administer oxygen to a patient using a nonrebreather mask. At this point you will be instructed to discontinue oxygen administration by the nonrebreather mask because the patient cannot tolerate the mask and start oxygen administration using a nasal cannula. Once you have initiated oxygen administration using a nasal cannula, you will be instructed to discontinue oxygen administration completely. You may use only the equipment available in this room. You have (5) five minutes to complete this skill station. Do you have any questions?

	Points Possible	Points Awarded
Takes or verbalizes body substance isolation precautions	1	
SCENE SIZE-UP		
Determines the scene is safe	1	
Determines the mechanism of injury	1	
Determines the number of patients	1	
Requests additional help if necessary	1	
Considers stabilization of spine	1	
INITIAL ASSESSMENT		
Verbalizes general impression of patient	1	
Determines responsiveness	1	
Determines chief complaint/apparent life threats	1	
Assesses airway and breathing — Assessment	1	
Assesses airway and breathing — Initiates appropriate oxygen therapy	1	
Assesses airway and breathing — Assures adequate ventilation	1	
Assesses airway and breathing — Injury management	1	
Assesses circulation — Assesses for and controls major bleeding	1	
Assesses circulation — Assesses pulse	1	
Assesses circulation — Assesses skin (color, temperature, and condition)	1	
Identifies priority patients/makes transport decision	1	
FOCUSED HISTORY AND PHYSICAL EXAM/RAPID TRAUMA ASSESSMENT		
Selects appropriate assessment (focused or rapid assessment)	1	
Obtains or directs assistant to obtain baseline vital signs	1	
Obtains SAMPLE history	1	
DETAILED PHYSICAL EXAMINATION		
Assesses the head — Inspects and palpates the scalp and ears	1	
Assesses the head — Assesses the eyes	1	
Assesses the head — Assesses the facial area including oral and nasal area	1	
Assesses the neck — Inspects and palpates the neck	1	
Assesses the neck — Assesses for JVD	1	
Assesses the neck — Assesses for tracheal deviation	1	
Assesses the chest — Inspects	1	
Assesses the chest — Palpates	1	
Assesses the chest — Auscultates the chest	1	
Assesses the abdomen/pelvis — Assesses the abdomen	1	
Assesses the abdomen/pelvis — Assesses the pelvis	1	
Assesses the abdomen/pelvis — Verbalizes assessment of genitalia/perineum as needed	1	
Assesses the extremities — 1 point for each extremity includes inspection, palpation, and assessment of pulses, sensory and motor activity	4	
Assesses the posterior — Assesses thorax	1	
Assesses the posterior — Assesses lumbar	1	
Manages secondary injuries and wounds appropriately **1 point for appropriate management of secondary injury/wound**	1	
Verbalizes reassessment of the vital signs	1	
TOTAL:	40	

CRITICAL CRITERIA

___ Did not take or verbalize body substance isolation precautions
___ Did not assess for spinal protection
___ Did not provide for spinal protection when indicated
___ Did not provide high concentration of oxygen
___ Did not find or manage problems associated with airway, breathing, hemorrhage, or shock (hypoperfusion)
___ Did not differentiate patients needing transportation versus continued on scene assessment
___ Did other detailed physical examination before assessing airway, breathing, and circulation
___ Did not transport patient within ten (10) minute time limit

PATIENT ASSESSMENT/MANAGEMENT—MEDICAL

	Points Possible	Points Awarded
Takes or verbalizes body substance isolation precautions	1	
SCENE SIZE-UP		
Determines the scene is safe	1	
Determines the mechanism of injury/nature of illness	1	
Determines the number of patients	1	
Requests additional help if necessary	1	
Considers stabilization of spine	1	
INITIAL ASSESSMENT		
Verbalizes general impression of patient	1	
Determines responsiveness/level of consciousness	1	
Determines chief complaint/apparent life threats	1	
Assesses airway and breathing — Assessment	1	
Initiates appropriate oxygen therapy	1	
Assures adequate ventilation	1	
Assesses circulation — Assesses/controls major bleeding	1	
Assesses pulse	1	
Assesses skin (color, temperature, and condition)	1	
Identifies priority patients/makes transport decision	1	
FOCUSED HISTORY AND PHYSICAL EXAM/RAPID ASSESSMENT		
Signs and Symptoms (Assesses history of present illness)	4	

Respiratory	Cardiac	Altered Mental Status	Allergic Reaction	Poisoning/ Overdose	Environmental Emergency	Obstetrics	Behavioral
•Onset? •Provokes? •Quality? •Radiates? •Severity? •Time? •Interventions?	•Onset? •Provokes? •Quality? •Radiates? •Severity? •Time? •Interventions?	•Description of the episode •Onset? •Duration? •Associated symptoms? •Evidence of trauma? •Interventions? •Seizures? •Fever?	•History of allergies? •What were you exposed to? •How were you exposed? •Effects? •Progression? •Interventions?	•Substance? •When did you ingest/become exposed? •How much did you ingest? •Over what time period? •Interventions? •Estimated weight? •Effects?	•Source? •Environment? •Duration? •Loss of consciousness? •Effects— General or local?	•Are you pregnant? •How long have you been pregnant? •Pain or contractions? •Bleeding or discharge? •Do you feel the need to push? •Last menstrual period? •Crowning?	•How do you feel? •Determine suicidal tendencies •Is the patient a threat to self or others? •Is there a medical problem? •Interventions?

	Points Possible	Points Awarded
Allergies	1	
Medications	1	
Past pertinent history	1	
Last oral intake	1	
Events leading to present illness (rule out trauma)	1	
Performs focused physical examination — Assesses affected body part/system or, if indicated, completes rapid assessment	1	
VITALS (Obtains baseline vital signs)	1	
INTERVENTIONS — Obtains medical direction or verbalizes standing order for medication interventions and verbalizes proper additional intervention/treatment	1	
TRANSPORT (Re-evaluates transport decision)	1	
Verbalizes the consideration for completing a detailed physical examination	1	
Ongoing ASSESSMENT (verbalized)		
Repeats initial assessment	1	
Repeats vital signs	1	
Repeats focused assessment regarding patient complaint or injuries	1	
Checks interventions	1	
TOTAL:	34	

CRITICAL CRITERIA

___ Did not take or verbalize body substance isolation precautions if necessary
___ Did not determine scene safety
___ Did not obtain medical direction or verbalize standing orders for medication interventions
___ Did not provide high concentration of oxygen
___ Did not evaluate and find conditions of airway, breathing, circulation
___ Did not find or manage problems associated with airway, breathing, hemorrhage, or shock (hypoperfusion)
___ Did not differentiate patients needing transportation versus continued assessment at the scene
___ Did detailed or focused history/physical examination before assessing airway, breathing, and circulation
___ Did not ask questions about the present illness
___ Administered a dangerous or inappropriate intervention

CARDIAC ARREST MANAGEMENT/AED

	Points Possible	Points Awarded
ASSESSMENT		
Takes or verbalizes body substance isolation precautions	1	
Briefly questions rescuer about arrest events	1	
Directs rescuer to stop CPR	1	
Verifies absence of spontaneous pulse *(skill station examiner states "no pulse")*	1	
Turns on defibrillator power	1	
Attaches automated defibrillator to patient	1	
Ensures all individuals are standing clear of the patient	1	
Initiates analysis of rhythm	1	
Delivers shock (up to three successive shocks)	1	
Verifies absence of spontaneous pulse *(skill station examiner states "no pulse")*	1	
TRANSITION		
Directs resumption of CPR	1	
Gathers additional information on arrest event	1	
Confirms effectiveness of CPR (ventilation and compressions)	1	
INTEGRATION		
Directs insertion of a simple airway adjunct (oropharyngeal/nasopharyngeal)	1	
Directs ventilation of patient	1	
Assures high concentration of oxygen connected to the ventilatory adjunct	1	
Assures CPR continues without unnecessary/prolonged interruption	1	
Re-evaluates patient/CPR in approximately one minute	1	
Repeats defibrillator sequence	1	
TRANSPORTATION		
Verbalizes transportation of patient	1	
TOTAL:	20	

CRITICAL CRITERIA

___ Did not take or verbalize body substance isolation precautions
___ Did not evaluate the need for immediate use of the AED
___ Did not direct initiation/resumption of ventilation/compressions at appropriate times
___ Did not assure all individuals were clear of patient before delivering each shock
___ Did not operate the AED properly (inability to deliver shock)

BAG-VALVE-MASK
APNEIC PATIENT

	Points Possible	Points Awarded
Takes or verbalizes body substance isolation precautions	1	
Voices opening the airway	1	
Voices inserting an airway adjunct	1	
Selects appropriate size mask	1	
Creates a proper mask-to-face seal	1	
Ventilates patient at no less than 800 ml volume *(The examiner must witness for at least 30 seconds)*	1	
Connects reservoir and oxygen	1	
Adjusts liter flow to 15 liters/minute or greater	1	
The examiner indicates the arrival of second EMT. The second EMT is instructed to ventilate the patient while the candidate controls the mask and the airway.		
Voices re-opening the airway	1	
Creates a proper mask-to-face seal	1	
Instructs assistant to resume ventilation at proper volume per breath *(The examiner must witness for at least 30 seconds)*	1	
TOTAL:	11	

CRITICAL CRITERIA

___ Did not take or verbalize body substance isolation precautions
___ Did not immediately ventilate the patient
___ Interrupted ventilations for more than 20 seconds
___ Did not provide high concentration of oxygen
___ Did not provide or direct assistant to provide proper volume/breath
    (more than 2 ventilations per minute are below 800 ml)
___ Did not allow adequate exhalation

SPINAL IMMOBILIZATION
SUPINE PATIENT

	Points Possible	Points Awarded
Takes or verbalizes body substance isolation precautions	1	
Directs assistant to place/maintain head in neutral in-line position	1	
Directs assistant to maintain manual immobilization of the head	1	
Assesses motor, sensory, and distal circulation in extremities	1	
Applies appropriate size extrication collar	1	
Positions the immobilization device appropriately	1	
Directs movement of the patient onto device without compromising the integrity of the spine	1	
Applies padding to voids between the torso and the board as necessary	1	
Immobilizes the patient's torso to the device	1	
Evaluates the pads behind the patient's head as necessary	1	
Immobilizes the patient's head to the device	1	
Secures the patient's legs to the device	1	
Secures the patient's arms to the device	1	
Reassesses motor, sensory, and distal circulation in extremities	1	
TOTAL:	14	

CRITICAL CRITERIA

___ Did not immediately direct or take manual immobilization of the head
___ Released or ordered release of manual immobilization before it was maintained mechanically
___ Patient manipulated or moved excessively, causing potential spinal compromise
___ Patient moves excessively up, down, left, or right on the device
___ Head immobilization allows for excessive movement
___ Upon completion of immobilization, head is not in the neutral in-line position
___ Did not reassess motor, sensory, and distal circulation after immobilization to the device
___ Immobilized head to the board before securing torso

SPINAL IMMOBILIZATION
SEATED PATIENT

	Points Possible	Points Awarded
Takes or verbalizes body substance isolation precautions	1	
Directs assistant to place/maintain head in neutral in-line position	1	
Directs assistant to maintain manual immobilization of the head	1	
Reassesses motor, sensory, and distal circulation in extremities	1	
Applies appropriate size extrication collar	1	
Positions the immobilization device behind the patient	1	
Secures the device to the patient's torso	1	
Evaluates torso fixation and adjusts as necessary	1	
Evaluates and pads behind the patient's head as necessary	1	
Secures the patient's head to the device	1	
Verbalizes moving the patient to a long board	1	
Reassesses motor, sensory, and distal circulation in extremities	1	
TOTAL:	12	

CRITICAL CRITERIA

____ Did not immediately direct or take manual immobilization of the head

____ Released or ordered release of manual immobilization before it was maintained mechanically

____ Patient manipulated or moved excessively, causing potential spinal compromise

____ Device moves excessively up, down, left, or right on patient's torso

____ Head immobilization allows for excessive movement

____ Torso fixation inhibits chest rise, resulting in respiratory compromise

____ Upon completion of immobilization, head is not in the neutral position

____ Did not reassess motor, sensory, and distal circulation after voicing immobilization to the long board

____ Immobilized head to the board before securing the torso

IMMOBILIZATION SKILLS
LONG BONE

	Points Possible	Points Awarded
Takes or verbalizes body substance isolation precautions	1	
Directs application of manual stabilization	1	
Assesses motor, sensory, and distal circulation	1	
NOTE: The examiner acknowledges present and normal.		
Measures splint	1	
Applies splint	1	
Immobilizes the joint above the injury site	1	
Immobilizes the joint below the injury site	1	
Secures the entire injured extremity	1	
Immobilizes hand/foot in the position of function	1	
Reassesses motor, sensory, and distal circulation	1	
NOTE: The examiner acknowledges present and normal.		
TOTAL:	10	

CRITICAL CRITERIA

___ Grossly moves injured extremity

___ Did not immobilize adjacent joints

___ Did not assess motor, sensory, and distal circulation before and after splinting

IMMOBILIZATION SKILLS
JOINT INJURY

	Points Possible	Points Awarded
Takes or verbalizes body substance isolation precautions	1	
Directs application of manual stabilization of the injury	1	
Assesses motor, sensory, and distal circulation	1	
NOTE: The examiner acknowledges present and normal.		
Selects proper splinting material	1	
Immobilizes the site of the injury	1	
Immobilizes bone above injured joint	1	
Immobilizes bone below injured joint	1	
Reassesses motor, sensory, and distal circulation	1	
NOTE: The examiner acknowledges present and normal.		
TOTAL:	8	

CRITICAL CRITERIA

___ Did not support the joint so that the joint did not bear distal weight
___ Did not immobilize bone above and below injured joint
___ Did not reassess motor, sensory, and distal circulation before and after splinting

IMMOBILIZATION SKILLS
TRACTION SPLINTING

	Points Possible	Points Awarded
Takes or verbalizes body substance isolation precautions	1	
Directs application of manual stabilization of the injured leg	1	
Directs the application of manual traction	1	
Assesses motor, sensory, and distal circulation	1	
NOTE: The examiner acknowledges present and normal.		
Prepares/adjusts splint to the proper length	1	
Positions the splint on the injured leg	1	
Applies the proximal securing device (e.g., ischial strap)	1	
Applies the distal securing device (e.g., ankle hitch)	1	
Applies mechanical traction	1	
Positions/secures the support straps	1	
Re-evaluates the proximal/distal securing devices	1	
Reassesses motor, sensory, and distal circulation	1	
NOTE: The examiner acknowledges present and normal.		
NOTE: The examiner must ask candidate how he/she would prepare the patient for transportation.		
Verbalizes securing the torso to the long board to immobilize the hip	1	
Verbalizes securing the splint to the long board to prevent movement of the splint	1	
TOTAL:	14	

CRITICAL CRITERIA

____ Loss of traction at any point after it is assumed
____ Did not reassess motor, sensory, and distal circulation before and after splinting
____ The foot is excessively rotated or extended after splinting
____ Did not secure the ischial strap before taking traction
____ Final immobilization failed to support the femur or prevent rotation of the injured leg
____ Secured leg to splint before applying mechanical traction

NOTE: If the Sager splint or Kendrick Traction Device is used without elevating the patient's leg, application of manual traction is not necessary. The candidate should be awarded 1 point as if manual traction were applied.

NOTE: If the leg is elevated at all, manual traction must be applied before elevating the leg. The ankle hitch may be applied before elevating the leg and used to provide manual traction.

	Points Possible	Points Awarded
Takes or verbalizes body substance isolation precautions	1	
Applies direct pressure to the wound	1	
Elevates the extremity	1	
NOTE: The examiner must now inform the candidate that the wound continues to bleed.		
Applies an additional dressing to the wound	1	
NOTE: The examiner must now inform the candidate that the wound still continues to bleed. The second dressing does not control the bleeding.		
Locates and applies pressure to appropriate arterial pressure point	1	
NOTE: The examiner must now inform the candidate that the bleeding is controlled.		
Bandages the wound	1	
NOTE: The examiner must now inform the candidate that the patient is showing signs and symptoms indicative of hypoperfusion.		
Properly positions the patient	1	
Applies high-concentration oxygen	1	
Initiates steps to prevent heat loss from the patient	1	
Indicates need for immediate transportation	1	
TOTAL:	10	

CRITICAL CRITERIA

___ Did not take or verbalize body substance isolation precautions
___ Did not apply high concentration of oxygen
___ Applied tourniquet before attempting other methods of bleeding control
___ Did not control hemorrhage in a timely manner
___ Did not indicate a need for immediate transportation

AIRWAY, OXYGEN, AND VENTILATION SKILLS
UPPER AIRWAY ADJUNCTS AND SUCTION

OROPHARYNGEAL AIRWAY

	Points Possible	Points Awarded
Takes or verbalizes body substance isolation precautions	1	
Selects appropriate size airway	1	
Measures airway	1	
Inserts airway without pushing the tongue posteriorly	1	
NOTE: The examiner must advise the candidate that the patient is gagging and becoming conscious.		
Removes oropharyngeal airway	1	

SUCTION

	Points Possible	Points Awarded
NOTE: The examiner must advise the candidate to suction the patient's oropharynx/nasopharynx.		
Turns on/prepares suction device	1	
Assures presence of mechanical suction	1	
Inserts suction tip without suction	1	
Applies suction to the oropharynx/nasopharynx	1	

NASOPHARYNGEAL AIRWAY

	Points Possible	Points Awarded
NOTE: The examiner must advise the candidate to insert a nasopharyngeal airway.		
Selects appropriate airway	1	
Measures airway	1	
Verbalizes lubrication of the nasal airway	1	
Fully inserts the airway with the bevel facing toward the septum	1	
TOTAL:	13	

CRITICAL CRITERIA

___ Did not take or verbalize body substance isolation precautions
___ Did not obtain a patent airway with the oropharyngeal airway
___ Did not obtain a patent airway with the nasopharyngeal airway
___ Did not demonstrate an acceptable suction technique
___ Inserted any adjunct in a manner dangerous to the patient

MOUTH-TO-MASK WITH SUPPLEMENTAL OXYGEN

	Points Possible	Points Awarded
Takes or verbalizes body substance isolation precautions	1	
Connects one-way valve to mask	1	
Opens patient's airway or confirms patient's airway is open (manually or with adjunct)	1	
Establishes and maintains a proper mask to face seal	1	
Ventilates the patient at the proper volume and rate *(800–1200 ml per breath/10–20 breaths per minute)*	1	
Connects mask to high-concentration oxygen	1	
Adjusts flow rate to 15 liters/minute or greater	1	
Continues ventilation at proper volume and rate *(800–1200 ml per breath/10–20 breaths per minute)*	1	
NOTE: The examiner must witness ventilations for at least 30 seconds.		
TOTAL:	8	

CRITICAL CRITERIA

___ Did not take or verbalize body substance isolation precautions
___ Did not adjust liter flow to 15 L/min or greater
___ Did not provide proper volume per breath
 (more than 2 ventilations per minute are below 800 ml)
___ Did not ventilate the patient at 10–20 breaths per minute
___ Did not allow for complete exhalation

OXYGEN ADMINISTRATION

	Points Possible	Points Awarded
Takes or verbalizes body substance isolation precautions	1	
Assembles regulator to tank	1	
Opens tank	1	
Checks for leaks	1	
Checks tank pressure	1	
Attaches nonrebreather mask	1	
Prefills reservoir	1	
Adjusts liter flow to 12 liters/minute or greater	1	
Applies and adjusts mask to the patient's face	1	
NOTE: The examiner must advise the candidate that the patient is not tolerating the nonrebreather mask. Medical direction has ordered you to apply a nasal cannula to the patient.		
Attaches nasal cannula to oxygen	1	
Adjusts liter flow to 6 liters/minute or less	1	
Applies nasal cannula to the patient	1	
NOTE: The examiner must advise the candidate to discontinue oxygen therapy.		
Removes the nasal cannula	1	
Shuts off the regulator	1	
Relieves the pressure within the regulator	1	
TOTAL:	15	

CRITICAL CRITERIA

___ Did not take or verbalize body substance isolation precautions
___ Did not assemble the tank and regulator without leaks
___ Did not prefill the reservoir bag
___ Did not adjust the device to the correct liter flow for the nonrebreather mask
   (12 L/min or greater)
___ Did not adjust the device to the correct liter flow for the nasal cannula (up to 6 L/min)

VENTILATORY MANAGEMENT
ENDOTRACHEAL INTUBATION

NOTE: If a candidate elects to initially ventilate with a BVM attached to a reservoir and oxygen, full credit must be awarded for steps denoted by "**" if the first ventilation is delivered within the initial 30 seconds

	Points Possible	Points Awarded
Takes or verbalizes body substance isolation precautions	1	
Opens airway manually	1	
Elevates tongue and inserts simple airway adjunct (oropharyngeal or nasopharyngeal airway)	1	
NOTE: The examiner now informs the candidate no gag reflex is present and the patient accepts the adjunct.		
**Ventilates the patient immediately using a BVM device unattached to oxygen	1	
**Hyperventilates the patient with room air	1	
NOTE: The examiner now informs the candidate that ventilation is being performed without difficulty.		
Attaches the oxygen reservoir to the BVM	1	
Attaches BVM to high-flow oxygen	1	
Ventilates the patient at the proper volume and rate (800–1200 ml per breath/10–20 breaths per minute)	1	
NOTE: After 30 seconds, the examiner auscultates and reports breath sounds are present and equal bilaterally and medical direction has ordered intubation. The examiner must now take over ventilation.		
Directs assistant to hyperventilate patient	1	
Identifies/selects proper equipment for intubation	1	
Checks equipment / Checks for cuff leaks	1	
Checks laryngoscope operation and bulb tightness	1	
NOTE: The examiner must remove the OPA and move out of the way when the candidate is prepared to intubate.		
Positions the head properly	1	
Inserts the laryngoscope blade while displacing the tongue	1	
Elevates the mandible with the laryngoscope	1	
Introduces the ET tube and advances it to the proper depth	1	
Inflates the cuff to the proper pressure	1	
Disconnects the syringe from the cuff inlet port	1	
Directs ventilation of the patient	1	
Confirms proper placement by auscultation bilaterally and over the epigastrium	1	
NOTE: The examiner must ask, "If you had proper placement, what would you expect to hear?"		
Secures the ET tube (may be verbalized)	1	
TOTAL:	21	

CRITICAL CRITERIA

____ Did not take or verbalize body substance isolation precautions
____ Did not initiate ventilations within 30 seconds after applying gloves or interrupts ventilations for greater than 30 seconds at any time
____ Did not voice or provide high oxygen concentrations (15 L/min or greater)
____ Did not ventilate patient at a rate of at least 10/minute
____ Did not provide adequate volume per breath (maximum of 2 errors/minute permissible)
____ Did not hyperventilate the patient prior to intubation
____ Did not successfully intubate within 3 attempts
____ Used the patient's teeth as a fulcrum
____ Did not assure proper tube placement by auscultation bilaterally and over the epigastrium
____ If used, the stylette extended beyond the end of the ET tube
____ Inserted any adjunct in a manner that would be dangerous to the patient
____ Did not disconnect syringe from cuff inlet port

VENTILATORY MANAGEMENT
DUAL LUMEN AIRWAY DEVICE (PTL OR COMBI-TUBE) INSERTION
FOLLOWING AN UNSUCCESSFUL ENDOTRACHEAL INTUBATION ATTEMPT

	Points Possible	Points Awarded
Continues body substance isolation precautions	1	
Confirms the patient is being properly ventilated with high-percentage oxygen	1	
Directs assistant to hyperventilate the patient	1	
Checks/prepares airway device	1	
Lubricates distal tip of the device *(may be verbalized)*	1	
Removes the oropharyngeal airway	1	
Positions the head properly	1	
Performs a tongue-jaw lift	1	
Inserts airway device to proper depth	1	
COMBI-TUBE / PTL		
Inflates pharyngeal cuff and removes syringe / Secures strap	1	
Inflates distal cuff and removes syringe / Blows into tube #1 to inflate both cuffs	1	
Ventilates through proper first lumen	1	
Confirms placement by observing chest rise and auscultating over the epigastrium and bilaterally over the chest	1	
NOTE: The examiner states: "You do not see rise and fall of the chest and hear sounds only over the epigastrium."		
Ventilates through the alternate lumen	1	
Confirms placement by observing chest rise and auscultating over the epigastrium and bilaterally over the chest	1	
NOTE: The examiner confirms adequate chest rise, bilateral breath sounds, and absent sounds over the epigastrium.		
Secures tube at appropriate step in sequence	1	
TOTAL:	16	

CRITICAL CRITERIA
___ Did not take or verbalize body substance isolation precautions
___ Interrupted ventilation for greater than 30 seconds
___ Did not direct hyperventilation of the patient prior to placement of the device
___ Did not assure proper placement of the device
___ Did not successfully ventilate patient
___ Did not provide high-flow oxygen (15 L/min or greater)
___ Inserted any adjunct in a manner that would be dangerous to the patient

VENTILATORY MANAGEMENT
ESOPHAGEAL OBTURATOR AIRWAY INSERTION FOLLOWING AN UNSUCCESSFUL ENDOTRACHEAL INTUBATION ATTEMPT

	Points Possible	Points Awarded
Continues body substance isolation precautions	1	
Confirms the patient is being properly ventilated	1	
Directs assistant to hyperventilate the patient	1	
Identifies/selects proper equipment	1	
Assembles airway	1	
Tests cuff	1	
Inflates mask	1	
Lubricates tube *(may be verbalized)*	1	
Removes the oropharyngeal airway	1	
Positions head properly with neck in the neutral or slightly flexed position	1	
Grasps and elevates tongue and mandible	1	
Inserts tube in the same direction as the curvature of the pharynx	1	
Advances tube until the mask is sealed against the face	1	
Ventilates the patient while maintaining a tight mask seal	1	
Confirms placement by observing chest rise and auscultating over the epigastrium and bilaterally over the chest	1	
NOTE: The examiner confirms adequate chest rise, bilateral breath sounds, and absent sounds over the epigastrium.		
Inflates the cuff to the proper pressure	1	
Disconnects the syringe	1	
Continues ventilation of the patient	1	
TOTAL:	18	

CRITICAL CRITERIA

____ Did not take or verbalize body substance isolation precautions
____ Interrupted ventilation for more than 30 seconds
____ Did not direct hyperventilation of the patient prior to placement of the device
____ Did not assure proper placement of the device
____ Did not successfully ventilate the patient
____ Did not provide high-flow oxygen (15 L/min or greater)
____ Inserted any adjunct in a manner that would be dangerous to the patient